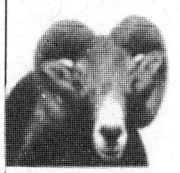# SHEEP PRODUCTION AND MANAGEMENT

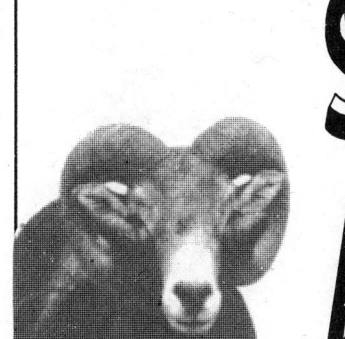

SHEEP PRODUCTION AND MANAGEMENT

J.L. Gupta

Former Director,
Sheep Husbandry Department,
Jammu, J & K

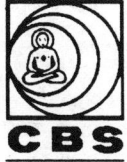

CBS

CBS PUBLISHERS & DISTRIBUTORS PVT. LTD.

New Delhi • Bengaluru • Pune • Kochi • Chennai

ISBN : 81-239-1312-5

First Edition : 2006
Reprint : 2007
Reprint : 2012

Published by Satish Kumar Jain and produced by V.K. Jain for
CBS Publishers & Distributors Pvt. Ltd.,
CBS Plaza, 4819/XI Prahlad Street, 24 Ansari Road, Daryaganj,
New Delhi - 110002, India.　• Website: www.cbspd.com
e-mail: delhi@cbspd.com, cbspubs@airtelmail.in
Ph.: 23289259, 23266861, 23266867　• Fax: 011-23243014

Branches:
• **Bengaluru:** Seema House, 2975, 17th Cross, K.R. Road,
  Bansankari 2nd Stage, Bengaluru - 560070　Ph.: +91-80-26771678/79
  • E-mail: cbsbng@gmail.com, bangalore@cbspd.com
• **Pune:** Bhuruk Prestige, Sr. No. 52/12/2+1+3/2,
  Narhe, Haveli (Near Katraj-Dehu Road By-pass), Pune - 411051
  Ph.:+91-20-64704058/59, 32342277　• E-mail: pune@cbspd.com
• **Kochi:** 36/14, Kalluvilakam, Lissie Hospital Road,
  Kochi - 682018, Kerala • Ph.: +91-484-4059061-65
  Fax: +91-484-4059065　• E-mail: cochin@cbspd.com
• **Chennai:** 20, West Park Road, Shenoy Nagar, Chennai - 60003ſ
  Ph.: +91-44-26260666, 26208620　E-mail: chennai@cbspd.con

Printed at :
India Binding House, Noida (UP)

In
reverence and sweet memory of
my inspiring mentor
and brother

Ram Chand Gupta

"They have condemned me as shepherd,
  But aren't thou, O Lord the great shepherd
    and we the meek sheep ?
Woun't thou protect the lamb against the
    wicked bisons and sinful goats ?
Would any caste count when the
    reckoning is to be made ?
Forsake me not thou shepherd Lord
    because of my lowly birth."

— *Sri Sri Paramahamsa Anjanappa Swamiji*

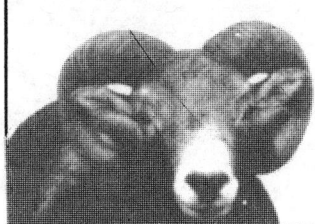

FOREWORD

Livestock products account for around 26 per cent of India's agricultural output. The proportionate contribution of small ruminants to the rural economy is quite significant and a source of sustainable livelihood and employment to millions of poor people. Sheep in particular is a bonhomie friend of poor sections of the society and the tribal. Besides lamb and mutton, sheep, provide wool, skin and other byproducts for cottage and organised industry. Of late, the ecologists too appear convinced of the symbiotic relationship of sheep to vegetation and forestation.

We in India have a diverse sheep germplasm of almost 40 breeds. Though well adapted to the local environment, their genetic quality and productivity is poor in general. Over the last fifty years wide ranging measures have been initiated to improve sheep production. Infrastructure and superior sheep germplasm centres have been created in different states and regions of the country. Various ICAR institutions and Agricultural/Veterinary universities have drawn out programmes and syllabus to train students and research workers to impart knowledge in sheep husbandry. Research and development in wool and mutton/lamb production is gaining momentum.

Under such a developing scenario, the availability of suitable literature and books is considered imperative. It is a matter of great satisfaction that Dr J.L. Gupta an expert in sheep husbandry and a teacher has ventured to compile the treatise *Sheep Production and Management* to bridge the gap. His long experience and association for almost four decades with small ruminant production and management systems especially in the state of Jammu and Kashmir finds a vivid reflection in the book.

Besides covering status of sheep production, breeds and breeding, pasture and nutrition, rearing and management, the salient aspects of development are encapsulated in this book. Constraints in sheep production and approach to varied related problems on one hand and offering 'food for thought' for the investigators and researchers on other, is another interesting feature of the book.

While appreciating the publication of such a text cum referral book and its presence on the shelves of libraries, I feel confident of its usefulness for the sheepmen, farm managers, students of animal sciences and agriculture, teachers and budding scientists in sheep husbandry and many others in the allied fields.

V. K. TANEJA
Deputy Director General (Animal Sciences)
Indian Council of Agricultural Research
Krishi Bhawan, New Delhi-110 001

PLATE 1

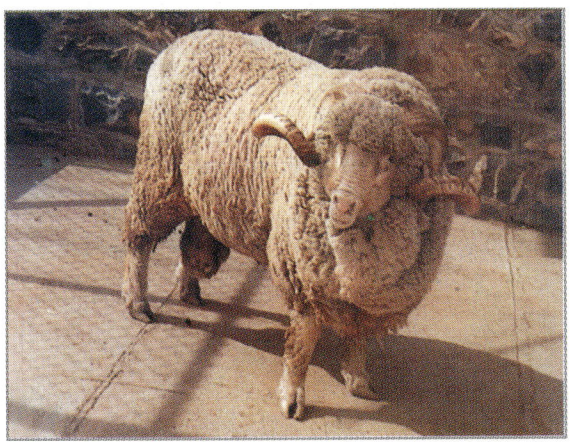

Fig. 1: Kashmir merino ram from Dacchigam Farm, Kashmir.

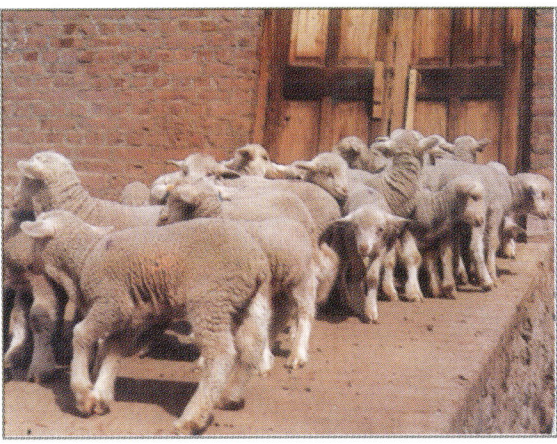

Fig. 2: Kashmir merino crop.

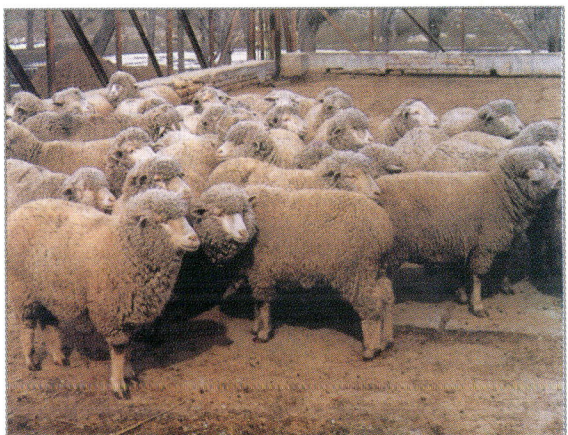

Fig. 3: Flock of Kashmir merino ewes.

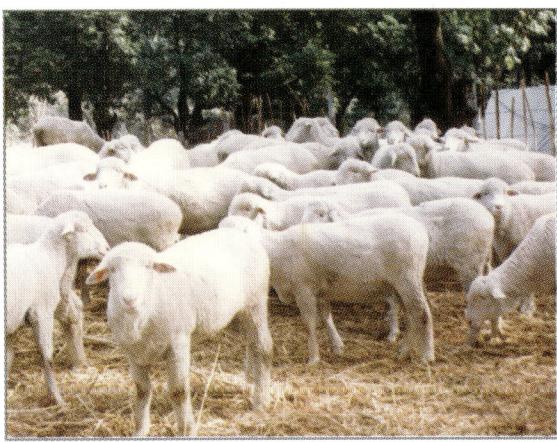

Fig. 4: Flock of Rambouillet crossbred sheep (ewes).

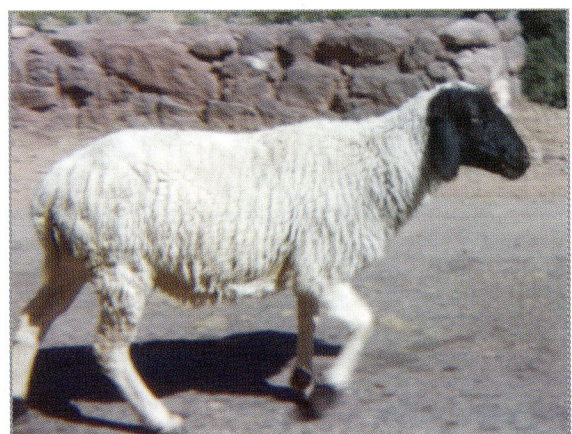

Fig. 5: Bakerwali sheep (ewe).

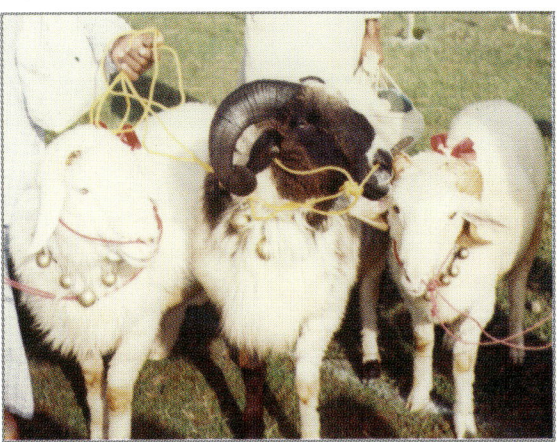

Fig. 6: Rams of Bakarwali (centre) and Gaddi (sides) sheepbreeds at a sheep show.

PLATE 2

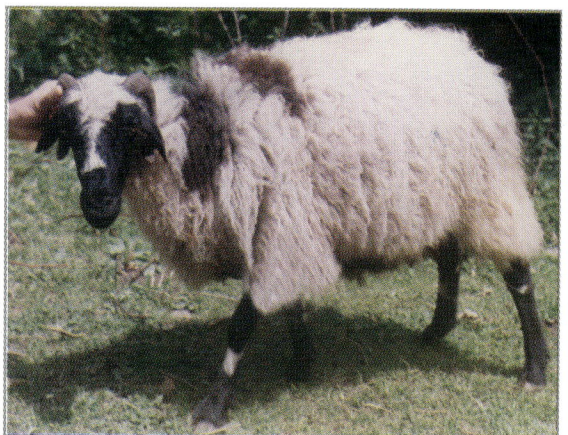

Fig. 7: *Changthang (Changluk) sheep.*

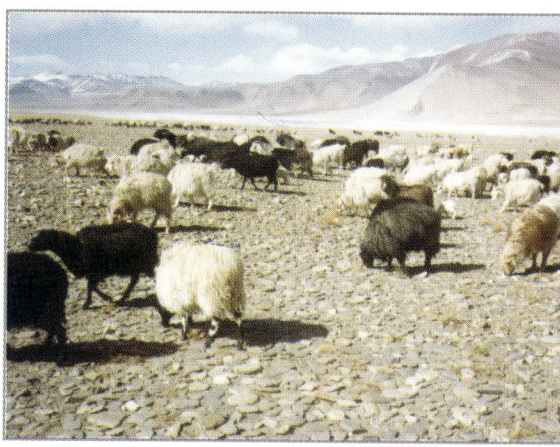

Fig. 8. *A flock of Changthang (Changluk) sheep.*

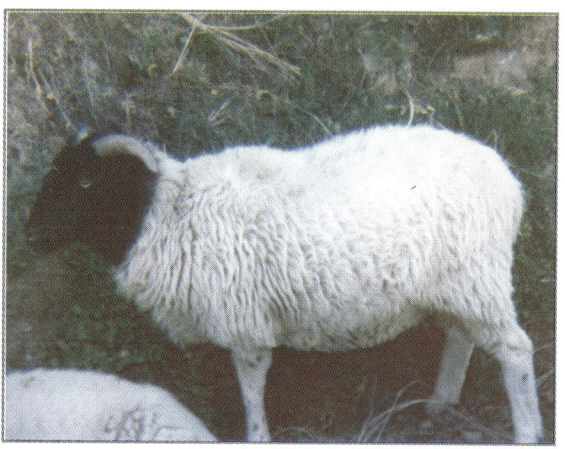

Fig. 9: *Gurez sheep: A ram lamb.*

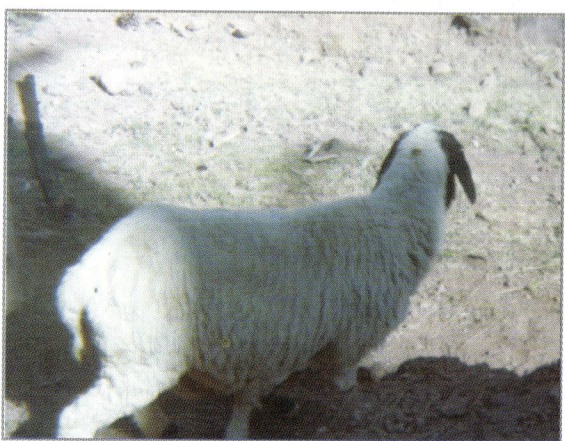

Fig. 10: *Gurez sheep: An ewe.*

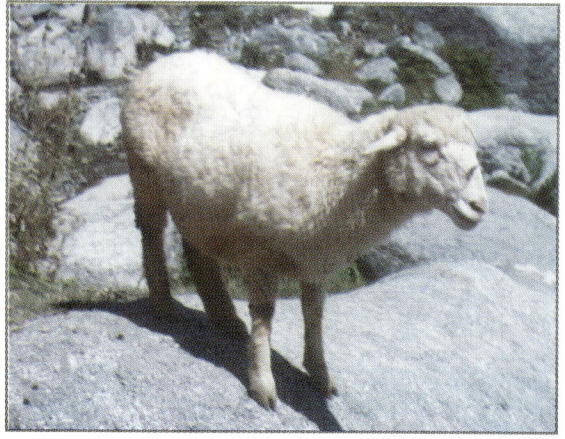

Fig. 11: *Gaddi sheep (ewe).*

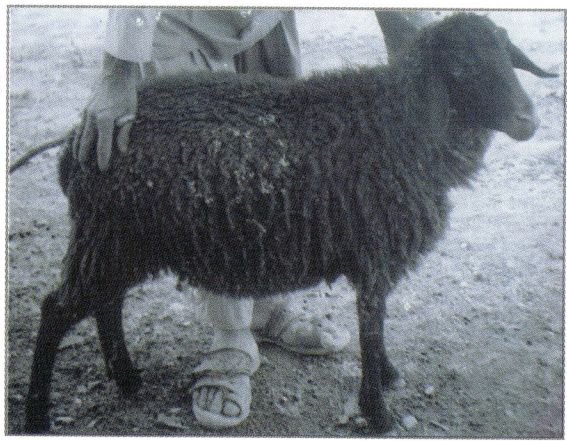

Fig. 12: *Kashmir Valley adult ewe.*

PLATE 3

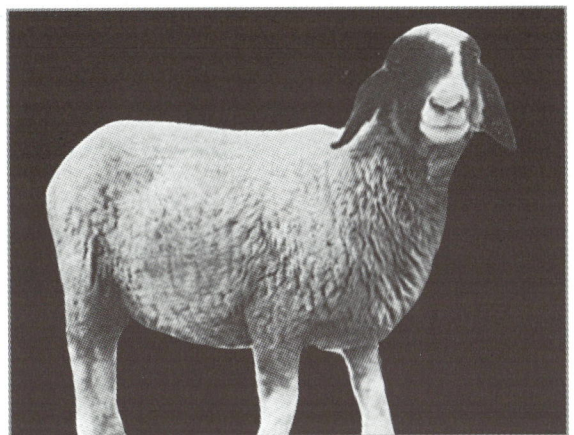

Fig. 13: Karnah sheep (ewe).

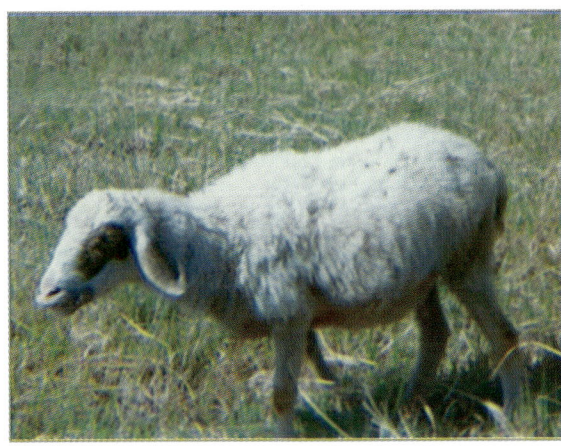

Fig. 14: Rampur Bushair sheep (ewe).

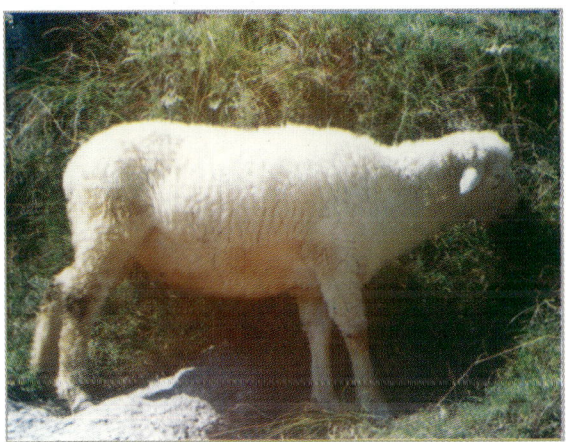

Fig. 15: Poonchi sheep (ewe).

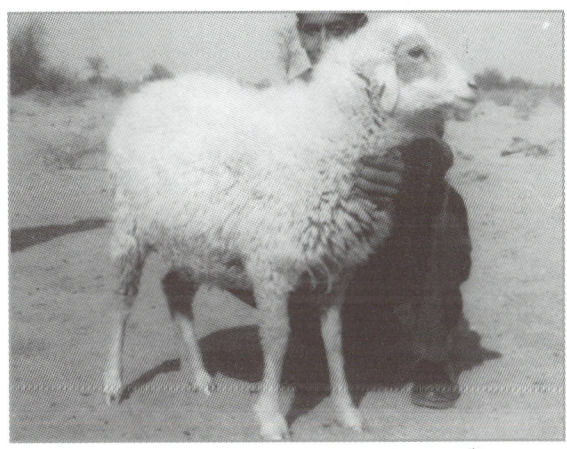

Fig. 16: Chokla sheep (ewe).

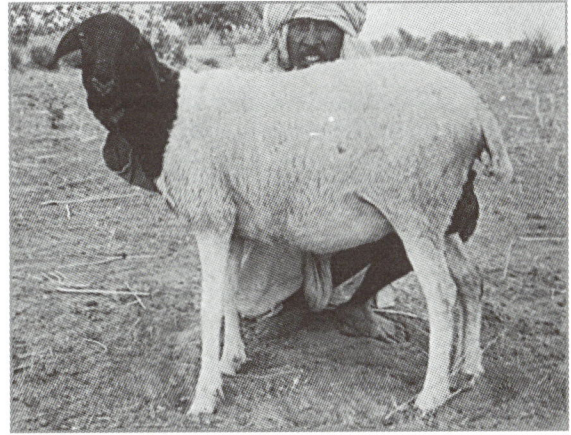

Fig. 17: Jalauni sheep (ewe).

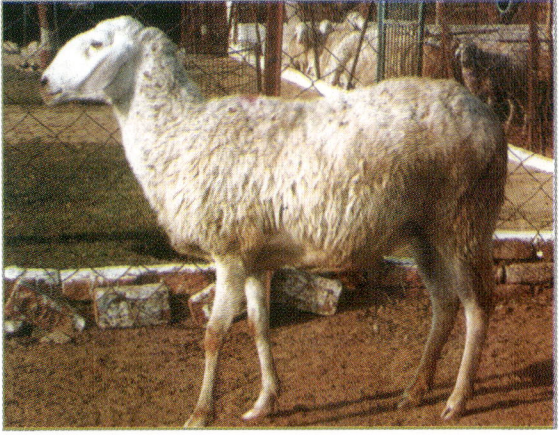

Fig. 18: Muzzafarnagri sheep (ewe).

PLATE 4

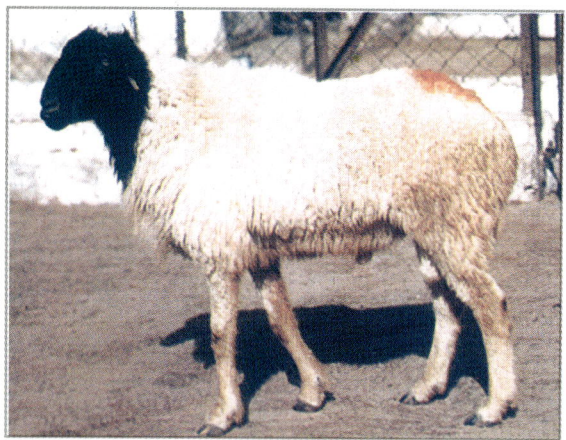

Fig. 19: Marwari sheep (ram).

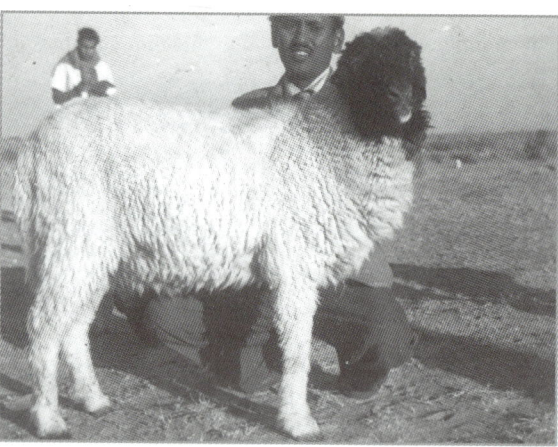

Fig. 20: Malpura sheep (ewe).

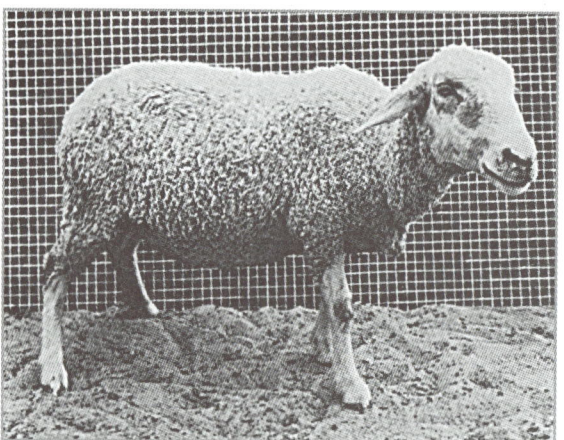

Fig. 21: Magra sheep (ewe).

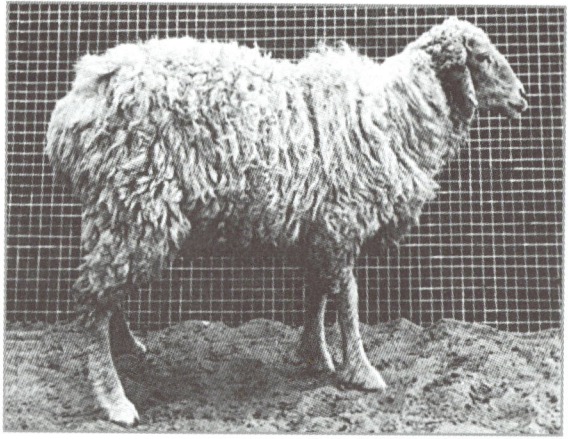

Fig. 22: Nali sheep (ewe).

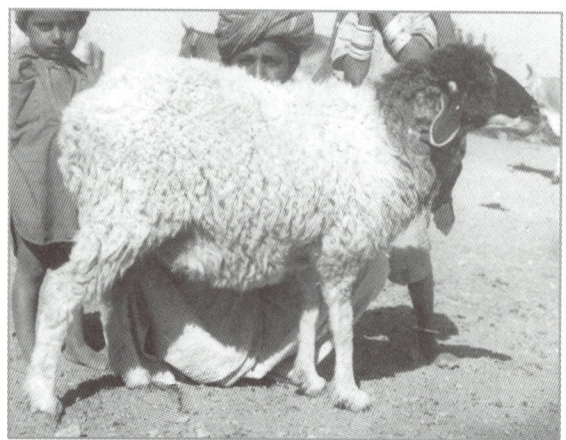

Fig. 23: Pugal sheep (male).

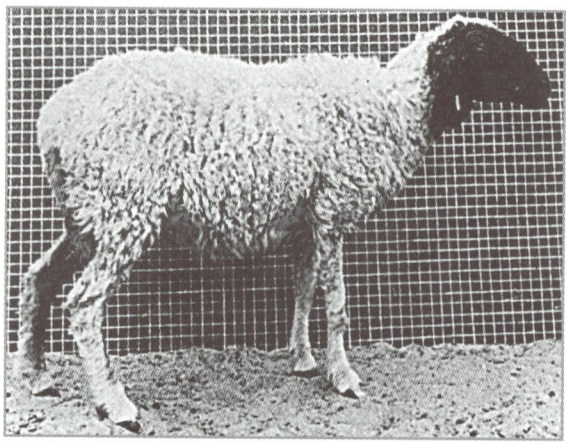

Fig. 24: Jaisalmeri sheep (ewe).

PLATE 5

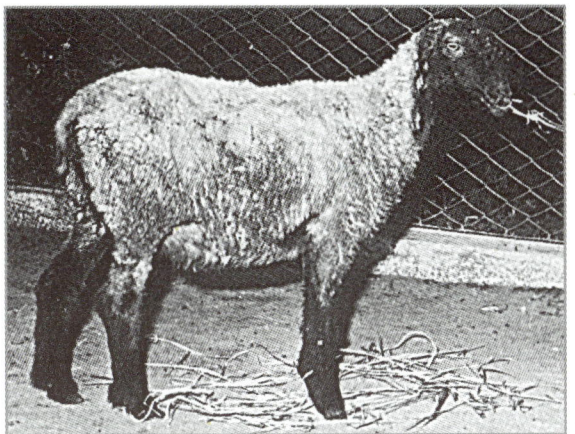

Fig. 25: Patanwadi sheep (ewe).

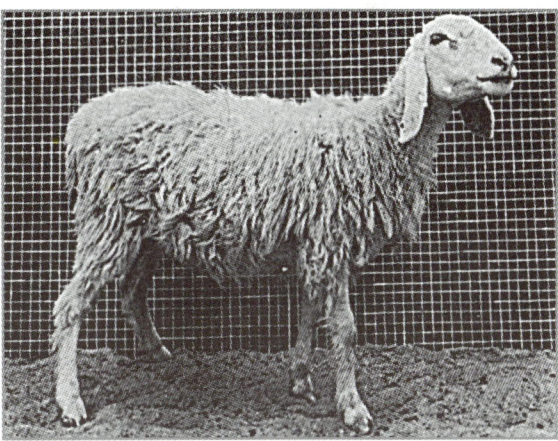

Fig. 26: Sonadi sheep (ewe).

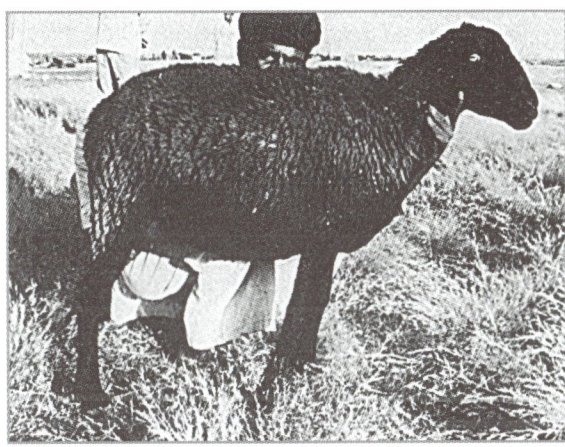

Fig. 27: Deccani sheep (ewe).

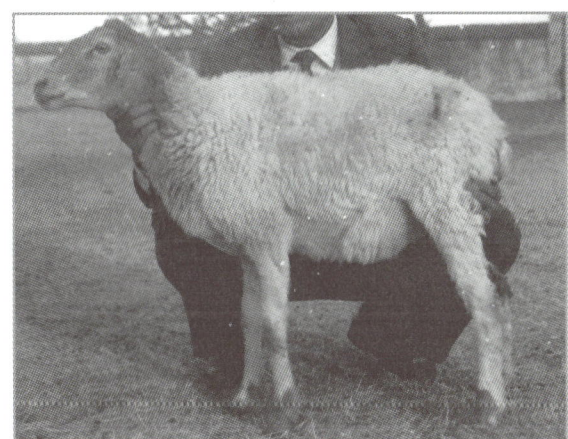

Fig. 28: Hassan sheep (ewe).

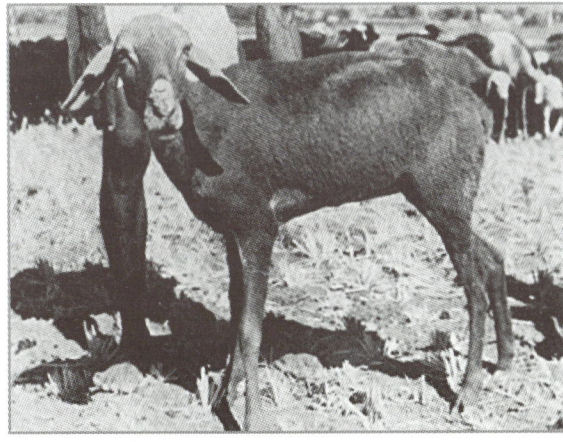

Fig. 29: Madras red sheep (ewe).

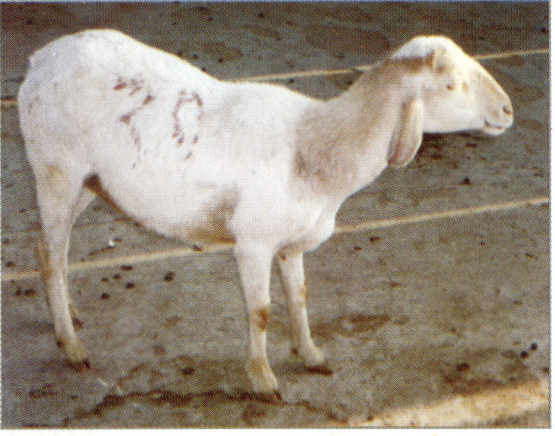

Fig. 30: Mandya (Bannur) sheep (ewe) at Panthal Sheep Farm, J&K.

PLATE 6

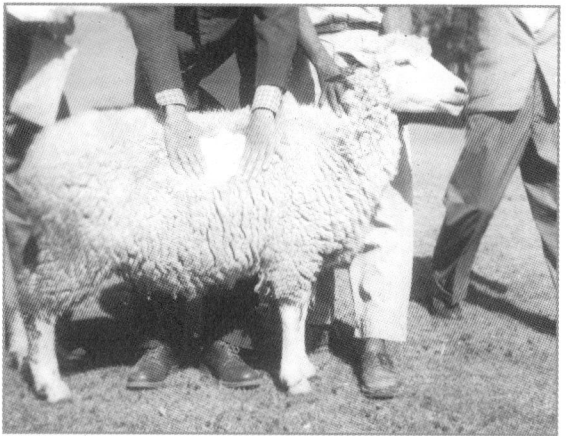

Fig. 31: Nilgiri sheep (ewe).

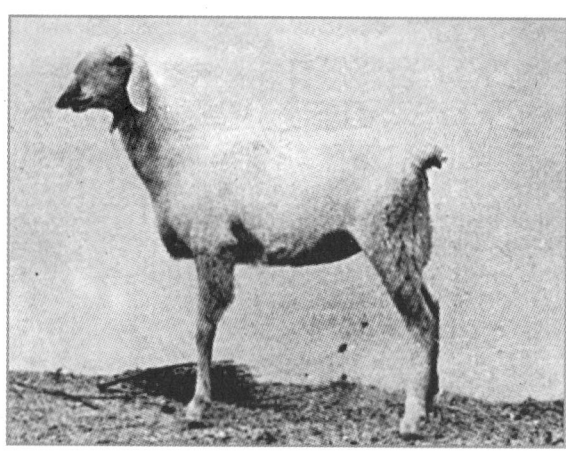

Fig. 32: Nellore sheep (ewe).

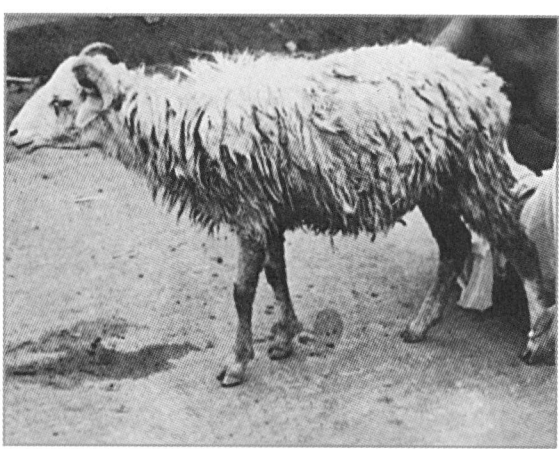

Fig. 33: Belangir sheep (ewe).

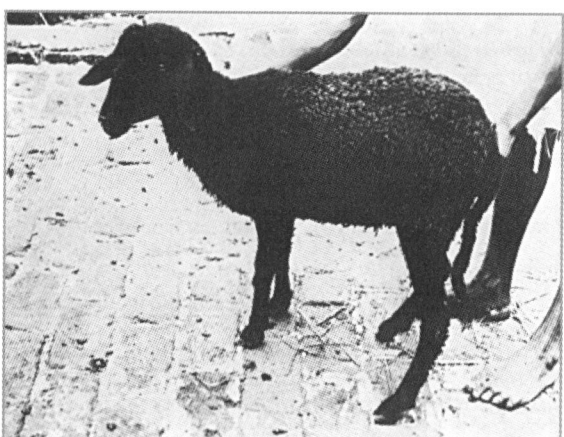

Fig. 34: Chotanagpuri sheep (ewe).

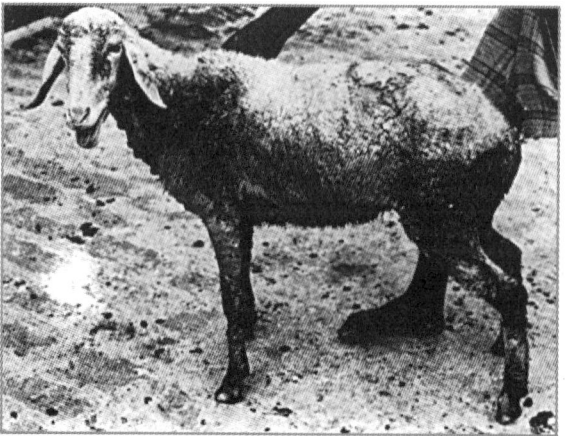

Fig. 35: Shahabadi sheep (ewe).

PLATE   7

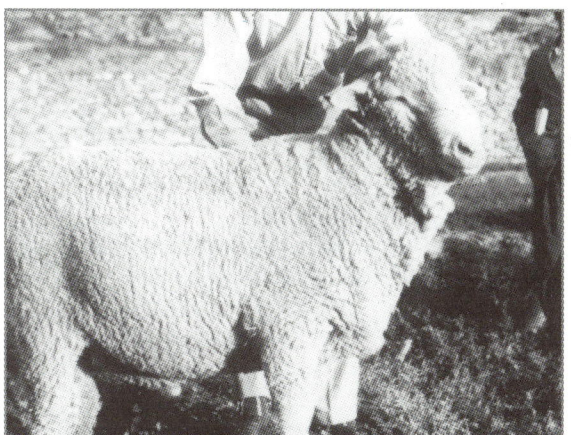

Fig. 36: Caucassian ram, S.B.F., Jeory, H.P.

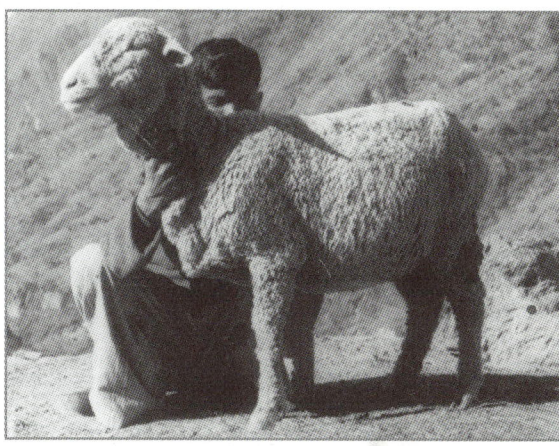

Fig. 37: Merino crossbred ram, S.B.F., Jeory, H.P.

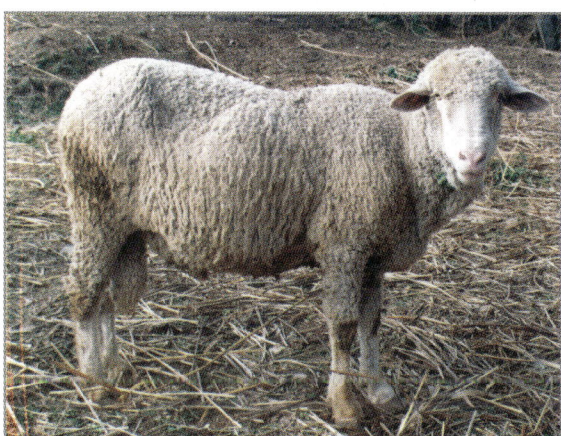

Fig. 38: Three-fourths bred Rambouillet graded ram, Rearing Centre, J&K.

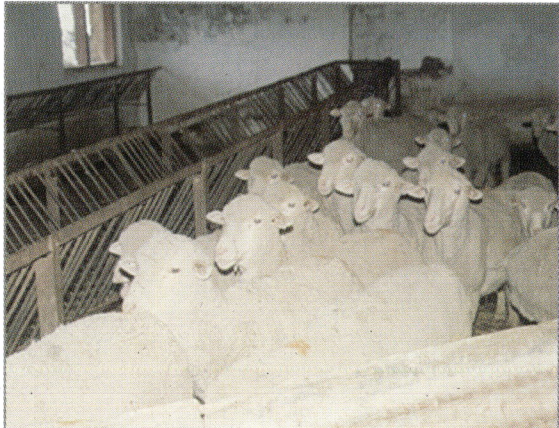

Fig. 39: Inside view of an improvised sheep shed: young lambs with mothers in a sheep pen.

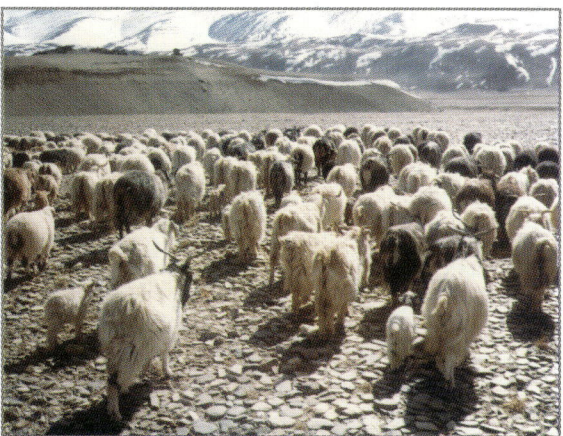

Fig. 40: Changluk sheep and Changra goat in open Changthang region, Ladakh.

PLATE 8

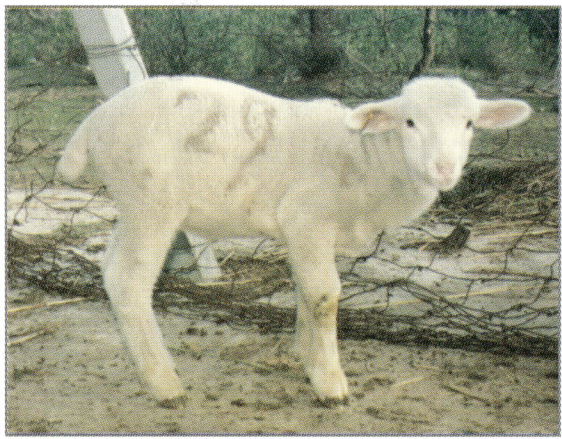

Fig. 41: Young lamb with identification marking, i.e. paint number and subsequent ear tagging at one week age.

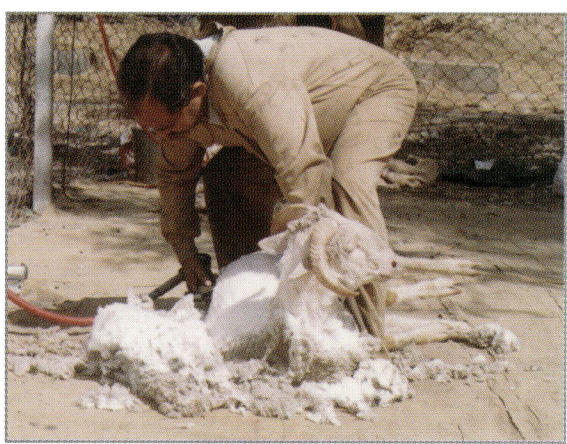

Fig. 42: The operation of machine shearing.

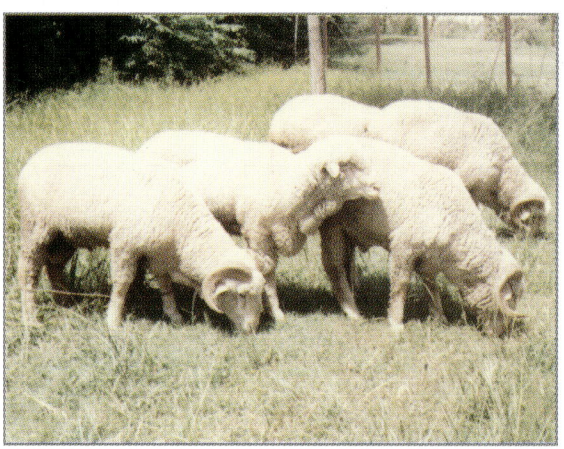

Fig. 43: Rams at the Open Nucleus Breeding Station.

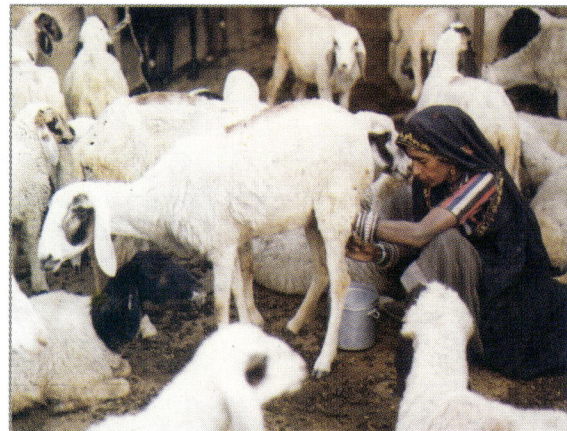

Fig. 44: Milking sheep — valuable for shepherd's family.

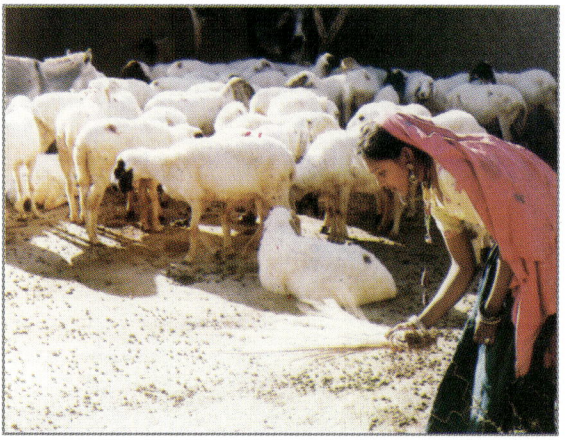

Fig. 45: Sheep dung pellets being collected by the farmer's family — more valuable is sheep manure for the land.

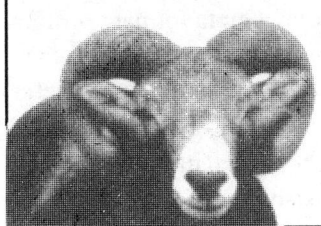

PREFACE

Most of the books about sheep husbandry available in India are of trans-Asia origin. The sheep rearing conditions and practices in Asian countries and India in particular are widely different from the countries of Europe, America and Australia. Hence, the dearth of a textbook relevant to Indian sheep rearing conditions was felt at times. My sheep farm career extended to almost two decades. Batches of fresh veterinarians and other trainees arrived at those sheep breeding and research projects for introductory training and grooming in sheep farming. In absence of required books they had to feel contented with the knowledge contained in the books of foreign authors.

This deficiency became further apparent during my teaching stint at the Veterinary College of Sher-i-Kashmir University of Agriculture Science and Technology (SKAUST) from 1996 to 2001. The demand from the students and the teaching staff for a suitable book on the shelves of library was ever pressing. This inspired me to take up the present venture. The class notes compiled by me as per syllabi for the various Animal Science courses of BVSc and AH degree laid the foundation of the book.

In this direction, the lectures of my revered teachers and professors during post graduate studies in the fields of sheep and wool production, sheep management, breeding and reproduction at ICAR institute Pune, HAU (Hissar) and Jaipur (Rajasthan) respectively have been of immense help. During the years 1959 to 2001, I had ample occasions to move across the livestock rearing areas of Rajasthan, Gujarat, Maharashtra, Karnataka, Andhra Pradesh, Tamil Nadu, Uttar Pradesh, Punjab, Himachal Pradesh and of course Jammu and Kashmir extensively. These visits afforded the needed eye appraisal of the sheep breeds, rearing practices and sheep and wool development in various regions.

The study and research work at a couple of small ruminant farms enabled the collection of a voluminous data and information. The liberal access to the libraries of Haryana Agricultural University, Punjab Agricultural University, Tamil Nadu University of Veterinary Sciences, Chennai, and the Departmental Library of Sheep Husbandry, Jammu, has proved a boon and is acknowledged with extreme gratitude. My sincere thanks are due to the authors of the literature cited and Food and Agriculture Organisation of the United Nations for reproduction of data from yearbooks and other information/photographs of sheep breeds from their other publications.

In addition to personal observations recorded in the treatise, lecture notes and literature of outside authors and recent publications of Indian authors have been relied upon for the account of exotic and Indian sheep breeds. The chapters on

Sheep Nutrition and Ruminal Digestion are the salient contribution of Dr. R.K. Sharma, Associate Professor (Nutrition), SKUAST, Jammu. Likewise Dr. R.K. Taggar and Dr. D.K. Karna, Assistant Professors (Ani. Breeding), SKUAST, Jammu, assisted in the preparation of the chapter 'Application of Breeding Principles'.

I am thankful to Dr. S.B. Bakshi, Assistant Professor, and Dr. S.K. Kotwal, Associate Professor of Veterinary Faculty, SKUAST, Jammu, for regular checking, rearranging of contents of the book and valuable suggestions towards improving the text material.

Appreciation is due to Mr Chaman Lal and Mr Surinder Kumar for the initial typing and subsequent computerization of the manuscript. The assistance of Mrs. Monika Mahajan for the drawings and Mr. Narjay Gupta for data scrutiny and conversion, etc. need a special mention here. My wife Mrs. Promila Gupta shared the anxieties in the compilation of this endeavour all through.

I hope the future editions shall make good the deficiencies and omissions as a part of regular improvement in the contents of this book in the times to come. Suggestions from the students, teachers, scientists and readers shall be most welcome.

Last but not the least, I place on record my sincere thanks to CBS Publishers and Distributors, Darya Ganj, New Delhi, for bringing out this book in the shortest time.

J.L. GUPTA

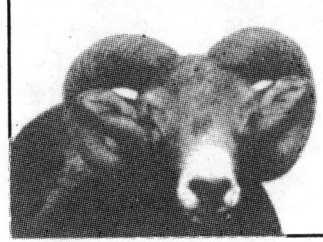

CONTENTS

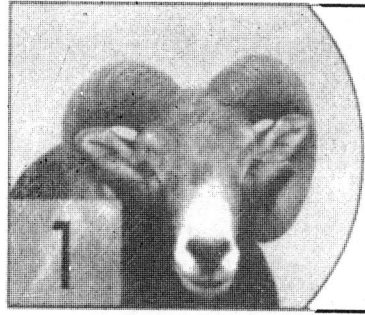

GLOBAL OVERVIEW OF SHEEP FAUNA

ORIGINAL SHEEP FAUNA

The prehistoric sheep inhabited various parts of the world, viz. Asia, Africa, Europe and America in wild state before domestication. The multitude of primitive *ovine* germ plasm is believed to have originated from these very progenitors. The wild fauna of *Ovis viginei* (the Urial) once roamed about in the mountains and plains of south west Asia, the *Ovis ammon* (the Argali) in the Asiatic highlands and the *Ovis musimon* (the Mouflon) in the south eastern Europe. The big horn, *O. canatensis* is believed to have existed in western and north America and the Audad, *O. tragalaphus* in north Africa.

Available evidence, genetic inferences and morphological relationship have more or less established origin of domestic sheep, *Ovis aries,* from the wild Urial, the Argali and the Mouflon. Fossil remains and findings of bones of domestic sheep recovered from Ammon in Turkey point to early existence of sheep in the countries of western Asia. The archaeological discoveries made there and in China, Egypt and Greece further establish a close relationship of neolithic man with sheep. Though the evidence of it are far numerous in Europe than in Asia, many a naturalist believe that the domestic sheep in all probability originated in Afro-Asian region.

Ladakh (India) and Tibetan plateau still do provide a glimpse of flocks of wild sheep types struggling for survivability in the inhospitable and remote terrains. Farther from the human habitation, more secure they appear to be.

SHEEP DOMESTICATION

Taxonomy

In the animal kingdom (Animalia) the domestic sheep is assigned the following zoological lineage.

Phylum	Chordata	Vertebrates
Class	Mammalia	Having suckling and hairy young ones
Order	Ungulate	Hoofed animals
Suborder hooves	Artiodactyla	Cloven footed
Section	Pecora	True ruminants
Family	Bovidae	Having hollow horns
Subfamily	Caprinae	Sheep and goat
Genus	Ovis	Sheep
Specie type	*O. aries*	Domestic sheep

Symbiotic relationship

The association of wandering man with the wandering sheep dates back to almost 12,000 years. For the survival of Stone-age man sheep was a highly prized gift of nature. Subsequent to early discovery of man about food value of sheep before wool, he learned that to protect his body from freezing cold, the sheep could be worth more alive than dead (Nina Hyde, 1988).

The early civilization thus developed a partial to complete dependence on sheep. Vulnerability of it in the hands of predators and the element of protection and propagation in the house holds further strengthened the mutual bondage of existence between man and sheep. Exploitation of such a symbiosis by mankind is considered to have resulted in the evolution of varied sheep races. The protracted process of domestication and sustained pressure of forces of genetic mutation, migration, natural selection and genetic assimilation over the ages, have all contributed to an unimaginable diversification. As a consequence, the number of sheep breeds has increased enormously over the past 8,000 to 10,000 years. However, the complex development of wild germ plasm into varietal domestic sheep types and breeds is hard to conjecture, or conclude in absence of detailed morphological and DNA studies. The mention of use of wool and woollens in the *Rigveda, Mahabharta* and many other old testaments lends enough credence to the fact that association of sheep with the Indian society dates back to far earlier period than the recent age projections of historical background of sheep rearing in India.

DOMESTICATION CHANGES

A remarkable change in the choice traits and parameters leading to specialized genotypes has come about and resulted in the formation of widely different types. But in the entire history of sheep domestication and breed origin a couple of evolutionary changes have remained unreconciled.

1. While the wild sheep have horned males and occasionally polled ewes, a number of breeds of domestic sheep are invariably polled.

2. All wild sheep possess short tails, but the domestic breeds have medium to long tails. Explanation generally cited for the appearance of polled trait in the domestic sheep includes the genetic mutation, where as the long tail development is attributed to a gradual evolutionary change. This further might have got preserved under domestication.

3. The third controversial feature of wild sheep is its possession of hairy coat with or without an inner short and finer coat. But for, perpetuation of hairy coat in certain primitive types, the hairy coat has almost disappeared in domestic sheep by and large. Density and length of fibres rather increased in the covering to the extent of fleece formation. The emergence of maximum woolly undercoat in the sheep of drier southern Europe and least soft undercoat development in the Asiatic humid region sheep is a striking feature.

4. Yet another issue is the seasonal shedding of hairy or fibre coat in spring by the primitive sheep. Soay* and wild Indian sheep varieties show shedding much alike the Tibetan antelope (*Chiru*), the Ibex or even Cashmere goat. The merinos and other modern varieties on the other hand do not exhibit such a seasonal behaviour.

ABORIGINAL SHEEP RACES

As cited by some investigators the evidence of Mesopotamian** civilization (4000-3000 BC) reveals a division of their domestic sheep into three types. Hairy sheep was the one that existed. The second was a broad tailed strain and the third a true fleece bearing type. Appearance of a broad tail is assumed to represent the first step in development. Apparently this type of sheep had many characteristics which persisted in several modern breeds of southwest Asia. But the particular type of sheep does not seem to have continued long with the Mesopotamian civilization. The sheep that remained in Asia were of coarse wool type suggesting their kinship to Argali sheep.

The fleece type or the third category subsequently emerged as a true domestic sheep, what actually was seen in the Egyptian sheep in the early centuries (3400 to 2400 BC). The sheep scientists infer that the evolution of definite types finally led to the development of three prominent races of sheep on this globe, viz.

---

* Soay sheep resemble the primitive sheep of Bronze Age Europe, found on the islands of Soay, off the West Coast of Scotland that shed their fleece annually.

** Mesopotamia-Syria, contemporary Iraq, i.e. country situated between the two rivers, the Tigris and Euphrates.

Egyptian sheep,

Thick and fat tail sheep, and

European sheep.

So intimately related was the sheep to various civilizations that it too suffered ups and downs with the rise and fall of dynasties. Wool was the chief source of wealth of traders and also the main revenue of the rulers.

Egyptian sheep

These are considered to have existed during prehistoric period about 5000 to 4000 BC. Apparently related to hairy Mesopotamian breed, these sheep were leggy with short spiral, transversely projected horns. Though these were predominant around 2400 to 1580 BC, the type gradually became extinct and fat tailed ones occupied the position. With the formation of a new empire in Egypt another breed with heavy horns and long thin legs appeared in 1580-1050 BC. The sheep scientists further believe that both these breeds and the hairy ones came originally from Syria. Probably hairy sheep could survive outside domestic control. The preservation of fat tailed and Ammon type could be entirely due to human protection. This latter variety was a real fleece sheep and eventually spread in most parts of North Africa.

The wandering man, hunters and herdsmen, inhabited the Nile valley in the pre-agricultural times. Their domestic animal possession included sheep and goat as well. Even before the Egyptian kingdom (3250 BC), Cyprus and other adjoining lands possessed reddish-brown Mouflon type domesticated sheep. Such animals show close resemblance to the modern breeds of European origin instead of any contemporary Egyptian or Asiatic ovine race.

Fat-tailed sheep

Fat-tailed and fat-rumped sheep have enormous fat accumulation at the rump region or on either side of tailbone. The lump of fat finds use in place of butter with the herdsmen. These sheep bear little kinship or appearance to the European sheep. Dumba sheep found in Iran, Afghanistan and NWFP. or the Dagroskaya of Balkan states are the descendants of these fat tailed sheep. Besides Central Asia these fat tailed/fat rumped sheep are also found in Africa and parts of China.

Ancient European sheep

Around Swiss Lake habitations, the remains of a small slender horned race of sheep were discovered around 1861 AD. Subsequently alive samples were also located in isolated mountain regions of Europe. The characteristics were that of a small black faced, black legged sheep with tail that reached the hocks. Sheep possessed goat like sharp horns, small mobile ears, short thick fleece, pigmented or glistening white. This type was named 'Torbary sheep'. Further evidence linked the origin of these sheep to wild Urial as per discoveries made in Turkestan, Cyprus and Asia Minor. A couple of investigators believe that the earliest domestic European sheep was derived from this stock. Massive spiral horns and other features of this race exhibited a close resemblance to the Mouflans.

The foregoing sheep types of Urial and Mouflan origin are further recognized as the forerunners of domestic breeds of northern Europe, southern Europe, fine woolled sheep or even the Iberian sheep.

North European sheep: A dark or mottled face sheep of moderate size was the first to exist in the northern part of the continent. It possessed a light coarse fleece and traits of Torbary sheep. Area of perpetration was in the north of Alps, the Ice lands or isolated fringes of Europe. Depending upon habitat and size, the northern sheep split into two types. A smaller variety thrived in the mountains and remote regions while the larger one proved thriftier in the low lands of Hungary, Germany, Scandinavia and Great Britain. Smaller strain sheep had mostly bare legs but better wool cover than the low land strains. Fleece was light, open, but with considerable pigmentation. Both the sexes were horned. Typical ones resembled the primitive 'Soay' sheep.

From the low land larger strains, the modern longwool breeds are considered to have originated, possibly following crossing with southern Europe sheep. Though there were black fibres dispersed in the fleece but the fleece appeared white because of more white fibres. Animals were usually bare face, bare legged and polled in majority of the cases.

South European sheep: The southern sheep was white faced, of medium size and of a relatively fine fleece. It was found throughout the Mediterranean zone in Rome, Spain, Greece, etc. As against the nature of northern sheep to scatter, these sheep had a strongly developed flocking instinct. Modern fine wool breeds are certainly, related to this type of sheep.

The Phoenicians and Mesopotamians are known to have developed a breed in which fibre fineness and density was markedly superior. Phoenician sheep and woollens used to be bartered by their mariners for other products as early as 600 years BC with Greece colonies. Carthegians drove out the Phoenicians around 350 years BC. Shortly thereafter, the Romans overthrew the Carthegians in 330 BC. Romans were active colonizers. They introduced sheep into Spain (Iberia) and Britain. All of the Roman colonies that raised sheep were encouraged and supervised in developing woollens.

The primitive fleece bearing sheep of the southern Europe provided the material for the future development of apparel wool.

ORIGIN OF FINE WOOL SHEEP

Wool was first worn in the form of a sheepskin. Because of the ease with which the wool fibres could be spun and thread woven and comfort derived from woven fibres, the wool probably became the first textile material to be used for clothing by the early man (Nina Hyde, 1988).

The credit for foundation of early Spanish Merino goes to Romans, who applied proper breeding systems and selection. With the over-running of Romans by Barbarians and subsequent set back to wool weaving at the hands of Barbarians and Moors, it were the monks who by their interest of agriculture prevented the loss of improved fine wool sheep. Two distinct breeds of sheep (the Merino and the Churos) appeared in Spain as a result of their work in the early Christian era. According to Ross (1989) Tarenton strain of superior fleece sheep developed by Romans lacked hardiness and required special care. These sheep were crossed by the Spanish during the reign of Claudius (1437-1440 AD) with the Laodician sheep of Asia minor and were the parent stock of Merino breed.

Development features of Spanish merino

A high degree of improvement was reached in the northern provinces of Spain, where vast and plentiful pasture was available. At the advent of winters these sheep were driven towards southern plains to travel back to their native northern grounds on the approach of summers. This system followed over many decades manifested into genetic assimilation resulting into behavioural reflection and instinct to change of pasture with the approach of season. They were consequently termed 'Transhumant' flocks.

The government applied a code of regulations for the transhument flocks and shepherds. This law regulated the periodical migrations. Winter pastures were reserved for them at a fixed rate. A strip of land of considerable width was left in grass along either side of the road for grazing and accommodation during to and fro movement from north to south and vice-versa. The sheep were kept in congenial temperature for better wool development. The wool of migratory flocks commanded nearly twice the price than that of the Estantes, i.e. the stationary flocks.

Merinos in Spain were then held as property by the Crown, the nobles or the clergies. Export of these sheep was prohibited but for royal decree or favour, or smuggling. Extreme attention was bestowed towards the fleece. Spain, therefore, exercised monopoly over fine wool until 19th century. Transhument flocks had the peculiar flocking instinct and gregariousness. These impulses and the tendency to follow a leader were so strong as to suggest a predominant descent from wild sheep Urial.

Scenario in other countries

Exceptional development in other countries like France, USA, Australia, New Zealand, Germany and Scandinavia took place by the middle of nineteenth century with complete dispersion of Merino blood in the virgin lands, through exportation thus breaking the Spanish monopoly over fine wool. A dissemination of merino was also witnessed in South Africa, Argentina, USSR and in some of the Asian and Latin American countries. The attempts to acclimatize merino in England did not succeed.

Argentina: Sheep was introduced in the 17th century and the Merino came late in the 18th century. Before 1880, the main trade of Argentina was wool, skin or hide and tallow. After 1880, Argentina and Uruguay became next only to New Zealand and Australia as a main source of mutton and lamb export to UK. It stood third only in the world in wool production in the middle of the 20th century and now continues to maintain a leading position after Australia, South Africa, USSR, New Zealand and China.

South Africa: The original native sheep of South Africa were fat tailed ones. Eastern parts proved suitable and these sheep predominated there. Merino sheep got introduced in 1812. Between 1904 and 1955 the population of woolly sheep increased from 11 million to 30 million. The number further soared steeply and majority of the sheep is Merino now. In the new environment of that country the development and selection has resulted into the upcoming of South African Merino. Almost all the wool is exported. Suitability of the country appears more for wool production than for mutton. As a producer and as an exporter of finest Merino wool South Africa is second in importance to Australia.

Australia: The entry of a few hundred fine wool sheep in Australia from Europe took place in ending eighteenth and early nineteenth century.

Vast grazing grounds and favourable climatic conditions resulted in Australia's growth, into world's biggest sheep country. Increase in population has been phenomenal. The sheep number has increased to 120 m within two hundred years. Over 90% of the sheep produce are available for export. Practically half of the sheep population is concentrated in south eastern parts of New South Wales. Despite refrigeration and active effort to build up frozen meat export trade; mutton and lamb have remained secondary to wool as a source of country's wealth. Presently Australia is the main exporter of Merino germ plasm to sheep rearing countries of the world despite export embargo on these sheep.

New Zealand: Sheep were introduced in this country in the year 1834 from New South Wales. Up to 1882, the merinos were the predominant sheep breeds of the country. Important export at that time was wool. After 1882, New Zealand switched over to lamb production. Favourable climate and pastures there helped the sheep enterprise to excel Australia and South Africa in fat lamb production. Another note worthy feature is that while developing her fat lamb industry New Zealand did not neglect wool export. Though quantum of Merino wool declined appreciably than the cross breed wool but wool export remained almost equal in value to lamb and mutton export.

United States of America: With the new settlers from Europe during 18th century, the sheep particularly the fine wool type found their entry into America. The rearing caught up initially but with subsequent development and industrialization, progress slowed down. Migratory sheep there used to be ranged in the central and inter-mountain Nevada desert. Sheep on the whole has not been so important industry despite existence and thriving of medium to big flocks in the ranches of Texas and Northwestern states. The main reasons being that mutton and lamb have never been popular among Americans who prefer beef. Secondly the woollen textile Industry of America remained dependent for its raw material from outside. This resulted into decrease in sheep numbers and thereby wool produced. The whole of wool production is consumed in the country. The reputed American Rambouillet is the predominant breed. Dorsets and many other sheep breeds are also maintained.

Russia: Erstwhile states of USSR had entirely coarse woolled sheep like other Asian countries. However, in the 20th century, the Russians through cross breeding with fine wool Merino from Australia and other countries evolved a number of fine woolled sheep of higher productivity like: Russian Merino and Stavropol, Grozenskaya, Caucasian, etc. This has been achieved through massive sheep imports, artificial insemination and strict management. Though former USSR occupies the position of 2nd highest wool producer in the world, yet it continues to be a major importer of wool.

Before the industrial revolution in Europe, UK, Germany and France had exceedingly good sheep. Spain was the abode of finest wool producing Merino and France the originator of Rambouillet. Germans too developed a heavyweight medium type of German merino, whereas England evolved large number of dual purpose and prolific sheep.

All the western industrialized countries like UK, France, Germany, Belgium, Italy, Russia, Czechoslovakia, Poland and even USA are importers of raw wool. In Asia Japan is the main importer of wool.

SHEEP DISTRIBUTION

The scatter of sheep types and population of the specie in various continents and countries of the globe presents a peculiar feature. A marked observation is the negligible presence of sheep in the hot humid regions. Coastal belt too is devoid of any appreciable sheep concentration. On the other hand, arid and semi arid zones whether cooler or warmer abound with sheep. The Nevada desert of America, the Thar desert of Rajasthan and the vast lands of Australia sustain a large sheep population. Temperate and sub-temperate areas of western Europe, USSR and Asia also support a sizeable number of sheep.

The mountain ranges of Alps, the Himalayas and the Karakurams are known to be the favourable abode of sheep fauna. A good number of excellent breeds still thrive on the sloppy terrains' of these mountains. For centuries now the diverse type of ovine fauna has survived under domestic and varied ecological conditions. Adaptation of sheep in the virgin lands and new environments further helped its proliferation. The number of sheep breeds existing in the world presently is estimated around 900.

Variable pattern of sheep survivability, production and population has attracted the attention of scientists. Transhument nature of flocks in Asia, Europe and American continents facilitated the acclimatization. The generations of improvised management have further helped the domestic sheep to gain foothold under diverse conditions. But the specie appears to have flourished in the areas that provided free movement and choice grazing. A close association is found to exist between 40 to 100 cm rainfall and density of sheep population. A consensus almost emerges about the existence of general levels of congenial environment and favourable climatic factors for sheep husbandry, viz.

1. Mean temperature to range between –2°C and +25° F. Range is wider under arid climatic conditions.
2. Annual rainfall ranging from 25 cm to 120 cm with a preferable monthly spread between 1.0 cm to 10.0 cm.
3. Relative humidity at lower environmental temperature to range between 65 to 95 percent and from 55 to 80 percent at higher limit of temperature.

Asia has the largest chunk of almost 37% of the total world sheep population (FAO 1997). This is followed by Africa 22%, Australian subcontinent 16%, Europe 15%, North America 2% and South America 8%. Based on 1991 sheep population statistics, Croston and Pollott (1994) indicated that Europe topped in sheep population density with 31 sheep per 100 hactares of land and 183 sheep/ 100 hac. of permanent pasture. In Asia the sheep population density was 12 sheep/100 hac. of land and 50 sheep/100 hac. of permanent pasture (Tables 1.1 and 1.2) .

IMPORTANT SHEEP REARING COUNTRIES

1. The early sheep rearing owes its existence in Northern hemisphere, particularly Asia and Europe. In the former, Afghanistan, Israel, Iran, India, Tibet and China possessed certain breeds having similarity to primitive wild sheep. Bulk of Asia's woolly and hairy sheep population is dispersed in China, India and Pakistan. The Central Asian countries are the abode of most of the fat-tailed and fat-rumped sheep (Table 1.3). Information about their further development in the Asian countries is obscure. However, the history of European sheep is better known, especially in the following three main areas.

   - Spain, where the development of fine wool sheep, the Merino took place.
   - Britain, the home country, where the evolution of excellent dual purpose and mutton sheep came into being.
   - South eastern Europe, particularly Italy and Balkan states, where flourished the mutton, wool and milk producing, triple purpose sheep.

2. Sheep concentration in the Southern hemisphere remained mainly confined between 20° to 60° latitude. A definite impact was visible in:

   - Argentina, Uruguay and some other parts of South America,
   - South African countries,
   - Australia, and
   - New Zealand.

During the 17th century the sheep industry was at peak in the Northern hemisphere. After exploration of Newlands, settlement of deported people came up. With them the sheep found entry in a couple of new countries like New Zealand, Australia and America and also started flourishing

Table 1.1: Sheep population (million)

Area	1960-62 (average)	1979-81 (average)	1988	1997	2001
World	1015	1092	1173	1064	1056
Asia	238	343	357	399	406
India	41	45	46.7	56.4	58.2

Source: FAO Production Year Books.

Table 1.2: Continental statistics of sheep population (000)

Continent	1979-81 (average)	1988	1997	2001
Africa	125517	138360	233585	250147
Asia	343429	357713	399546	406584
Australia + New Zealand (Oceania)	202264	217043	167248	164001
Europe	123288	166509	162951	144812
North America	13151	11466	16049	15327
South America	110660	112250	85034	75312

Source: FAO Production Year Book, Vol. 39 (1985), Vol. 53 (1999), and Vol. 55 (2001).

Table 1.3: Sheep population of important sheep rearing countries (000)

Sl. No.	Country	1979-81 (average)	1985	1995	1997	2001
1.	Afghanistan	18667	13600	14300	14300	11000 *
2.	Australia	134871	149747	120862	123333	120000 F
3.	Argentina	31473	28750	21626	17295	13500 F
4.	Bulgaria	10358	10501	3398	3020	2286
5.	China	101864	95194	117446	132691	133160
6.	Ethiopia	23205	23000	21750	21850	22500 F
7.	France	12133	12676	10320	10126	10000 F
8.	India	44987	46930	54131	56472	58200 F
9.	Italy	9120	11098	10682	10920	11089
10.	Iran	34740	40000	50898	52000	53000 F
11.	Kazakhstan	34162	35379	24273	13000	8939
12.	Mongolia	14261	13391	13787	13561	15667
13.	New Zealand	67393	67854	48816	43394	43987
14.	Pakistan	22580	25037	29065	30532	24200
15.	Romania	15766	18637	10897	9663	7800 *
16.	Russian Fed.	63566	61700	31818	21710	14000 *
17.	Somalia	10467	11800	13500	13500	13200 F
18.	South Africa	31625	30256	28784	29187	28800 F
19.	Spain	14721	17520	23018	21827	24400
20.	Sudan	17628	19709	23200	24500	47000 F
21.	Turkey	46199	40391	35646	33072	29435 F
22.	UK	21643	23946	42771	42559	33697
23.	Uruguay	19219	21196	20205	19770	13032 F
24.	USA	12670	10716	8886	7937	6965
25.	Former USSR	142591	142876	90653	63072	–

Source: FAO Production Year Book, Vol. 39 (1985), Vol. 53 (1999), and Vol. 55 (2001).

there. Suitable climatic conditions, vast pastures, cheap and abundant land and absence of competition for land favoured fast multiplication. Soon after, these countries possessed more than half the sheep population of the world. Relatively cheaper rates of wool and mutton led to immense export of the commodities. In the beginning of 20th century industrial revolution in Europe slackened the tempo of sheep production. The coming up sheep industry in Southern hemisphere gave a further setback in the Northern hemisphere owing to two reasons.

1. The entry of cheaply produced and abundant superior wool from Southern hemisphere in Europe checked the expansion of Merino sheep in Europe resulting in the steady decline in wool production.

2. The invention of refrigeration technology at the dawn of industrial revolution made the export of mutton and frozen lamb possible from Australia and New Zealand to European meat market. As a result some profound changes in the economy of sheep industry of sheep breeding countries took place. Unlike Asia where tribals mainly maintained sheep, in Australia, New Zealand, America and in some of the European countries the sheep rearing has been adopted as a part of elite farming. The big sheep properties occupy a status of honour and economic prosperity.

SHEEP—A PREFERRED ANIMAL

As compared to other classes of livestock the sheep possesses the following advantages:

- They are unexcelled in the utilization of more arid type of ground vegetation.
- They utilise wasteland. As excelled scavengers, sheep consume stubbles, clean fields and destroy weeds.
- Compared to cattle they produce more liberally in proportion to what they consume.
- Being ever productive, the two products wool and lamb (mutton) are available for market at two different periods. It seldom happens that both items sell at bottom price in any period.
- Sheep returns are quicker, lamb may be marketed within 18 months after the ewes are bred.
- Habit of bedding down on the raised areas of the range or grazing ground leaves the larger portion of droppings at spots where they are needed most.
- The way the manure pellets are dropped in the farmlands and trampled into the soil by gentle movement, ensure minimum wastage of pasture biomass.
- Dispersal of seed of pasture material through contact and defecation in the pasture offers the effortless advantages. Besides, moistening of seed in the pasture also takes place through urination.
- Wool clip is easily stored and transhipped.
- Sheep do not require expensive housing or equipment. Lambs born in cold weather may require warm shelter at lambing time. After that protection from wind and storm only and a dry place to lie down are needed.
- Rearing practices and feeding habits do not warrant intensive labour.
- Emerging concept compares sheep to a traveller's cheque, sell and cash it wherever, whenever required to meet exigencies.

FACTORS DETRIMENTAL TO SHEEP PRODUCTION

Following are some of the factors that are quite unfavourable to sheep production.

- Wool has always been a politicized matter and it is apt to remain so, thus making it rather difficult to predict prices over a long period of

Table 1.4: Comparative status of sheep and lamb production of various continents (000 tonnes)

Continent	Year	Gr. wool prod.	Mutton prod.	Skins prod. (dry wt.) sheep and lamb	Milk prod.
Africa	1989-91 *aver.*	227	900	34.9	1424
	1997 *est.*	210	1129	39.1	1603
Asia	1989-91 *aver.*	560	2056	98.6	3423
	1997 *est.*	619	3031	145.2	3520
Australia + NZ	1989-91 *aver.*	1370	1178	89.0	–
(Oceania)	1997 *est.*	981	1106	77.6	170
Europe	1989-91 *aver.*	307	1429	86.9	2920
	1997 *est.*	231	1255	78.2	2779
North America	1989-91 *aver.*	47	203	5.5	–
	1997 *est.*	28	153	4.2	–
South America	1989-91 *aver.*	302	289	19.8	33
	1997 *est.*	198	265	18.2	35

Source: FAO Production Year Book, Vol. 49 (1995) and Vol. 51 (1997). World Statistical Compendium for raw hides and skins (1998). FAO Commodities and Trade Div. of the United Nations.

Table 1.5: Sheep production status of major sheep rearing countries (000 tonnes)

Country	Greasy wool production		Mutton and lamb production		Skins (dry weight)	
	1989-91 average	2001	1989-91 average	2001	1989-91 average	1997
Argentina	143	58 F	85	50 F	4.8	3.2
Afganistan	15	17 F	113	88 F	3.5	3.7
Australia	1042	700 F	613	663 *	38.5	35.6
Bulgaria	26	8 F	66	41 F	3.4	1.2
China	239	305 F	551	1435 F	20.7	54.0
Ethiopia	12	11 F	–	83 F	–	5.6
France	22	22 F	171	135 F	8.7	8.0
India	42	48 F	181	230	12.9	13.5
Italy	14	11 F	79	60	8.0	7.2
Iran	45	74 F	233	280 F	16.3	28.8
Kazakhstan	3	23	–	88 F	–	10.2
Mongolia	21	22	108	90	2.7	2.0
New Zealand	318	250	565	562	50.4	42.6
Pakistan	47	39	189	39 *	6.9	8.3
Romania	35	22 F	92	54 F	6.4	5.7
Russian Fed	–	38 F	–	110 *	–	12.1
Somalia	–	–	32	38	2.2	2.4
South Africa	98	53 F	133	118 F	10.1	9.6
Spain	30	31 F	216	240	13.4	12.8
Sudan	21	46 F	70	144 F	2.6	3.2
Turkey	64	44 F	305	313 F	11.7	10.0
UK	75	47	374	258	20.4	21.8
Uruguay	90	54	60	50 F	5.5	4.6
USA	40	21 F	162	103	5.2	3.8
Former USSR	463	–	942	–	31.1	33.6

Source: World Statistical Compendium for Raw hides and skins (1998), FAO Commodities and Trade Divsiion of the United Nations.

FAO Production Year Book, Vol. 49 (1995), Vol. 51 (1997), Vol. 53 (1999), and Vol. 55 (2001).

F   FAO estimates.

*   Unofficial figures.

time. The International Exim Policies and trends within the country are prone to fluctuations.

- The increasing competition with synthetic fibres.
- Bias persists in certain quarters against sheep as an environmental degrader.
- Squeezing forage resources, urbanization and industrialization.
- Certain heart problems in the human beings are being attributed to high mutton intake.

- Sheep themselves are susceptible to parasitism. Lower disease resistance than other classes of livestock is deterrent to rearing a flock of sheep.
- Tending and shepherding are not particularly attractive. This results in the scarcity of satisfactory herders and knowledgeable hands.
- These animals fall an easy prey to the predators, which are innumerable, right from vultures, jackals, dogs, wolves to panthers, bears, etc.

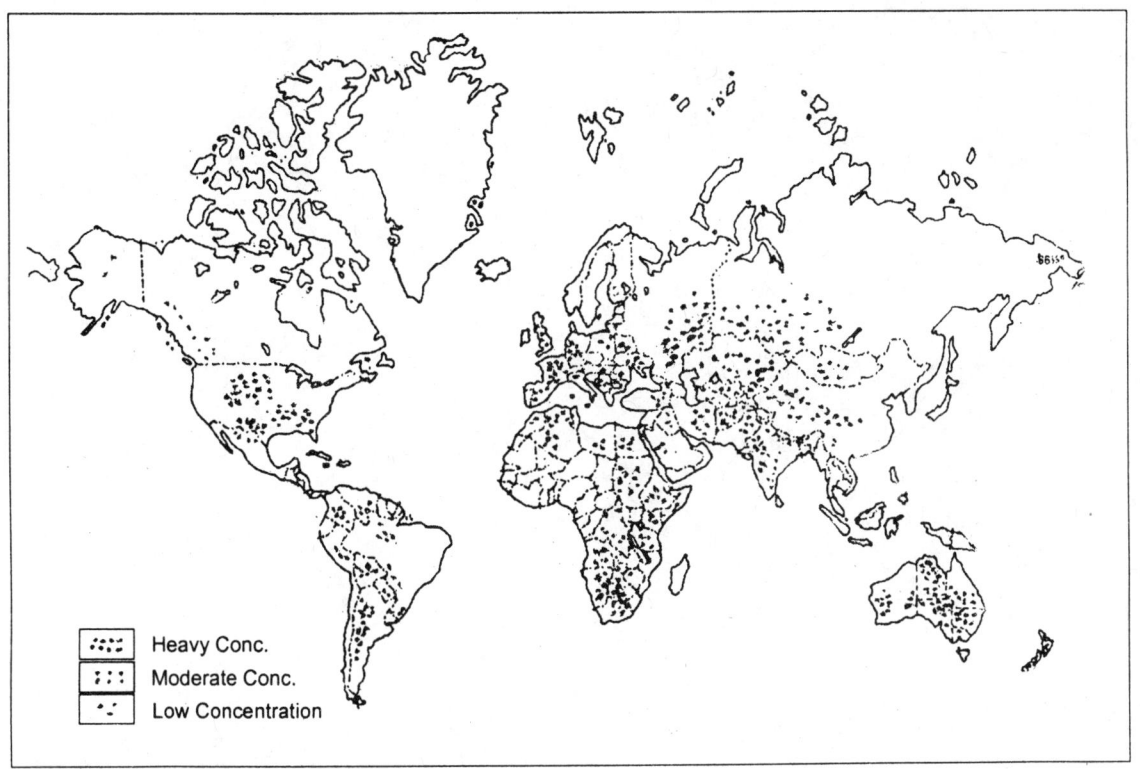

Fig. 1.1. Sheep distribution in world (important sheep rearing countries).

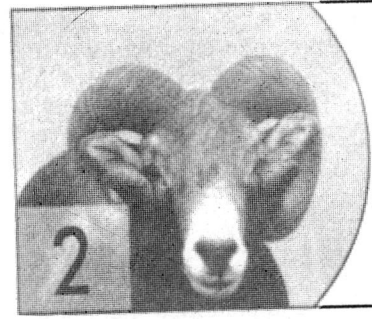

DOMESTIC SHEEP TYPES

BASIS OF CLASSIFICATION

For classification of sheep breeds varying yardsticks are employed. A universally considered basis is the wool quality or the nature of wool coat of the sheep. Categorization into various types is also practised as per genetic groups or on product utility aspects. Pattern of rearing system has also led to identification of sheep into migratory, semi-migratory and sedentary ones.

Wool coat

The domestic sheep world over has a wide range of body coat from hairy to fine wool variety. The nature of wool has served to classify sheep into various wool types.

Fine wool type: Like Merino, Rambouillet, Caucasian, Stavropol, Kashmir Merino, Bharat Merino, Polworth and a number of other Merino strains and Merino crossbreds.

Medium wool type: Particularly English Down breeds viz. South Down, Dorset Horn, Suffolk, Polled Dorsets and Indian Breeds like Chokla, Nilgiri, Karnah, Rampur Bushahr and Merino half-breds of Indian sheep breeds. The staple length in English breeds is shorter as compared to Indian breeds and cross breds.

Coarse carpet wool type: In this class are included the mixed wool breeds, Scottish black face, Navajo and most of the indigenous sheep of Rajasthan, Gujarat, Maharashtra and North temperate region.

Long wool breeds: Coarser than above but grow into longer staples. These sheep are further split into:
1. Lustrous wool: Leicester, Romney Marsh, Lincoln, Border Leicester, etc.
2. Demilustrous wool: Like Cheviot.

Hairy sheep breeds: Like Dumba, Chang-thangi and most of the India's Southern plateau sheep breeds.

Genetic basis

Pure breds: Original pure-breeds, like Merino, Lincoln, Down breeds, Dumba, Karakuls, Deccani, Nali, Gaddie and other indigenous Indian breeds.

Crossbreds: Corriedales, Polworth, Russian Merino, Kashmir Merino, Hissardale, and Bharat Merino.

Others: Triple or multiple breed crosses, though not a popular approach, yet remarkable results achieved in a couple of cases, viz. crosses of Nilgiri with fine wool breeds and development of Cormo and Targhee sheep.

Utility

Woolly sheep: Where primary emphasis is wool. Merino strains and Merino crossbred breeds, i.e. Kashmir Merino, Bharat Merino.

Mutton sheep: Sheep where emphasis is mainly on a muttonous conformation and mutton production, South Down, Polled Dorsets and Mandya sheep breeds are typical examples.

Dual and triple purpose sheep: The sheep breeds in the development of which more than one trait receives attention, i.e. wool and mutton or wool, lamb (mutton) and milk.

The example of former type is Corriedale or even Rambouillet. In the latter types are included the Patanwadi, Zeckel, Welshmore, Romanov type sheep breeds.

Special purpose breeds: The Karakuls for pelt; Dumba for fat. Changthangi for pack purpose. These are additional utility angles other than the usual wool, mutton, etc.

Exotic and indigenous sheep

The former types of sheep are the ones that exist or have been developed in other countries. These have a clear distinction over the latter 'the Desi sheep of Indian subcontinent from origin and habitation angles. Whereas, a visible genetic transformation has occurred in the exotic sheep over the centuries to excel in specialised traits, the indigenous varieties have remained almost genetically preserved until recent times. In both the types we come across diverse genotypes, breeds and even variations in nature, characteristics, productivity, adaptability, disease resistance, etc.

The exotic sheep being dealt in this chapter are generally classified further as:

Fine wool breeds

Fine wool crossbreds

Long wool breeds

Down breeds or mutton sheep

Milch sheep.

FINE WOOL EXOTIC TYPE

These mainly include Spanish merino descendants:

Saxon merino

The cousin of king of Spain in Saxony received a royal gift of 300 Escurial sheep in the year 1765 AD. Under the meticulous care, shelter and feeding by the German shepherds, a flock of superior wool merino came into existence in Saxony after selection. These sheep achieved an exquisite fineness of wool and marvellous fleece far better than the native Spanish.

French merino

With the permission of king of Spain, Louis XVI of France purchased 334 Merino ewes, 42 rams and 7 wethers in 1786 and stationed them at an experimental farm in village Rambouillet near Paris. It is said that the French maintained them on improved but undisclosed management practices and thus developed a fine wool sheep which subsequently came to be known Rambouillet sheep, after the name of the village.

It was bigger in size, sturdy, more prolific, fast maturing, possessing a better muttonous conformation and a plain body. Though more of a woolly sheep the Rambouillet presented the overall characters of a dual purpose sheep.

As it happened, the Rambouillet gradually disappeared from the progressive scenario of France. But in the virgin lands of America it flourished making it believe the USA particularly Northwest states and later Texas region of that country was in fact the home of Rambouillet. From America these sheep have been imported into India repeatedly in the second half of 20th century. Number far exceeds any other imported sheep. Right from the north temperate to arid region and Deccan plateau, this breed is the only one that has performed well.

Merino in England

Royal sheep of Spain attracted attention far and wide, especially that of nearby domains. King George IV of England too ventured to introduce Merino, but due to existing good breeds in England, the sheepmen there neither liked these sheep nor the merino thrived in the humid environment of England.

Merino in America

British settlers had carried with them the longwool English sheep. It was only in 1810 that Colonel Humphery brought the Merino to USA. Keeping the importance of wool in view, special attention was paid towards fineness of fleece, weight of fleece and length of wool. But the carcass quality was attended to the least. As a result a small sheep with many skin folds, producing dense fine greasy wool called Vermont Merino was produced. Wrinkles made the shearing difficult. Predisposition to fly strike was quite marked. Due to yolk impregnation of fleece, yield was too low.

Where as the Vermont Merino possessed folds on neck, head, thighs and legs, further selection among them produced medium type and still plainer bodied Merino, the Delaine sheep, having comparatively less fine wool than Vermont but of a longer staple.

Merino in Australia

About 100 sheep were first introduced in Australia by Captain Phillip in 1788 and some more by two other Naval officers in 1791. Attempts proved futile (Belschner, 1965) Another effort was made by Captain John McArther with a larger consignment soon after. To get heavier fleeces he imported large number of Vermont sheep. This mistake was realized later as large-scale wrinkles were undesirable. A plainer body sheep carrying only three neck folds was developed by the Peppin sheepmen and named Peppin Merino. Many breeders suspect that some breeding manoeuvre must have been accomplished by the Peppin sheep breeders to avoid wrinkles. May be, they introduced some longwool blood. Spanish, German and French sheep also contributed to the development of Australian Merino. Recent observations by some investigators hint at the contribution of Indian sheep* in the development

of modern prolific merino sheep in Australia. These sheep are stated to have been exported via Calcutta to that country in the 18th century.

The Australian Merino has played a conspicuous role in the development of various crossbred types in various states of India in the 20th century. Hissardale, Deccan Merino, Nilgiri crossbred sheep, Kashmir Merino and Bharat Merino are such well-known Indian crossbred sheep that have Australian Merino blood.

Features of Australian merinos: Whole body of the sheep except eyes and muzzles is covered with dense white wool. Bare portion of muzzle is of pink fleshy colouration. White muzzle is objectionable. Eyes are light grey. Hoof and horns are of amber colour. Horns in male are well developed, spirally coiled. Ewes are invariably polled or may have insignificant buttons. Bare part of the face is covered with soft silky hair. Uniformity in wool is characteristic. The britch or thigh wool resembles the wool of the sides as much as possible. The back is thin fleshed, straight and only slightly elevated at the withers. The backbone is rather sharp.

Australian Merino development history reveals that it has been bred for quantity and quality of wool. Prolificacy, muttonous conformation or the dairy traits hardly found priority consideration of breeders. Till 1880 these merino in Australia produced just about 2 kg average greasy fleece. Selection, breeding manipulation, abundant pasturage, etc. raised the status from 3.5 kg average greasy wool in rams to 8 to 9 kg over a period of 120 years. A typical Merino fleece coat is firm and packed. On parting with fingers visible lumps of wool are discernible. Tips of wool are neither fuzzy, nor standing or straight and appear rex** type.

---

* The Booroola Merino flock situated near Cooma in Australia (reared by Seear's Brothers) is known for prolificacy. Turner (1982, 1993) and Ghalsasi et al (1993, 1994) reveal the possibility that the gene for high prolificacy got introduced to Australia with the Bengal microsheep Garole which were first shipped from Calcutta in 1792 and 1793. Besides prolificacy the Garole sheep have many other fleece and body chracteristics similar to those, reported for the early Bengal sheep in Australia. The DNA studies are reported under progress to establish the contribution of Garole sheep in the origin of Fec. B gene in Booroola flock. The latter sheep have an extended breeding season and can breed at most times of the year.

** rex: a fleece coat of uniform length of fibres and without any standing out fibres.

Merino in New Zealand

Introduction of Merino in New Zealand took place in 1834. Because of heavier rainfall in the North islands, the Merino did not thrive there. But performance was good in the uplands of South islands. Till the last quarter of 19th century wool had a good market. But then with the coming of refrigeration at the end of the century, subsequent wars in Europe and the demand for mutton, the wool trade took a change to mutton trade. Romney Marsh found a better favour with the farmer and the Merino was pushed out. In later years Corriedale sheep, a cross of Merino and long wool, mutton type sheep like Romeny and Lincoln occupied the centre stage of sheep breeding in New Zealand.

Merino in South Africa

Original sheep in the Union of South Africa were fat tailed type. But Merino got a quite congenial environment there and soon it came up into a second best homeland for Merino after Australia. The Merino germplasm had in fact come from the same source of Spain, France, Saxony and subsequently Australia. Tendency to go in for fine wooled and wrinkled Merino did not pay dividends and ultimately the Merino breeders preferred Peppin type. The Merino of South Africa today is of bigger frame producing less fine wool than the imported forefathers. Almost sixty years back (around 1940) Mysore state and present Maharashtra had imported South African Merinos for cross breeding trial in those states. For fine wool crossbreeding of temperate zone sheep of India this is viewed as a prospective alternative of Australian merino.

Merino in Argentina

In the South American continent, this is prominent Merino rearing country. The introduction of Merino followed after America. Vast natural pasture resources have helped to flourish the sheep and variety of merino germ plasm of comparable production has come up there.

CROSSBREDS OF FINE WOOL SHEEP

Beset with many international developments, the emphasis on sheep shifted in early 20th century from wool to mutton, as an item of income. Mutton industry afforded bonanza for some nations. This

Table 2.1: Important characteristic of exotic fine wool sheep breeds

Breed and home Country	Body weight (kg)		Greasy fleece weight (kg)		Wool yield %	Annual staple length (cm)	Wool count. ('s)	Lambing %
	Ram	Ewe	Ram	Ewe				
Merino								
Australia	68-91	45-64	8.2-12.7	3.6-6.4	45-65	7-12	60-80's	105-135
Argentina	70-80	50-60	10-14	4-6	60	5-8	60-64's	–
South Africa	52-91	36-54	6-9.5	4.5-8.2	45-55	7-12	62-70's	105-130
USA	68-102	36-72	4.5-11.4	3-8.2	45-60	6-9	64-70's	115-135
USSR	75-85	45-50	9.0-11.5	5-6	55-64	6-9	60-64's	120-130
Rambouillet								
USA	85-135	54-95	6.5-11.5	3.5-8	45-65	6-10	60-70's	105-160
France	80-85	45	–	–	45-60	6-9	64-72's	–
Delaine								
USA	68-90	54-65	6-9	4-6.5	50-60	6-10	64-72's	–

Source: (i) Dhamale and Mooley (1963-64); (ii) W.Von Bergen (1965); (iii) Personal collection (1988); (iv) Stan Dorman (1995)

trend resulted into many farmers trying at developing requisite type of animals. Merino when crossed with other breeds especially the long wool types produced progeny, which yielded maximum profits from both the items, viz. wool and mutton. Crosses further proved to be prolific, better milkers having superior carcass quality and fleece which was at least as valuable as superfine wool.

Corriedale

To achieve the objective of greatest economic return from both wool and meat, Australian breeders crossed Merino with well framed long wool breeds, then back crossed the progeny to pure Merino to produce a "come back" type similar to the Merino. The Corriedale was simultaneously evolved in both Australia and New Zealand around 1874 by selective breeding among crossbred offspring's of pure Merino and Romney/Lincoln sheep. The breed is now sufficiently fixed after a hundred years of line breeding.

1.   Romney Marsh rams × Merino ewes ↓ F_1

2.   Lincoln rams × Merino ewes ↓ F_1

Romney × Merino crosses were found least suitable but the Lincoln × Merino crosses proved satisfactory. This led to the abandoning of Romney as foundation of Corriedales.

As per official description it is a recognized breed, but no uniformity exists. It is believed that besides Lincoln as a chief stock, other longwool breeds like Romney, Leicester and Border Leicester rams may have also been used over Merino ewes. However heavy culling levels in the progeny and interbreeding amongst the best selected half breds for at least 15 years or 4 to 5 generations was resorted to for registration as a breed.

_____
* Lwj—Lambs weaned per ewe joined

The modern Corriedale is a large framed plain bodied, polled sheep producing heavy lamb carcasses and mutton, fleece is heavy, bright with good style, length and handle. Mean fibre diameter is 25 to 30 microns. Yield approaches 70%. Breed's popularity ranks second only to the Merino in the world. Corriedales account for almost 70% of sheep population in South America alone. *Lwj component to the extent of 1.40 can be achieved.

From time to time Corriedale sheep have been imported into India in the last forty years. Big consignments arrived in the Indo-Australian Project, Hissar in early seventies of twentieth century. Results on long-term basis reveal that these did not thrive or perform well except under orchard conditions of Kashmir and at a few other locations.

Polworth

Second such a crossbred sheep developed in late nineteenth century in Australia is Polworth. Reciprocal crosses between Merino and Lincoln were made and the F_1 back crossed to maintain three quarter Merino and one quarter Lincoln inheritance. To fix the characters interbreeding for three generations practised. These sheep are devoid of folds, have long stapled wool and proved suitable on mixed farms abroad. North-western states of this country particularly UP received good consignments of Polworth sheep but could not gain popularity at the Govt. farms where they were maintained in early sixties of twentieth century. Another big venture to rear Polworth sheep at Dhulia farm (Gujarat) was launched by M/s Raymonds soon after, but abandoned after a decade or so.

Bond sheep

By using Saxon/Peppin Stud Merino ewes and imported Lincoln rams Thomas Bond originated the said sheep in Lockhart, NSW. in 1909 through careful selection. Improvements have continued since then to raise this as Australia's best dual purpose sheep. Like Corriedale, the bond sheep are able to produce results in a wide climatic range. They are being managed successfully under 35 to 110 cm rainfall conditions.

Bonds are huge, long bodied heavy boned, open-faced sheep with robust constitution. In full wool and fattening state, a stud sire can weigh up to 150 kg and thereby appear as biggest breed currently available in Australia. They have big, bulky long stapled wool of 22-28 microns of a soft feel. Bonds are acclaimed for the production of long, lean, fast growing lambs with a sound ratio of lean meat to fat cover. Skin value is also stated more than any other traditional prime lamb. High fertility, high fleece weight and availability of lambs and wethers at very young age are characteristic of Bond sheep for big returns.

Other cross breds

By an identical breeding manoeuvre and by using other fine wool breeds too, a couple of more cross breds have been evolved in various countries, viz.

Panama	: Rambouillet rams x Lincoln ewes
Columbia	: Lincoln rams x Rambouillet ewes
Romaldale	: Romney Marsh x Rambouillet ewes
Cormo	: Corriedale rams x Merino ewes.
South dale	: South down rams x Corriedale ewes
Targhee	: Rambouillet rams x Triple cross ewe (of Lincoln, Rambouillet and Corriedale)

Indian crossbreeds of merino

Kashmir-merino is a product of Merino x local carpet wool sheep of Jammu and Kashmir. F_1 further crossed to fine wool merino strains to obtain a stabilised interbred of three fourth Merino and Delaine inheritance.

Hissardale, Deccan Merino, Bharat Merino and Nilgiri Merino are other fine wool crossbred sheep developed by various states in India by infusing Merino germplasm into local carpet wool breeds. The merino inheritance in all such crossbreds approaches 75%.

LONG WOOL BREEDS

England was once the home of most of the long coarse but lustrous wool sheep, particularly the Leicestershire, Lincolnshire, Romney Marsh and the Cotswool sheep. They were slow maturing and appear to have been bred exclusively for wool.

Lincoln

Originally belongs to Lincoln shire county in west England. Big in size, heavy, breed of poor mutton quality, but carrying the heaviest fleece of valuable long wool. Crossing the old Lincoln with Dishlay Leicester in the home country tended to fatten but the progeny reduced in size. This change was not much relished by the farmers. Lincoln is reckoned to produce heavier clip and mutton than other breeds. Wool is the strongest, lustrous and of the longest staple out of English breeds. Wool quality ranges from 36 to 44s. Leicester and a small British Lincoln appear identical. Head is long of medium width. Sheep have a forelock of wool hanging down the eyes. Face is otherwise dull, white and free of wool. A male yearling may weigh almost 80 kg and adult over 120 kg. Because of greater size, weight and long coarse wool, the Lincoln was much in demand for cross breeding the fine wool sheep in Australia and America. Improved Australian Lincoln sheep is heavier and produces 9 kg wool (10 month clip) of 30 to 40 micron fibre thickness and over 20 cm staple length. Annual wool production of adult rams may be 14 to 15 kg.

For improvement of fibre length and other traits of Indian fine wool crossbred sheep or their transformation into valuable lustrous wool variety the introduction of Lincoln blood has been suggested at times*. Rambouillet cross breds under sedentary and semi-migratory conditions in

---

* Recommended by Hafeq consultants (1978) Report Rajouri district J&K State; Golden Jubilee of Sheep Dev. in J&K (1992); Task Force Seminar to Review NCA recommendations for Northern States, held at Jammu (1993) and Gupta (1994).

Jammu and Kashmir state are sound foundation material to synthesize an indigenous Corriedale type by crossing these ewes with the Australian or New Zealand Lincoln sires.

Romney Marsh

English Romney is a tall and hardy breed adaptable to a wide range of pastoral conditions. These animals possess an outstanding degree of resistance to internal worm burden. Though the Romney Marsh sheep are capable of attaining good weight but are no match to Lincoln in this respect.

New Zealand Romney is low set with wide shoulders, well sprung ribs and with lighter bone. Wool is demi-lustrous suited for blankets, knitting yarn and tweed. Ten month clip grows to 12 to 15 cm. Carcass weight at yearling stage is around 32 to 35 kg and 40 to 45 kg for an adult animal. Fleece weight is 3.5 to 4 kg. These sheep were introduced in Bihar, Maharashtra and Tamil Nadu (erstwhile Madras State) four decades back. Breeding Nilgiri sheep with Romney resulted into staple and wool yield improvement. Definite observations about other stations are lacking. J&K State also imported 10 rams and 45 ewes from New Zealand in 1963. More than half died in acclimatization process and rest did not fare well.

Leicester

Once short fine wool was the pride of Spain and long coarse lustrous wool became the basis of England's industrial progress, Like other English breeds the Leicester sheep also used to be reared in the table lands of England. These were long legged lengthy animals possessing mutton traits to the dislike of butcher.

Appreciating the dire need to have a sheep of faster growth and fattening quality, a sheep farmer of Dishlay Grange in Leicester county England, Robert Bakewell (1725-1795) began improving his sheep in 1755. He was a keen observer and judged his sheep both by eye and hand. "By their fruits ye shall know them". With this concept in mind he used the sensitive and reliable approach of assessing the breeding value of the sire on one

hand and observing the quality of lambs they left. In his venture for a perfect symmetry and mutton quality sheep he took the advice of butchers too. He tried to find out the quality of small sized animal than the long legged ones. Instead of selling his rams, he introduced a system of letting out the rams to the neighbouring breeders on condition of taking them back when ever required. To study the breeding performance of these rams, he paid frequent visits to those flocks. Whenever he came across a ram, which threw progeny of desired qualities, he withdrew such ram and practised close inbreeding from those rams to fix the desired characteristics. Some people believe that he must have resorted to cross breeding or selection as well.

Bakewell thereby succeeded in establishing a New or the Improved Leicester. The new type was smaller in body and lighter in the fleece. Main innovation was the improved capacity to put on fat and to lay on this fat before reaching full maturity. This was with the aim of evolving an economical and efficient mutton-making machine under the backdrop of:

1. Increase of population and a rising standard of living in England of his time.
2. Abdundance of winter forage and root crops which enabled them to exploit the same for improving fattening abilities of their sheep.

Bakewell's society

Visualizing the need to enforce certain procedure, Bakewell organised a Dishlay Society of 12 members in 1790. Every member had to follow the rules framed by him.

1. No member to hire or use any ram that did not belong to the members of the society.
2. The members were not to let rams for a season below 12 guineas or to ram breeders at less than 40 guineas each.
3. The members were not to let any greater that 30 rams in any one year.
4. Unless a member disposed off the whole flock he was not allowed to sell these outside the society for breeding.

5. Ram progeny and the rams were to be maintained under the same nutritional level. At any season of the year, any other food than green vegetable, hay and straw was also stipulated.

New Leicester was later used to improve the Lincoln and Romney Marsh breeds. Breed became popular in Yorkshire and other breeders improved further towards a leaner carcass and heavy fleece. Coarse wool, presence of horns, dark poll, speckled face, ears, and legs and blue skin are undesirable qualification of the breed.

Border leicester

Has been evolved from Bakewell's Leicester by crossing with Cheviot and developed as a definite breed.

One of the Bakewell's colleagues was "Culleys". He used to carry the Dishlay rams to the border, where Cheviot and Black face hilly sheep were reared, but were not good for meat. When these hilly sheep came down from the hills, he bred the same to infuse the qualities of Border Leicester for obtaining rapid fattening and early maturity. Priority was lamb first and wool next.

Wool of Border Leicester is lustrous, long in staple and coarse. Fleece weight of males ranges from 5 to 8 kg and of females 3.5 to 5.5 kg. Mature rams attain a carcass weight of 80 kg and ewes from 40 to 50 kg.

Four Border Leicester rams were used for breeding in old Maharashtra in 1950-51. In UP also 50 ewes and 20 rams were introduced in 1954. However these failed to survive. On the recommendations of Prof. Alfred Barker of Leeds University, Jammu and Kashmir, state had also imported three Border Leicester rams from England in 1940. Four more were procured from Australia in 1942. These perished within three years of arrival in the state. Only 122 crossbred lambs of local ewes were born out of them. Survival of progeny also remained precarious throughout. No long-term inference was possible.

DOWN BREEDS

The fat lamb sire breeds include English short wool mutton sheep and the long wool sheep types.

Table 2.2: Measurement of characteristics of important long wool and mutton breeds

Breed	Type	Body weight (kg)		Av. fleece weight (kg)	Staple length of wool (cm)	Wool quality (count)
		Ram	Ewe			
Romney Marsh	Longwool (coarse)	90-115	68-90	4.0-6.5	20-25	32-36s
Lincoln	Longwool	100-120	70-90	5.0-9.0	25-35	36-40's
Border Leicester	Longwool	80-110	60-80	3.0-4.50	15-20	44-48's
Corriedale	Crossbred Medium	80-110	55-75	3.0-5.0	12-16	52-56's
Polwarth	Crossbred Fine	80-112	50-70	3.5-6.0	10-16	56-60's
Targhee	–do–	80-110	50-70	–	–	–
Bond Sheep	Crossbred Stud.	100-150	80-90	–	–	–
Dorsets	Muttonbreed Medium Wool	80-100	50-70	2-3	8-10	54-58's
Cheviot	–do–	70-90	50-68	1.5-3.5	10-12	50-56's
Hampshire	–do–	100-120	70-90	–	–	–
Suffolks	–do–	100-120	70-90	2.5-4.0	10-12	52-58's
South Down	–do–	60-80	50-55	–	–	–

Source: (i) Dhamale and Mooley (1963-64); (ii) Scott W.N. (1978); (iii) Stan Dorman (1995)

South Down

Till the middle of 18th century stress was mostly laid on wool. After the development of Leicester by 'Robert Bakewell', John Ellmen (1753-1832), another farmer of Sussex county embarked upon improving his speckle faced sheep on bare waste land pastures of Sussex which were growing shrubs.

He paid close attention to carcass quality in consultation with butchers. The sheep he developed are known as South Down. They are with minimum waste, maximum development of the cuts which consumer prefer and therefore an ideal type of sheep for the butcher.

Original scrub sheep	Developed South Down sheep
Long legged, slender boned, short wool	Low set, compact, blocky sheep, sire stamping the finest quality lamb.
Light in shoulder, high at withers, narrow face, speckled black and white face	Though world's premier mutton sheep yet carrying the finest and most valuable fleece of an English sheep.

A general consensus exists among sheep breeders that he attained this improvement entirely by selection, though it is also possible that the selection he made resulted in inbreeding or line breeding. South down wool is very short (hardly 3 to 5 cm on annual basis) demi-lustrous and 56 to 60s. quality and used in the manufacture of special felts. Fleece weight of an original breed ewe is 1.3 to 1.8 kg. It is a small sheep. At 3 months the lamb weighs about 14 kg and attains a weight of 25 to 28 kg at 9 months. South Down is a shy breeder.

Breeds like Suffolk, Oxford, Hampshire, Dorset Horn, etc. have evolved by the use of South Downs. The folding system is practised to allow availability of fodder crop within a defined area to save the energy expenditure and help conserve the same. Animals are not to move to long distances. An acre may accommodate 10 sheep.

Dorset Horn and Suffolks

Both the breeds are better placed in their qualities over South Down. Early maturity, higher fecundity, and better productivity are usual. Ewes are good milkers. They some times lamb thrice in two years and give over 150% lambing. Wool is short staple, demi-lustrous and of 50 to 56s. quality. Annual clip is 2 to 3 kg.

All the Down breeds require a high plane of nutrition. Quite often these breeds were recommended for introduction in India. Dorset Horns came to Bihar. South Down and Poll Dorsets arrived in Jammu and Kashmir, Punjab, Uttar Pradesh, Rajasthan, Bombay (Maharashtra), Mysore (Karnataka), Andhra Pradesh, Madras (Tamil Nadu) and some other states in the past fifty years. Results have not been encouraging under Indian conditions. To produce better mutton synthetics Dorsets have been introduced in Nellore, Mandya and Madras Red sheep in peninsular region and in arid zone sheep recently.

Down breeds have very good carcass shape with well-developed hindquarters and backs. They are further divided into two groups.

1. Early maturing but with slower growth rates like South Down, Ryeland and South Suffolks, etc.
2. Late maturing but with faster growth rate like Suffolks, Dorset Down, Polled Dorsets, Dorset Horn, Hampshire, Shropshire, etc.

MILCH SHEEP

Besides wool and mutton, the sheep milk is an important commodity for the shepherd in India, especially under migratory condition. In most of the countries mutton is paid better attention than wool. In Italy and Balkan states sheep milk occupies great economic importance. It is converted into cheese by adding rennet. Texel and West Fresion sheep breeds in Denmark and Holland are reared for milk. Sardinia and Piedmont in Italy. Romanov and other dairy trait sheep in Bulgaria are known to contribute almost one-third of the whole milk production of that country. Awasi is a dual-purpose breed in Palestine. Israel and

Egypt too have such type of milk sheep. Incidentally all these sheep have a potential for high lambing rate and lamb survival. Welsh mountain breed of England is said to be a highly prolific sheep giving above 200% lambing and sufficient milk to support the progeny.

Certain exotic dairy sheep yield 2 to 3 litres of milk per day. This is without suckling lamb.

Usually the lambs are allowed to suckle for 50 to 60 days. Milk yield as high as 400 lit. has been recorded in a lactation period of 200 days in some ewes abroad. Average butterfat is 6.8%. Milch sheep do well when maintained in small flocks of 5 to 8 animals and kept under stall fed condition.

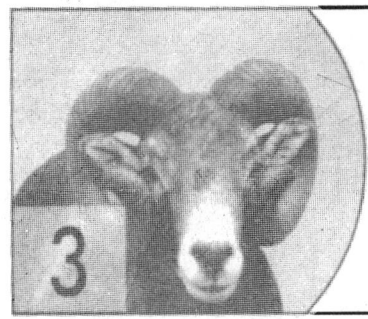

SHEEP SCENARIO IN INDIA

SHEEP DISPERSAL

Sheep is run on the big private properties in sheep advanced countries of USA, Australia, New Zealand and at organised State farms in USSR. In India, however the rearing of sheep and goat is a traditional vocation of most of the nomadic tribes in states like J&K, HP, UP, Rajasthan, Gujarat, Maharashtra, Karnataka, Andhra Pradesh, etc. Over the centuries the tribesmen have acquired excellent professional expertise. These small ruminants constitute the sole or at least a major source of livelihood of the tribals. A large population of small, marginal farmers and landless or poor sections of the rural society also derive their sustenance through the rearing of sheep and goat. At a couple of State and Central farms or Research institutions the sheep flocks are also maintained for multiplication, research, ram production and germ plasm conservation.

Against big flock holdings of a few thousand sheep on commercial farms and ranches in countries abroad the strength of sheep holding in India varies from a few animals to a few hundred per family only. Managing of big size flocks in this country is constrained by the small land holdings and limited pasture resources of the sheep farmers. Recent observations reveal that barring certain public and institutional farms the flocks' size is dwindling in the private properties in the country. Sheep distribution pattern in the country is presented in the Fig. 3.1 and statewise sheep population is given in Table 3.1.

CONTRIBUTION STATUS

Population

But for minor fluctuations the sheep population of India has remained static around 40 million for thirty years after independence. It is only after 1977 that a marked upward trend in sheep number was visible and crossed a mark of 50 million after 1992.

The contribution of sheep rearing to the GNP is over Rs. 8000 million in the form of wool, mutton, skins, milk and manure. Through wool and woollen products, leather and leather products, meat and meat products and other items the sheep constitute a sizeable share out of rupees 50,000 crores, total contribution of Livestock sector. Directly or indirectly sheep provide employment to almost 5 million population of the country.

Production

During the period from 1970 to 1995 the sheep population of India has increased from 40.4 million to 50.7 m. Wool and mutton production increased from 35.17 m kg to 45.6 m kg and 125 m kg to 173 m kg respectively. Even the availabiilty of raw sheep skins for the industry improved to 40 thousand tonnes against earlier 32 thousand tonnes.

Wool

India possesses 4.5% of the world sheep population and the wool production constitutes only 1.4% of world wool production. The average wool production per sheep in India stood at 0.70 kg in

Table 3.1: State wise sheep population of India (in lacs)

State	1951	1972	1982	1992	1997	Wool prod (000' kgs)	
						1999–2000	2001–02 est.
Andhra Pradesh	101.9	83.43	75.19	77.87	97.43	3136	3392
Arunachal Pradesh	–	–	–	00.30	00.27	59	59
Assam	–	00.51	00.46	01.50	00.84	–	–
Bihar	09.1	09.83	13.22	16.90	19.56	1274	1338
Goa	–	–	–	–	–	–	–
Gujarat	36.4	17.22	23.57	20.27	21.58	2646	2709
Haryana	–	04.59	07.58	10.44	12.75	2202	2403
Himachal Pradesh	06.3	10.40	10.90	10.79	10.80	1576	1596
Jammu and Kashmir	09.8	10.73	19.09	29.47	31.70	5440	6460
Karnataka	43.5	46.62	47.92	54.32	80.03	5441	5904
Kerala	–	00.10	00.07	00.29	00.03	–	–
Madhya Pradesh	06.9	10.09	09.59	08.36	06.57	798	827
Maharashtra	–	21.28	26.71	30.74	33.68	1610	1643
Manipur	–	00.02	00.14	00.14	00.08	–	–
Meghalaya	–	00.18	00.26	00.23	00.17	–	–
Mizoram	–	–	–	00.01	00.01	–	–
Nagaland	–	–	–	00.03	00.02	–	–
Orissa	06.8	13.69	19.90	18.40	17.65	–	–
Punjab	08.5	03.88	06.11	05.26	04.36	957	957
Rajasthan	53.9	85.56	134.31	124.97	145.85	19202	20060
Sikkim	–	–	00.11	00.16	00.05	8	35
Tamil Nadu	79.3	53.93	55.37	58.49	52.59	646	625
Tripura	–	00.02	00.05	00.05	00.06	–	–
Uttar Pradesh	16.4	19.56	23.07	24.04	19.05	2245	2059
West Bengal	06.2	–	–	14.90	14.42	636	642
Chhatisgarh	–	–	–	–	01.96	–	–
Uttaranchal	–	–	–	–	03.11	–	–
Delhi	–	–	–	–	00.11	–	–
Pondicherry	–	–	–	–	00.02	–	–

Source: Livestock census reports GOI.

Note: (i) Separate sheep population figures for newly carved states of Jharkhand not available.

(ii) UTs of Nicobar, Chandigarh, Haveli, Daman and Diu and Lakshadweep have no sheep population.

1951. Over the last four decades it has risen to 0.90 kg against the current world average of 2.4 kg per sheep. As a solitary note however an improvement in wool production to 1.45 kg per sheep has been achieved in Jammu and Kashmir state. This is believed to be due to successful implementation of the sheep cross breeding programme in the state. Annual wool production of some of the sheep breeds of Rajasthan is above 1.5 kg, but the rest are low yielders. The far low average wool production of India's sheep accounts for the meager overall wool production of the country. Wool production in India in 1951 was 27.5 m kg. An increase of 60% has been witnessed by the close of 20th century. Almost 31% of the wool produced is suitable for coarse material. Another 35% finds utility for superior carpets, hosiery blankets and apparel. Quality carpet wool is also less in production. Thus in recent years huge imports of wools particularly from Australia, Italy, Turkey, New Zealand and other countries have taken place. Country is short of fine wool by over

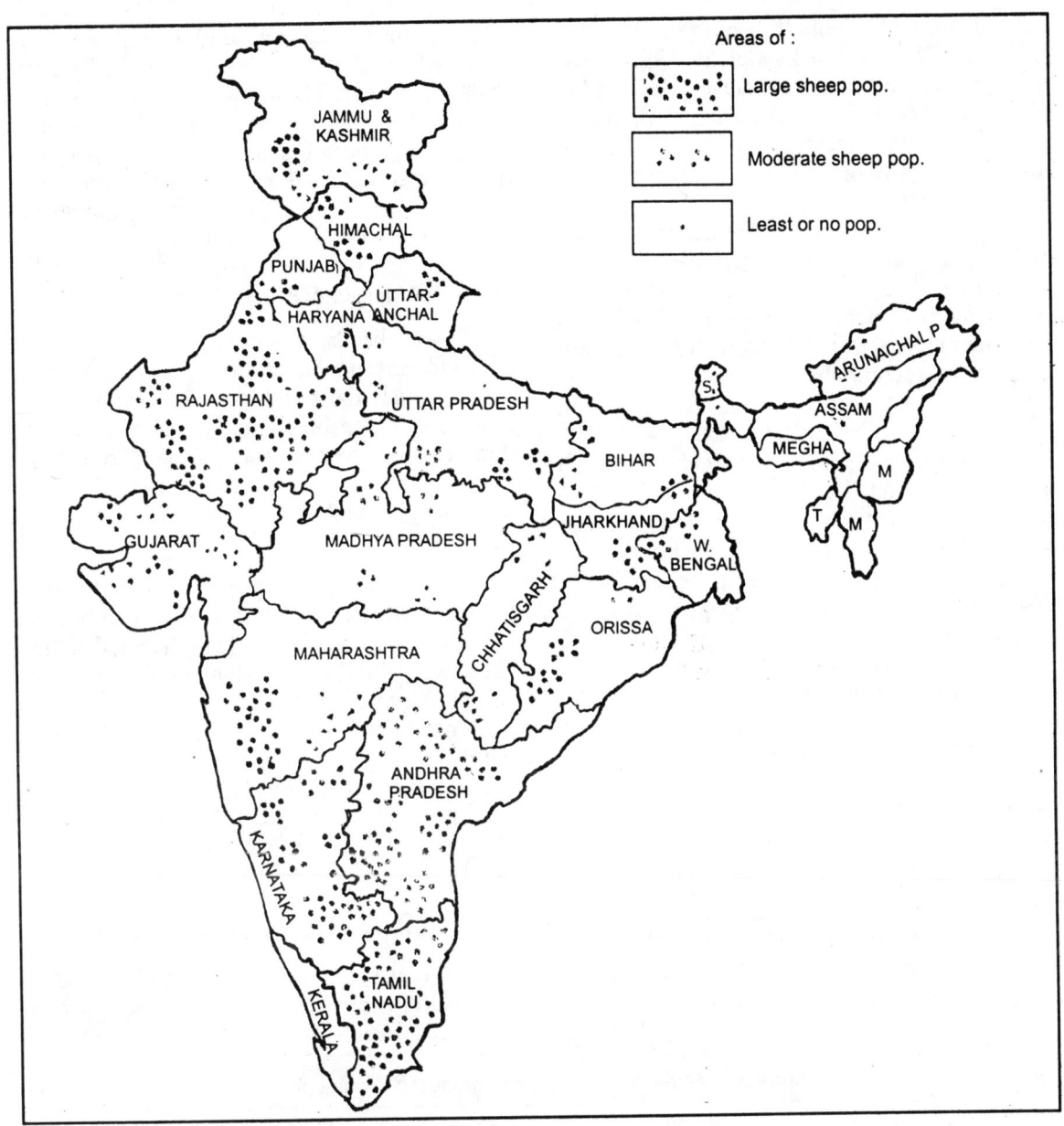

Fig. 3.1: Pattern of sheep distribution in India

5.0 million kg as far as internal requirement is concerned. The organised sector needs 34.5 million kg more for its worsted sector installations. Roy (1999) indicated that the consumption of wool in Indian carpet industry is 45 m. kg. Out of that 20 m. kg are imported. For quality carpets and woollens the New Zealand wool imports alone have crossed a mark of 15 m kg.

Mutton

Mutton production of the country was 118 million kg in 1979-80. This increased to 130 million kg in early eighties of twentieth century and further soared to 173 million kg during 1995 (FAO estimates). Export of mutton during 1993-94 has been to the extent of 3.6 million kg. worth Rs. 40 crores. The export increased to Rs 61.57 crores during 1997-98 in addition to casings and processed meat.

An annual increase of 0.5% in sheep population has lead to corresponding increase in mutton production. The heavier crossbred sheep and relative improvement of carcass weight of cross bred sheep in J&K from 12 kg to 15 kg and overall increase in the country from 10 kg to 12 kg average is cited another reason for increase in mutton production.

Earlier estimates placed the yearly sheep slaughter rate around 25% of the population. The improved health cover, better survivability and augmented sheep population over the last decades have tended to make available a higher component of 30 to 32% sheep population for slaughter annually to meet the increasing demand for mutton. The per capita consumption of meat in India works out to only 1.57 kg per annum. The country falls short of almost 256.4 million kg meat against the requirement of 423.4 million kg.

Skins

Sheep and goat skins provide an invaluable raw material for the leather industry. Quantum of annual skin production in India is about 40 million kg. Almost 90% of it are recovered at slaughter. The one collected from dead sheep is inferior and often not fit for processing.

Approximately 22.5 million pieces of skins are available from sheep which value around Rs. 350 crores in raw state. The dry weight of these sheep and lamb skins is estimated around 13.5 thousand tonnes. After processing, the value addition to this finished material is about Rs. 700 crores. The exports of sheep leather and leather goods fetch over Rs 990 crores to the country.

SHEEP REARING ZONES

Based on husbandry practices and agro-climatic regions the sheep germ plasm is divided into four zones. Besides the usual classification adopted earlier, the sheep breeds in India are at times referred to after their respective zones (Table 3.2).

North temperate (Himalayan) zone

Comprises of Jammu and Kashmir, Himachal Pradesh, Uttaranchal and part of Punjab, Sikkim and Arunachal Pradesh. Important sheep breeds of this zone are Bakerwali, Changthangi, Gaddie, Gurez, Karnah, Poonchi, Rampur Bushair and Kashmir Merino. Indigenous sheep of the north bordering states viz Tibetan, Biangi, Gaddie and even the extinct Purik present a similarity while-as, Changthangi in the western part of this region seems closer to Dumba, Karakul type sheep as far as body coat, features and comformation are concerned.

North western (arid and semi-arid) zone

This zone covers the states of Rajasthan, Gujarat, Haryana, Western parts of Punjab and Uttar

Table 3.2: Sheep distribution and production zonewise

Zone	Sheep population (Lacs)	Population contribution (%)	Wool production (Lac kg.)	Wool contribution (%)
North Temperate	36.3	07.15	47.9	10.50
North Western	214.5	42.23	298.2	65.40
Southern Peninsular	208.6	41.07	91.2	20.00
Eastern	48.5	9.54	18.7	4.10

Source: Singh, R.N. (1998).

Pradesh and Madhya Pradesh. Chokla, Jaisalmeri, Magra, Malpura, Marwari, Muzaffarnagri, Nali, Pattanwadi, Pugal, Sonadi and the developed Hissardale and certain synthetic sheep are the breeds of consequence in this zone.

Southern peninsular zone (the Deccan plateau)

This includes the states of Maharashtra, Andhra Pradesh, Karnataka, Tamil Nadu and part of Madhya Pradesh. Except the fine wool Nilgiri sheep all other sheep breeds of this zone namely, Deccani, Bellary, Coimbatore, Hassan, Kilakarsal, Madras Red, Mandya, Macheri, Nellore, Ramnad white and Tiruchy Black are coarse to hairy mutton type sheep.

Eastern zone

Eastern Uttar Pradesh, Bihar, Orissa, West Bengal, Assam and other North Eastern states fall in this zone. From sheep and wool point of view this zone is not of much significance. Some of the important sheep breeds in the area are Balangir, Chhotanagpuri, Ganjam and Shahbadi. These are mainly mutton and carpet wool types. Bonpala and Tibetan sheep inhabit the northern hills of this zone falling under temperate climatic environment.

In the last few years keen interest has been evinced in the states of Bihar, Orissa and Arunachal Pradesh by small and marginal farmers in sheep rearing after the introduction of the state and central sponsored schemes under poverty alleviation programme.

Union territories of Chandigarh and Pondicherry have negligible sheep numbers, while Andaman and Nicobar, Dadara and Nagar Haveli, Delhi, Lakshadweep, and Daman and Diu have no sheep population.

INDIGENOUS SHEEP BREEDS

Some sheep scientists have identified 42 local sheep breeds in the country. The possibility of existence of a couple more identical strains can not be ruled out.

The crossbreeding of indigenous sheep breeds for fine wool production undertaken in temperate zone in particular has transformed the local sheep into cross breds. This leaves little scope for finding many true to type sheep of main local breeds in the temperate region. However, Changthangi and some other peripheral area sheep are still outside the ambit of cross breeding and exist in pure state.

Restricted cross breeding trials have been initiated in other zones as well. But due to a general policy of selective breeding, most of the local breeds of north western and southern region are unaffected by and large.

North temperate zone breeds

Home tracts and characteristics of breeds

1. Bakerwali: It is a completely migratory sheep, reared by a nomadic tribe of Bakerwals in J & K State. Heavier built than Gaddie and sturdy in appearance. Invariability producing pigmented wool; tan or black face, ears, fetlock and even whole body; spotted lambs are common. Roman nose is typical of the breed (Figs 5 and 6, PLATE 1).

2. Biyangi (Biangi): Rearing tract is Kinnaur and partly Lahaul Districts of HP. Sheep are bigger in size than Gaddie. Wethers and rams, like Gaddie and Changthangi sheep are used as a beast of burden and carry 8 to 10 kg weight tied to their back over the high and difficult mountain ranges. In fact these sheep appear a conglomeration of the Gaddie sheep and medium wool Tibetan sheep. Biangi of Kinnaur possesses fine coat.

3. Changthangi: Habitat is Changthang plateau of Ladakh (J&K). These sheep are bigger in size than any other sheep of J&K. Mostly coloured and the dark pigmentation extends to hooves. Wool is coarse and long like Karakuls. They thrive well under cold desert conditions of Changthang. Annual wool production is 1.0 to 1.6 kg. Wethers are used as pack animals for the transport of salt and other commodities over the inhospitable and high terrain of Ladakh (Figs 7 and 8, PLATE 2).

4. Danpuri: Inhabits Almora Division of Uttranchal. They have appearance like Gaddie. Animals are woolly type but smaller in size than the latter. Not recognized as a separate breed.

5. Gurez: This is a heavy built sheep breed of the rugged mountainous Gurez area in Kashmir valley. Eyes, ears, muzzle or even fetlocks may be tan or black. Annually the animals are shorn twice and total clip weights 0.8 to 1.1 kg. Wool is medium quality (Figs 9 and 10, PLATE 2).

6. Gaddie: Home tract is hills of Kathua, Udhampur and Doda Districts of Jammu and Kashmir State; Chamba, Kangra and Kulu districts of Himachal Pradesh. Gaddie sheep are migratory or semi migratory. White in colour, tan, brown face, ears, around the eyes is also common.

Usually medium size but strain to strain differences exist. Wool is of medium quality and annual clip comes to 0.9 kg. Around 1½ year age an average ram weighs 30 to 32 kg and an ewe 22 to 24 kg (Fig. 11, PLATE 2).

7. Kashmir Valley: Habitat is Kashmir valley. Sheep are small in size and mostly coloured; fawn or black. Produce about 600 to 700 g wool in two clippings in a year (Fig. 12, PLATE 2)..

8. Karnah sheep: Mountainous Karnah tehsil of Kashmir valley is the home tract. These sheep are of medium size and possess medium to fine white wool coat. Two shearing in a year are practised. Length of each clip is 5 to 6 cm. Average annual wool production is 0.9 to 1.0 kg (Fig. 13, PLATE 3).

9. Rampur-Bushair: Shimla, Rampur-Bushair, Kinaur District of HP and adjoining areas of Uttranchal is the home tract of the breed. Animals are of medium size, mostly white with colour spots on face and ears at times; migratory in nature and produce a medium to fine quality fleece. Adult ewes weigh 24 to 28 kg and rams 30 to 35 kg. Fleece weight is 0.9 kg to 1.2 kg (Fig. 14, PLATE 3).

10. Poonchi: Resembles Gaddie but is invariably white and of finer wool than Gaddie.

Maintained in Rajouri and Poonch Districts of J&K on semi migratory pattern (Fig. 15, PLATE 3).

North western region

1. Chokla: Home tract is Churu and Jhunjhunu districts of Rajasthan. Medium size, tan face with or without black patches, colour may extend upto middle of neck. Medium ears and medium tail. Rams and ewes hornless. Wool is relatively fine and annual clip is 1.4 to 2.0 kg in two shearing. Ewes weigh 20 to 28 kg and rams 28 to 36 kg (Fig. 16, PLATE 3).

2. Jalauni: Found around Jalaun, Jhansi and Kanpur District of UP and Tikamgarh and Shivpur districts of MP. Animals are medium size and woolly type. Like Muzaffarnagari, Jalauni sheep are also polled, have long flat ears, coarse body coat and dependent areas without wool (Fig. 17, PLATE 3).

3. Lohi: Only a limited number is found in Ferozepur District of Punjab. Major rearing tract is western Punjab (Pakistan). Big size and long trailing ears. Good mutton breed but has a potential as milch sheep. Quite prolific.

4. Muzaffarnagari: Muzaffarnagar, and other adjoining areas of Saharanpur and Meerut districts of Uttar Pradesh is the home tract. Larger in size than other sheep breeds of UP White body with black or brown spots. Fleece is white and coarse. Legs are bare. Though produces wool but is considered better for mutton. Both sexes are invariably polled and possess long drooping ears (Fig. 18, PLATE 3).

5. Munjal (kanjli): Reared by farmers in Punjab and Haryana areas bordering Rajasthan, Ludhiana, Sangrur, Ferozpur, Abohar and Bhatinda Districts of Punjab and adjoining belt in Haryana have the main population of such type sheep. The origin is assumed from Bikaneri (Magra-Nali) and Lohi breeds. Possess the valuable characteristics of the latter as far as wool, mutton, milch and even fertility rates are concerned. Wool is white carpet type tending to yellowing in summer. Tail and ears are long. Like Lohi these fatten well in stall fed conditions and puberty sets in early. These sheep constitute about 75% of total 5 lac sheep population of Punjab.

6. Marwari: It is typical nomadic sheep of Marwar taking up inter-state migration. Reared in Jodhpur division and adjoining areas of Ajmer and Udaipur divisions of Rajasthan and adjacent part of Gujarat. Hardy breed,' stockily built, medium size animal. White body and black face. Ears are twisted; tubular and medium or short and tail is also short to medium. Both the sexes are polled. Animals are shorn twice in March and October. Wool is carpet type. Rams yield 1.5 to 2.5 kg and ewes 0.7 to 1.2 kg of wool per annum (Fig. 19, PLATE 4).

7. Malpura: Found in Jaipur, Tonk, Malpura and Sawai Madhopur Districts of Rajasthan. Mostly stationary in nature. Light brown faced. Appears white bodied from a distance. Short tubular ears, medium to long tail. Wool production in the ewes is 0.7 to 1.2 kg and rams 0.9 kg to 1.5 kg per head in two shearing of a year and it is of coarse hairy type. Body weight ranges from 20 to 28 kg in ewes and 28 to 34 kg in rams (Fig. 20, PLATE 4).

8. Magra: Mainly reared in Bikaner District and in small numbers in Churu, Nagaur and Jhunjhunu Districts of Rajasthan. Well built; white face, light brown patches around eyes; medium size, medium tail and medium twisted ears. Wool yield is 1 to 2 kg in three shearings. Body weight of an ewe is 22 to 28 kg and that of ram 25 to 32 kg. Wool quality is medium to coarse, lustrous and suitable for carpet production (Fig. 21, PLATE 4).

9. Nali: This breed inhabits Ganganagar, Jhunjhunu, Churu Districts (north and north-eastern part of Bikaner Division) extending to Haryana state. Medium size, light brown face with long leafy ears, short tail. Fleece quite greasy and often both clips show yellowing or canary stain. In 2 to 3 shearing in a year the sheep produces 1.5 to 2.5 kg wool of medium to coarse (carpet) type (Fig. 22, PLATE 4).

10. Pugal: Pugal area in western Bikaner and north of Jaisalmer district of Rajasthan is the home

area of the breed. Animals are compact and well built. Uniform black or light brown face; characteristic white streaks on either side of nose and above eyes. Short tubular ears and medium tail. Annual fleece weight is 1.2 to 2 kg in two to three shearings and wool is of medium to coarse variety (Fig. 23, PLATE 4).

11. Jaisalmeri: Found in Jaisalmer, Barmer and northwestern parts of Jodhpur district. Heavy built, black or brown faces and this colour extends upto neck. Long ears, long tail and Roman nose. Fleece is white and medium (carpet) variety. Shearing is done in March and October, Ewes yield 1.2 to 2 kg wool and rams 1.6 to 3 kg wool annually in adult age. Body weight of a ram ranges around 34 to 40 kg and that of ewe 28 to 34 kg (Fig. 24, PLATE 4).

12. Patanwadi: Also known as Kutchi or Deshi sheep locally. Derives its name from Patan in Mehsana District in Gujarat. Mostly reared by Bharwads in Kutch, Sourashtra and Mehsana area of Gujarat on sedentary footing; at times, along the coastal line. Patanwadi sheep is of medium to large size; white with brown face; Roman nose; ears medium with tassels having a tuft of hair, tail is short. Animal is delicate in constitution. Ewe is a good milker, next to Lohi, giving 400 to 500 ml milk. These are woolly sheep. Ewes give about 0.8 kg and rams 0.9 kg wool of carpet type per annum. Body weight of ewes varies from 22 to 28 kg that of rams from 32 to 40 kg. Chanotri is another strain of sheep of Gujarat of unrecognised type and of lesser importance (Fig. 25, PLATE 5).

13. Sonadi: Home tract is Udaipur Division; mainly Udaipur, Dungarpur and Chittorgarh districts. Good specimens may also be found in northern Gujarat. Animals are long, well built with white or light brown faces, long bare legs, long tails and ears. Both sexes are hornless. Wool coat is white but very coarse and hairy. Annual wool production is 0.5 to 1.0 kg in ewes and 0.7 kg to 1.3 kg in rams. Rams generally weigh from 35 to 40 kg and ewes 22 to 30 kg (Fig. 26, PLATE 5).

South peninsular zone breeds

1. Deccani: Main sheep breed of Deccan plateau (Maharashtra, Karnataka and Andhra Pradesh). Particularly found in the Districts of Kolahpur, Sholapur, Sitara, Sangli, Poona, Ahmednagar, etc. A medium sized woolly sheep of semi-arid zone of Peninsula. Mostly black or brown appearing greyish and has white patches. Decades of selection in the past has resulted in the evolution of a white fleece sheep producing 0.7 to 0.9 kg medium to coarse wool in two shearings. Sheep have Roman nose and long ears. Shepherding communities of Dhangars and Kurbars rear them in Maharashtra and Karnataka respectively. Two types, short blocky very coarse one and other leggy and slightly better woolled one are available. Body weight of a Deccani ewe is 22 to 24 kg and that of a ram 35 to 38 kg (Fig. 27, PLATE 5).

2. Bellary: Home tract is Bellary district of Karnataka. Also found in south east area of Andhra Pradesh. Medium size and very similar to Deccani. Produces coarse and hairy fleece of white to black with grey or roan mixtures. Rams horned; ewes polled. Wool weighs 400 to 600 g in two shearings. Adult ewes weigh 25 to 27 kg and rams from 33 to 36 kg.

3. Coimbatore: Part of Madurai and Coimbatore districts of Tamil Nadu is the rearing belt. White, but the coat is hairy. Black or tan spots may also be present. Ears are medium and directed backwards. Ewes are polled but rams may be polled or horned. Body weight range of Coimbatore sheep is 20 to 25 kg.

4. Dhormundhi: A high rainfall area sheep of Chanda District (Sironcha Tehsil) of Maharashtra. Number is small. Medium type, white in colour, brown patches on head. Mutton type, non-woolly with hairy body. Body weights are identical to Deccani.

5. Hassan: Found in Hassan and Shimoga Districts of Karnataka. Small in size; colour varies from white to light brown with black spots. Fleece is coarse; hardly 400 to 500 g annual clip in two shearings. Males are horned and females polled.

Body weight range is from 20 to 25 kg (Fig. 28, PLATE 5).

6. Kilakarsal (Ramnad): Thanjavur, Ramnad, Ramnathpuram and Madurai districts of Tamil Nadu are the home of the breed. It is also hairy and dark brown with black or brown spots on belly and legs. Clean face and Roman nose are characteristic of the breed. Animal possesses tassels and males have well developed and outward twisted horns. But for body coat colour and some other feature differentiation, the Ramnad white and Kilkarsal are identical. Kilkarsal has at times been referred to as Ramnad breed. In both the breeds the body weight of ram is around 28 to 30 kg and ewe 20 to 22 kg.

7. Kenguri: Raichur district of Karnataka. Not a recognised breed. Number small. Medium size, colour varies from dark brown to black.

8. Madras Red: Found in Madras, Chingalpat and North Arcot district of Tamil Nadu, medium in size, brown in colour, without wool, possessing short goat like hair, usually polled, mutton of average quality, skin (pelt) fetches good price. Tail is short, ears are medium. Rams have twisted horns. Body weight of ewes is 20 to 24 kg and that of rams 32 to 36 kg (Fig. 29, PLATE 5).

9. Macheri: Occurring in North Arcot, Chingalpat districts and Tirunalvelli in Tamil Nadu. Hairy, small in size, colour varies from grey to white, with or without brown patches or brown streak on top line. Pair of tassels is characteristic. Polled males and females, medium ears and short tail. Ewes weigh 20 to 22 kg and rams 28 to 32 kg.

10. Mandya: Also called Bannur or named after the village Bandur where best specimens are available. Rearing area is Mallavalli Taluka of Mandya district of Karnataka. Breed samples exist in other areas in Karnataka, Maharashtra, Andhra and Tamil Nadu. White, with tan face and head, brown colour extending to neck, relatively small sized sheep, hardy, hairy and mutton type. Both sexes polled (Fig. 30, PLATE 5).

Named South Down of India by Mr. Khot (S.S.) former Liaison Officer Sheep, to Govt. of India due to muttonous conformation and excellent mutton quality. Quite prolific breed. Generally reared by Kurbar community in a batch of 10 to 15 sheep. This sheep is known for adaptability under higher rainfall as well. Consignments have reached in northeast India and even Sri Lanka. In Orissa, UP and J&K these sheep faired well. But small size, slow maturity and hairy coat are the impediments in acceptability by farmers. Adult rams weigh between 30 to 36 kg and ewes from 20 to 25 kg.

11. Nilgiri: Home of this breed is hilly tract of Nilgiri district of Tamil Nadu. It is the only woolly breed of South. (Appears to have originated as a result of crossing of indigenous sheep with exotic sheep). Colour white, sometimes brown patches may be found. Roman nose, ears flat and drooping. Tail medium, both sexes polled, wool is medium to fine but short and annual clip is around 500 to 600 gm Body weight ranges from 25 to 30 kg (Fig. 31, PLATE 6).

12. Nellore: Home tract is Nellore district of Andhra Pradesh, may be seen in adjoining districts also. Entirely mutton type, hairy, wattles, i.e. tassels are a common feature, colour is fawn brown, white or grey samples may also be found. Leggy than Bannur. Rams are horned and ewes polled. Ewes weigh 26 to 28 kg and rams around 32 to 36 kg (Fig. 32, PLATE 6).

12. Ramnad white: Found in Ramnad, Madurai and part of Coimbatore districts. Predominantly white and similar to Macheri except that the belly has black streak and grey hairy growth on thighs, extending to fetlock. Rams have twisted horns and ewes are polled.

13. Tenguri or Yalag: Home is east Bijapur district. Mutton type, long legged, colour white to brown, but no wool. Rams horned, ewes polled. Rams weigh around 35 kg and ewes 25 kg.

14. Trichi (Tiruchi black): Trichurapally, Salem, Coimbatore, South Arcot and Dharmpuri districts of Tamil Nadu are the home area of the breed. Small size, black in colour, coarse woolled or hairy and mutton type. Hardly, produces 300 grams of coarse hairy wool annually. Males are horned and ewes polled. Ears short and turned downwards. Body weight range is 17 to 20 kg.

15. Vembur: Found in Tirunalvelli district of Tamil Nadu. Bigger size and tall animal. White with tan sprinkling (patches) over the whole body. Hairy coat of short length. Ears are drooping. Ewes weigh 26 to 28 kg and rams 35 to 40 kg.

Eastern zone breeds

1. Belangir: These sheep are found in Sambalpur, Belangir and some other districts of Orissa. Animals are medium in size, white and varying levels of tan and black colouration exist. Rams are horned and ewes polled. Body coat is hairy and not fit for shearing. Body weight ranges from 15 to 25 kg (Fig. 33, PLATE 6).

2. Bonpala: Found in Southern Sikkim. Well built but leggy animal, white as well as black colour or even an admixture is there. Both the sexes are horned. Body coat is coarse, hairy. Dependent parts are without the coarse covering. Animals attain a body weight of 40 to 45 kg.

3. Chottanagpuri: This sheep breed is found in Chottanagpur, Ranchi, Hazaribagh, Palamau and Santhal Parganas of Bihar and Bankura district of West Bengal. Small weight and size. Grey or tan in colour. Body coat is hairy. Both sexes are polled. Ears and tail short. Adult males and females range between 16 to 20 kg only (Fig. 34, PLATE 6).

4. Ganjam: Found in Ganjam, Koraput and Phulbani districts of Orissa. Medium in size and tan brown colour, white spots quite common. Rams are horned and ewes polled. Wool coat is hairy. Body weight ranges from 20 to 30 kg.

5. Shahabadi: The home tract is Shahbad and Gaya districts of Bihar. Medium sized animal. Grey to dark grey in colour. Wool coat very coarse and hairy. Both sexes are polled. Medium ears, and long tail. Body weight of adult males and females usually ranges between 25 to 35 kg. Both the above sheep breeds of Bihar are not considered important for wool, being hairy (Fig. 35, PLATE 6).

6. Tibetan: Found in Northern Sikkim and Arunachal Pradesh. Animal medium in size, colour is white, black or brown spots on body, brown face may also be seen, Both sexes are horned. Roman nose. This is the only local variety in this eastern region, which is woolly, and medium in quality. Body weight ranges from 20 to 30 kg.

The production characteristics of local sheep breeds are given in Table 3.3.

EXOTIC SHEEP IN INDIA

First introduction of exotic sheep in India took place about two hundred years back. In the beginning of 19th century, the East India Company brought Cape Merino and South Down sheep with the possible objective to introduce in the local sheep of southern region and some other states. Madras government purchased Australian Merino rams in 1838 for trial in private sheep of Nilgiries. Record of performance of imported sheep and these experiments are unknown except that improvement in wool and carcass size was apparent in the cross breds. Rulers of certain erstwhile states of the country also obtained English sheep as gifts or through purchase in late 19th and early 20th century. But for serving as fancy and show animals, definite record of their performance is difficult to make out from the old narrations. Some crossbred varieties are shown in Figs 36, 37 and 38, PLATE 7.

Table 3.3: Production characteristics of local sheep breeds

Sl. No.	Name of sheep breed	Birth weight (kg.)	Adult body weight (kg)		Gr. fl. weight kg.	Staple length (cm) 6 monthly	Fibre diameter (mi)	Medul-lation (%)	Wool quality and spinning count('s)
			M	F					
1	2	3	4	5	6	7	8	9	10
1.	Chokla	2.26	25-35	21-30	1.3-2.2	5.0	26	5.5	Medium to fine 54 to 60's
2.	Magra	2.98	32-34	22-30	1.3-2.1	6.4	31	36.7	Medium 46 to 50's
3.	Nali	2.48	30-36	27-32	1.3-2.7	6.0	28	36.5	Med. to coarse 40 to 50's
4.	Pugal	–	30-34	25-30	1.3-2.2	8.9	30	39.9	Medium 46 to 50's
5.	Marwari	2.49	27-36	22-30	0.9-1.8	4.5	33	45.1	Medium 46 to 50's
6.	Jaisalmeri	–	32-45	30-36	1.8-3.1	5.6	32	41.5	Medium 50 to 54's
7.	Malpura	2.51	30-34	25-30	0.6-1.3	7.3	39	67.8	Coarse 40 to 44's
8.	Sonadi	2.40	30-39	25-30	0.9-1.3	6.6	55	83.2	Very Coarse Below 40's
9.	Patanwadi	–	32-40	22-28	0.8-1.0	5.0	28	34.1	Medium 46 to 50's
10.	Lohi	2.81	30-38	–	1.1	6.6	33	24.2	Coarse to Medium
11.	Muzzafar-nagri	2.86	30-36	–	1.5	3.7	45	69.9	–do–
12.	Rampur Bushair	2.30	30-35	24-28	1.2	7.7	34	23.8	Medium 46 to 52's
13.	Gaddie	2.02	30-32	22-24	0.9	5.7	29	25.7	–do– 46 to 50's
14.	Karnah	–	32-36	24-28	1.0	6.0	28	13.5	Medium to fine 48 to 52's
15.	Deccani	2.80	35-38	20-24	0.7-0.9	7.0	35	24.2	Coarse to med. 40 to 44's
16.	Bellary		33-36	25-27	0.4-0.6	3.2	59	43.4	Very coarse 32 to 36's
17.	Nilgiri	2.73	25-30	–	0.5-0.7	4.4	24	21.3	Fine 56 to 60's
18.	Coimbtore		20-25	–	0.4	5.7	41	58.3	
19.	Chotta Nagpuri	–	16-20	–	0.4	3.2	53	83.6	
20.	Shahbadi	–	25-35		0.5	3.7	50	87.0	
21.	Tibetan	–	20-30		0.9	7.2	–	19.3	

Source: Kaul (1942-43); Acharya (1972), Gupta (1972), Basuthakur and Acharya (1981), Acharya (1982), Devendra and Faylon (1988), Gupta (1994)

Punjab (undivided) and UP (the then United Provinces) procured Australian Merino and Romney Marsh sheep in 1906. Eight Merino consignments arrived in the next two decades. In Punjab these were stationed at Hissar Livestock Farm. Attempts had been made there to improve Dumba and local sheep since 1867. But the real crossbreeding work was undertaken by Mr. Branford on the importation of Merinos in 1906. The indigenous foundation stock then selected was Bikaneri ewes for crossbreeding with Merino rams. Efforts of over twenty years led to the development of a desired sheep named 'Hissar Dale'. In UP Merino cross breeding attempted in 1912 gave favourable indication about wool production body weight and thrivability but the trials were not carried to any logical end on grounds of financial constraints. Similar attempts made in the North Western Province (now in Pakistan) exhibited improvement in body weight, wool quantity and quality of the desi sheep of that terrain.

In early thirties of 20th century, Imperial Council of Agricultural Research took the initiative of introducing a number of exotic sheep breeds, viz. Merino, Romney Marsh and English breeds like Cheviot, Border Leicester. Wensleydale, etc. in Deccan Plateau, Punjab, J&K, Bihar, NWFP and UP. The British sheep did not give encouraging results. Attempts, however, yielded dividends as far as Merino cross breeding was concerned. These limited experiments with inadequate germplasm and imperfect scientific backup could not produce lasting impact. It was in fact after independence only that under the auspices of Indian Council of Agricultural Research, a systematic programme of sheep development was suggested and launched countrywide. In more eager states the organised work took off right in 1950. Since then lot many exotic sheep breeds found their way in various states of the union.

The salient details of importations of the exotic sheep breeds are given in Table 3.4.

Table 3.4: Salient importations of exotic sheep breeds

S.No.	Exotic sheep breed	States where introduced
1.	Delaine Merino	J&K (1951)
2.	Spanish Merino	H.P. (1961-62)
3.	German Land Merino	H.P. (1963-64) (57-58, 70-71, 80-81, 87-88)
4.	Rambouillet	J&K, H.P. U.P., Rajasthan, Haryana, Punjab, Maharashtra, Gujarat, Karnataka, Andhra, Tamil Naidu and Bihar. (during 1950-1995).
5.	Australian Merino	J&K, H.P., U.P. Haryana, Rajasthan, Gujarat, Maharashtra. 1940-1943, 1960-1988.
6.	Russian Merino, Stavropolskaya	J&K, H.P., Gujarat, U.P., Rajasthan, Arunachal Pradesh. (1966-1972)
7.	Polworth	H.P., U.P, (Prior 1963), Rajasthan, Gujarat (1968-69).
8.	Corriedale	J&K, H.P., U.P., Punjab, Haryana, Rajasthan, Gujarat, M.P., AP, Karnataka, Tamil Nadu, Assam, Bihar (1960 onwards).
9.	Suffolk	J&K, Rajasthan, (CSWRI.), Karnataka (After 1963).
10.	Border Leicester	Maharashtra, U.P., J&K. (Around 1940)
11.	South Down	J&K (1960's)
12.	Dorsets	J&K, Punjab, Haryana, Maharashtra, AP, Karnataka, Tamil Nadu (After 1960).
13.	Hampshire	J&K
14.	Romney Marsh	J&K, Tamil Nadu
15.	Karakul	Rajasthan, Gujarat, J&K. (1970 onwards)
16.	Caucasian	J&K, H.P. (1957-58)
17.	Grozen	J&K (After 1968)

Isolated imports of Kuibyshev and Gissarkayi (for Tamil Nadu) Scottish Black Face (for HP) Dumba (for Gujarat) and Somali sheep (for Maharashtra) had also materialised earlier. Five Border Leicester rams were introduced in old Maharashtra in 1950-51. Likewise 50 ewes and 20 rams of Border Leicester breed were tried in UP in 1954, but they did not do well.

The sheep imports primarily comprised of three types:

- Merino and its descendant fine wool sheep breeds.
- South Down and its collaterals — Mutton types.
- Long coarse wool breeds and their crossbreds to improve fibre length and to impart dual conformation on the analogy of some excellent crossbreds developed by sheep advanced countries.

The main objectives of introduction were to:

- Study the adaptability of these superior breeds under our conditions and to propagate them.
- Exploit their qualities of production through transforming local breed progenies into better producing crossbreds.

CROSSBRED SHEEP DEVELOPMENT

From the sheep development aspect, the period of last eighty years is split into three salient portions.

Phase I : Pre-Independence stage

The first phase is marked by an initial groundwork in isolated pockets. There was hardly any public sector sheep farm in the country till 1930 where any organised sheep breeding manoeuvre for improving the productivity of local sheep could have been made. Some states and the Union Government appreciated the need for sheep development to ameliorate the economic condition of tribals and rural poor. In 1933, a subcommittee of Imperial Council of Agricultural Research

considered sheep and goat breeding schemes and recommended that distinct indigenous breeds be taken up for systematic and selective breeding. The centres and the sheep breeds so selected were:

1. Hissar (Livestock farm) and Hingoli for Bikaneri breed.
2. Hasur, Bhamburda (Bombay), Mahbubnagar (Hyderabad) and Mysore for the Deccani breed.
3. Bharkhand (Baluchistan) for the Dumba breed.
4. Kangra (then in Punjab) for the Gaddie breed.

Importation of sheep breeds from abroad including Merino materialised. But for the work in progress at Hissar no tangible result of sheep and wool improvement was visible anywhere. The upcoming of the fine wool crossbred 'Hissardale'* appeared promising.

1. *Hissardale:*   Originated by selective cross breeding of Bikaneri sheep (presumably Nali and Magra) with Merino. Hissardale sheep possess three-fourths Merino blood. They are medium in size, white body coat, wool cover extends to fore head and base of ears. Body is without wrinkles, skin and muzzle are pink and hooves are amber colour. Both sexes are polled. Ears are short to medium and tail is long.

Animals produce 1.5 to 2.5. kg fine wool annually of 60 to 62's quality and 4 to 6 cm staple. Medullation of the indigenous breed almost disappeared. A large number of Hissardale rams were introduced in Kangra and Kulu districts. Their survivability remained precarious. Due to loss of germplasm and the subsequent neglect, the number of Hissardale decreased.

2. Erstwhile Bombay state (Maharashtra) has the distinction to lead the sheep research work in the country right from the time of S.J. Bruen, Livestock Advisor of Bombay state in early thirties of twentieth century. Even the first wool testing laboratory was established in the country at Poona. The cross breeding of Deccani sheep with Merino also got on way in this period in Bombay state, to develop a 'Deccan Merino'.

---

* Further work in this direction was organised by Rai Bahadur (Dr.) P.N. Nanda who subsequently became Director, Punjab Veterinary Services and later Animal Husbandry Commissioner to Govt. of India.

3. Jammu and Kashmir state under the patronage of the then state ruler (Maharaja Hari Singh) got a sheep and wool survey conducted by Professor Alfred Barker of Leeds University (England) in early 1930's. A sheep concern, 'Kashmir Sheep Farm (Pvt.) Ltd.' was established in 1937. Later on, the research work was partly financed and guided by the Imperial Council of Agricultural Research. The crossbreeding of local sheep with a number of exotic sheep breeds was undertaken.

Phase II : Post Independence

The next twenty years after independence of India witnessed augmented sheep improvement activities.

1. Indian Council of Agricultural Research took up the scheme 'Sheep and Wool development on regional basis' in the different agro-climatic and sheep rearing areas, viz. crossbreeding of:

    - Deccani × Merino/Rambouillet at Sheep Breeding Station Poona (Maharashtra).
    - Rampur Bushairi with Rambouillet at Jeori farm (HP).
    - Gaddie and other local breeds with Rambouillet at Banihal/Reasi, J&K.
    - Chottanagpuri with Romney Marsh at Gaya (Bihar).
    - Nilgiri with Romney Marsh at Ooty (Tamil Nadu).

2. Importation of varied and superior exotic sheep breeds materialised.
3. Scientific breeding plans were drawn up by experts and introduced.
4. More sheep germplasm production centres/ farms were added.
5. The ICAR set up a postgraduate training institute in Sheep and Wool Production and Management at Poona (Maharashtra) in 1962.
6. The Indian Veterinary Research Institute initiated research in health, nutrition, breeding aspects, etc. of small ruminants in a big way. Disease investigation and new vaccines brought a sea change.

7. The concept of independent department/ sections for small ruminant development took shape in some of the states, i.e. Rajasthan, J&K, etc. and extension services also received a fillip. Thrust on infrastructure development was visible in many sheep rearing states.
8. Agricultural Universities that sprung up in some of the states did add Sheep Breeding and Research sections to the animal science faculty.
9. The Central Sheep and Wool Research Institute at Avikanagar, Rajasthan, started functioning, after 1962.
10. Sheep improvement through selective breeding was initiated in certain breeds of Rajasthan and other states.

The renewed efforts after independence led to the evolution of fine wool Deccani × Merino and Nilgiri × Merino cross bred and triple cross of Kuibyshev and Romney with local Nilgiri sheep. Their impact in private flocks did not linger, possibly on account of limited germplasm resource and imperfect stabilization. The outstanding achievement however took place in Jammu and Kashmir state where sustained scientific efforts resulted in the development of an acclimatised fine wool and heavier sheep the 'Kashmir Merino'

Kashmir merino

The work to produce a suitable sheep in Jammu and Kashmir environment started in the first phase period around 1938-39 at Banihal/Reasi stations. The disease problem in the beginning resulted in a set back and killed major lot out of 1000 local sheep. The Merino graded stock whatever available/developed by the time of dawn of independence was looted away by the Pakistani raiders in February, 1948.

Experiment restarted in 1951 with the partly recovered crossbred stock, the available old Merino and a Delaine (Wangenalla) Merino ram, received as gift through Government of India. Local sheep of Karnah, Bhaderwahi (Gaddie) and Poonchi strains were bred to Merino and then to Delaine to achieve 75% fine wool exotic inheritence. Subsequent interbreeding among three-fourths breds and rigid selection over a couple of generations was carried out. This uniform flock of fine wool sheep having around three-fourths Merino blood was then shifted from Banihal/Reasi stations to an ideal environment of Dachigam in Kashmir and named 'Kashmir Merino'. Caucasian Merino blood is also known to have found entry in a part of this flock at the evolution stage (Gupta, 1994). Figures 1, 2 and 3 in PLATE 1 depict Kashmir Merino variety of sheep.

Characteristics

It is medium to good size sheep, white in colour and appear like a Merino with minimum folds. Rams are invariably horned and ewes polled. Skin, muzzle, lips and inside of ears are pink in colour. Ears are short and tail long. Fleece is dense and fine, diameter of fibre is 20 to 24 microns. Belly and legs are also covered with wool. Forehead has a good tuft of wool. Greasy fleece weight of ewes is 2.5 to 3 kg and that of rams 3 to 4 kg. Length of annual clip is 7 to 8 cm. At 1½ year age the body weight of female sheep is 32 to 36 kg and of a male 40 to 50 kg.

Due to constraints in procuring adequate Merino, Rambouillet sheep have been imported and made use of, for producing stud stock and for cross breeding at private flocks. The Rambouillet inheritance is also stabilized at 75% in the cross bred and graded progeny. Because of inherent qualities of hardiness, plain body, heavy weight, muttonous conformation, etc. the developed sheep is suitable for the plain area flocks. These crossbred sheep withstand the rigours of long migrations as well. Adaptation under varied climatic conditions and different rearing systems has also been found satisfactory.

Phase III

The period from 1968-69 onwards witnessed a systematic and scientific thrust in sheep cross breeding. This is further marked by a better perception of sheep and wool improvement programme culminating into the evolution of a number of synthetic sheep types of diverse genetic make up and nature. The salient developments are as follows.

- An Indo-Australian Sheep Breeding Project with joint collaboration of two Governments (later on named as Central Sheep Breeding Farm Hissar) started near Hissar (Haryana). Centrally sponsored large farms at Fatehpur-Sikar (Rajasthan), Challakere (Karnataka), Mamidipally (AP), Daksum (J&K) and Bhaisora-Varanasi (UP) were also launched.

- Report of Ad hoc Committee on Sheep Breeding Policy (framed by the Ministry of Agriculture and Cooperation, Govt. of India) issued in March 1970.

- Report of National Commission on Agriculture (1976) provided necessary recommendations for sheep and goat breeding in the country.

- Large scale importation of outstanding sheep breeds like Russian Merino, Rambouillet, Corriedale, Australian Amerino, Dorsets, Karakul, etc. materialised for various regions.

- Over the 2nd and 3rd phase the number of Govt. Sheep Breeding farms cumulatively increased to over one hundred against a dozen only as existed in the first phase.

- Sheep and Wool Development and Marketing Boards/Corporations/Federations were created in some of the States.

- The All India Coordinated Research Project (including S and G) started. AICRP on Sheep is an improvised scheme over the earlier project. Crossing Gaddie with Rambouillet and Merino sheep at Tal (HP), Chokla, Nali and Jaisalmeri at CSWRI (Avikanagar) and Nilgiri sheep at Sandya nallah (TN) were taken up. Besides fine wool production cross breeding schemes for carpet wool and mutton improvement have also been introduced.

- The scheme of three tier ram production, i.e. Exotic Nucleus stations, Stud ram production farms and registered private flocks became functional for production and supply of improved rams. Open nucleus breeding system is the much favoured approach to sheep development now.

A number of improved sheep genotype have evolved in the 3rd phase period in India. Table 3.5 gives fleece characteristics of some Indian crossbred sheep.

1. Nilgiri synthetic: Produced by breeding Nilgiri ewes with the fine wool (Rambouillet and Soviet Merino) rams at Sheep Breeding Farm Sandya Nallah Ooty. Interbreeding at 50% exotic inheritance is followed by selection. Wool is fine; annual clip is around 2 kg in the Nilgiri synthetic sheep.

2. Patanwadi synthetic: Patanwadi sheep were crossed with Rambouillet and Soviet Merino rams by the Gujarat Agri. University at Dantiwara to produce fine wool crossbred sheep. Wool production is 2 to 2.5 kg per annum and fibre diameter is 22 to 25 micron. But for short staple, the required fibre fineness and medullation levels are met with in both the above synthetic sheep.

3. Bharat merino: CSWRI has evolved a crossbred sheep by breeding Nali and Chokla ewes with Rambouillet and Soviet Merino sires. Upgrading to 75% exotic inheritance was done and interbreeding-cum-selection practised in the progeny. These sheep are maintained at the CSWRI's Southern Regional Research Station, Mannavanur. Annual greasy fleece weight is around 3 kg, and fibre diameter 21 micron. Single annual shearing produces the required length of fibre for the worsted industry.

4. Avivastra: In this case Nali and Chokla crosses with Rambouillet/Russian Merino were maintained at 50% exotic level at Avikanagar. Interbreeding and selection has resulted into a strong fine woolly sheep, the 'Avivastra'.

5. Avikalin: At Avikanagar (CSWRI) the coarse and hairy Malpura sheep were crossed with Rambouillet rams. Such a crossbred sheep at 50% exotic inheritance produces a good carpet wool. Annual wool production is 1.5 to 2 kg. Staple is short and medullation within the range of carpet wool standards.

6. Mutton synthetics or avimaans: To meet the soaring demand for mutton in the country, attempts are being made to develop fast growing, feed efficient sheep of mutton conformation through cross breeding. In J&K State, local sheep and imported sheep like South Down, Polled Dorset, Corriedale, etc. have been used to produce suitable germ plasm of muttonous conformation

Table 3.5: Fleece characteristics of some Indian crossbred sheep

Breed/Genetic group		Greasy Fleece weight (kg)	Staple/Fibre length (6 monthly) (cm)	Av. fibre diameter (mi.)	Medulation %
Rambouillet x Nali Synthetic ½ bred		2.7	4.5	22.6	10.3
Rambouillet x Chokla Synthetic ½ bred		2.6	4.5	22.1	6.2
Rambouillet x Gaddie Synthetic ½ bred		1.5	6.2	24.8	1.0
Rambouillet x Poonchi	–do– –do–	1.5	7.1	25.4	1.0
Rambouillet x Patanwali	–do– –do–	1.6	5.2	23.2	20.8
Rambouillet x Niligiri	–do– –do–	1.1	4.6	20.6	3.2
Rambouillet x Chokla	3/4 Ramb. bred	2.7	4.9	19.8	3.0
Rambouillet x Gaddie	–do– –do–	1.7	5.2	21.7	Nil
Rambouillet x Poonchi	–do– –do–	1.6	5.2	22.5	Nil
Kashmiri Merino Stabilized 3/4th interbred		2.8	5.6	20.4	Nil
Avivastra	Stabilized CB	1.9	3.6	21.6	7.6
Avikalin	–do–	1.6	4.2	25.2	22.1
Avimaans	Mutton Synthetic	1.0	4.4	28.0	39.8

Source: As for Table 3.3.

at the farms of Sheep Husbandry Department and SK University of Agriculture Science and Technology Kashmir.

The production characteristics of local mutton type sheep are given in Table 3.6.

At Avikanagar (CSWRI) the Malpura and Sonadi sheep have been bred with Dorset and Suffolk rams. The progeny was interbred and a sheep (with 50% exotic blood) possessing good mutton qualities developed and named 'Avimaans'

Likewise at Palamner and Nellore (AP), Mandya (Karnataka) and Kattupakkam (TN) Nellore, Mandya and Madras Red sheep have also been bred with Dorset and Suffolk rams to synthesise a sheep that attains a weight of 25 kg at six month age and shall weigh above 30 kg in the same period under feed lot conditions. Under intensive system of rearing in parts of Punjab and Jammu villages the feed lot maintained crossbred lambs gained more than 40 kg weight at one year age, thus opening up new hopes for the sedentary sheep rearing.

Varied types of trials in the direction of carpet wool, dual type or heavier sheep production are under way at many other stations, namely Veterinary College, Bikaner; MPKV, Rahuri; HAU, Hissar; CIRG, Makhdoom; Central Sheep Breeding Farm, Hissar; and elsewhere.

SHEEP BREEDING POLICY

In the earlier decades a general approach was to emphasise 'produce wool in hills and mutton in plains'. ICAR in its initial years suggested broad outlines for breeding of sheep on the requisition of states. It was not until two decades after independence that the scientific trials and the data originating there-from made it possible for the experts to evolve definite line of action and propose a proper breeding policy.

Report of the Ad hoc Committee on Sheep Breeding Policy (1970) set up by the Ministry of Agriculture and Cooperation, Govt. of India

The committee had kept in view the geographical, agro-climatic and ecological factors and the scope for the development and demand for wool and mutton, while proposing the breeding policy.

Table 3.6: Production characteristics of local mutton type sheep

Breed/Crossbred	Feed lot performance			Carcass traits		
	Body weight at 6 month age (kg)	Av. daily Live weight gain (g)	Feed effici-ency %	Slaughter (hot) carcass weight (kg)	Dressing* %	Bone: Meat Ratio
Malpura	22.3	107	12.7	9.8	49.4	1:8.1
Sonadi	19.8	92	12.2	8.7	48.3	1:7.4
Mandya	18.1	87	13.5	8.2	49.0	1:4.8
Nellore	20.0	90	14.6	8.7	48.3	1:5.1
Muzzafarnagri	31.2	129	23.8	18.3	55.0	1:3.1
Deccani	32.2	167	14.7	10.3	45.1	1:6.7
Madras Red	18.5	101	12.5	8.6	51.6	1:3.3
Malpura and Sonadi Synthetic	26.6	139	15.0	11.6	50.1	1:8.4
Mandya Synthetic	23.7	110	14.5	10.6	49.0	1:5.1
Nellore Synthetic	26.5	134	14.5	11.4	50.2	1:4.6
Deccani Synthetic (x Dorset)	34.7	188	16.2	14.2	49.9	1:8.8

*On pre-slaughter weight basis.
Source: As for Table 3.3.

Specific recommendations about the individual states were made and it was suggested to undertake a periodic review. General suggestions about various regions embody the abstract policy.

- That the temperate region comprising Jammu and Kashmir, Himachal Pradesh and Uttar Pradesh offered opportunities for fine wool production. A large scale programme of cross breeding of local sheep with exotic fine wool rams of Rambouillet or Merinos from USSR be undertaken. It would be necessary to set up a large sheep breeding farm for a continuous supply of fine wool rams in this region.

- Some other exotic breeds of sheep, such as Corriedale, Dorsets and Romney Marsh may also be utilized for cross breeding of indigenous sheep in other states on limited trial basis, in selected pockets, where they have not given successful results earlier, as certain sheep breeds are known to suit to areas with high rainfall.

- The committee also recommended that where such cross breeding of local sheep with exotic sheep is to be taken up, the existing farms be reorganised or the state departments should set up sheep breeding farms with necessary facilities for breeding exotic sheep for maintaining a continuous supply of acclimatized rams.

   The state departments were further advised to estimate their requirement for exotic sheep and import sufficient number and continue to import additional rams for some more period.

- For the adequate supply of selected rams of indigenous sheep breeds, the committee further stressed that facilities at the other sheep breeding farms be also improved. As over-stocking of farms leads to low productivity and high mortality, so the committee emphasised the need to increase the forage production at the farms.

- The committee generally recommended the level of cross breeding with exotic breeds upto 50%, except for sheep breeding farms and certain selected areas in temperate region the exotic inheritance to increase beyond 50 per cent in the progeny.

Sheep Breeding Policy as laid down by the National Commission on Agriculture (1976)

- The level of exotic fine wool inheritance should be stabilized around 50 per cent in arid and semi-arid areas and the crossing of exotic fine wool breeds with black faced indigenous breeds should be avoided.

- The total sheep population in Jammu and Kashmir, Himachal Pradesh, hilly regions of Uttar Pradesh, sheep of Chokla and Nali breeds in Rajasthan, Nali sheep in Haryana, Pattanwadi sheep in Gujarat, Nilgiri sheep (TN) and better woolly sheep of Arunachal Pradesh may be brought under cross breeding for fine wool production using Rambouillet or Merino rams.

- Selective breeding among sheep of important carpet wool breeds and other woolly sheep except Pattanwadi in Gujarat should be undertaken.

- A few large sheep breeding farms of Marwari, Jaisalmeri, Pugal and Magra breeds should be established in their respective home tracts.

- The population of woolly sheep in Haryana, Punjab, western Uttar Pradesh, Rajasthan, Maharashtra, Andhra Pradesh, Karnataka, Tamil Nadu and Bihar should be crossed with exotic dual purpose breed like Corriedale or medium fine wool Rambouillet to evolve a dual purpose sheep for producing better carpet quality wool, better live-weight and higher dressing percentage.

- The hairy breeds other than Mandya and Nellore should be graded up with Nellore and Mandya. In Mandya and Nellore selective breeding based on six monthly body weight should be practised.

- It would be advisable to establish four large exotic sheep breeding farms in different regions of the country for undertaking cross breeding with Corriedale/Rambouillet.

The National Commission on Agriculture further suggested avoiding frequent modifications of the breeding programme.

The advancing scientific knowledge, the international trends, need for conservation of indigenous germ plasm, faster productivity requirements, findings of various surveys and the fast changing socioeconomic conditions however, necessitated a review of the policies so that the sheep production programme fits in well with the changing scenario. The Central Government framed a Task Force in 1993 to go into various aspects of sheep, goat and rabbit production and make appropriate recommendations about the additions and changes in the existing sheep breeding policies.

PRECAUTIONS IN EXOTIC SHEEP INTRODUCTION

While introducing the foreign sheep breeds in the country whether for propagation or cross breeding, certain vital aspects need to be taken care of. A fair knowledge of breed, its habitat, nature, environment of the home region, rearing system adopted, type of forage and disease problem is essential. Exotic sheep have restricted breeding season. Once they pass through a oestrus period, they seldom breed further. If at all they breed out of season, the results may not be uniform.

The introduction of a foreign breed of livestock involves shifting of an adapted germ plasm from its home tract to a new environment and thus is prone to numerous new genotype-environment interactions. Such situations call for advance care and managerial action:

- An ideal location and shelter shed plan is desirable.
- Open airy sheds are preferred where essential. Pucca flooring is avoided. Soil and lime are good for flooring. Stone flooring is not good.
- Plinth wall be raised at least a foot or two above the ground level.
- In case of soiling of earth floor with urine and dung, it should be scrapped and composted or applied in the crops. Regular cleaning of habitation area is warranted.

- Where pucca flooring is essentially required, the clay brick flooring shall be enough.
- No grass or any vegetation should be permitted to grow in and around the pen and the shed.
- Unless inclement weather prevails the sides of the shed should not be closed or covered. For the exit of gases, the top ventilation provision is essential.
- Racks for hay and separate trough for feed (concentrates) water, salt licks, etc. need to be provided in the sheds or elsewhere in the paddocks.
- Open ground around the shed kept for exercise may be covered with gravel and sand in places where rainfall is heavy or the soil is clayey. Larger paddocks around the shed may have a few shady trees.
- It is better not to keep the breeding rams together. Stud rams should be kept in a separate compartment with attached open ground for exercise.
- Ewes should be kept together in a bigger shed without compartments to reduce excitement.
- The imported sheep should not be permitted to graze on grass-lands or fields till they get acclimatised.
- Provision of clean dry hay of good quality grasses needs to be ensured. Other forage such as lucerne, alfa-alfa (Berseem) green oats mixed with peas, turnips, kale, etc. if grown at the farm are very helpful. Oat fodder as fresh or baled hay serves the purpose well. Standard pellet concentrates/feeds are the best.
- Greens though essential should be fed in limited quantity only.
- A pasture with at least 6 months rest and sufficient exposure may be allocated.
- The best time to introduce the imported sheep is November to February in a major portion of the country.
- Fresh supply of clean water must be ensured.
- Dosing sheep (just after entry) with medicines be avoided unless circumstances clearly prove the existence of internal worms.
- Vaccination be permitted/conducted where necessary.

- Sudden changes and repeated handling be discouraged.
- Imports of Rambouillet, Merino, Corriedale or mutton sheep are mostly from ranches, where they do not see many persons. Arrival of unfamiliar persons or even attendants near the livestock frightens and makes them restless rather wild at times.
- Quarantine period of 2 to 3 weeks is essential to ward off the chances of new diseases.
- A further period of adaptation before breeding in a particular environment is desirable.
- Finally every precaution and restraint is to be observed while importing sheep and goats from countries and flocks having history or incidence of diseases like caprine angio-encephlomyelitis (CAE), bovine spongiform encephlopathy (BSE), blue tongue, scrapie, brucellosis and other communicable infections.

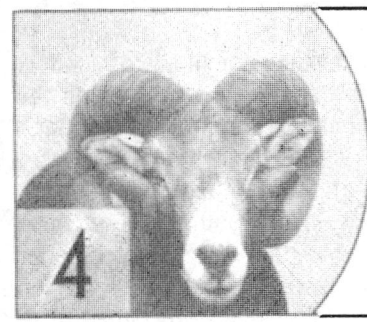

NATURE AND BEHAVIOUR OF SHEEP

4

NATURE

Varied types of sheep exist in the world and even within this country. Differences among them are present in size, body conformation, type and colour of body coat and even production patterns. Notwithstanding these differentiating features, the sheep possess some inherent commonalties, which assign the specie a unique position in the animal kingdom. These special endowments have permeated from wild stage to the domestication and further to the present day developed sheep with the same intensity and increasing social relevance. The proverbs like 'as meek as a sheep' or 'as timid as a lamb' find beautiful expression in a greatman's quotation: "Confront a child, kitten and a lamb to a sword, the child gets frightened, the kitten scares away out of danger, and the lamb licks the sword".

For the humanity at large, the same sheep message is that of humility, love and extreme sacrifice. In fact sheep has placed itself on the alter of man and surprisingly used to have significance in obsolete rituals and offerings. Right from stone age to the modern society every part of sheep stands out in utility for the mankind, whether it is wool, fur, skin, mutton, bones; viscera, glands; hooves, horns, blood or the dung and other excreta.

GRAZING, FEEDING AND DRINKING HABITS

1. Sheep by nature is a pastoral animal and prefers roaming about in the open.

2. It is a close grazier preferring short herbage. While browsing, sheep trim leaves of a plant, but usually spare the growing tip and leave the stem standing. Mobile lips, sharp incisors below and a tough dental pad above are the natural provision for feeding of short grasses. The upper lip is very mobile due to a vertical fissure in the centre. This permits one half of the lip to move some what independent of the other half. Mobile lips and sensory dental pad further help in selection of forage by touch. The inherent love which sheep have for change of grazing ground is always visible from the playful and absorbing interest that they envince just after they are turned into a fresh pasture.

3. The flock responds instantaneously to the sound of a lopping axe or the whistle of the shepherd for watering or offering of salt licks. The usual scene is one of simultaneous bleating and hysterical running of flock towards the site. Being ruminants, sheep are adapted not only to the consumption of grains but also to bulky feed such as hay and grasses though reject the very coarsest and bitterest varieties. They make use of senses of taste, smell and vision in the pasture or at the feeding trough. Cultivated leguminous fodders *such as clovers, berseem, lucerne, cowpeas, field beans, etc.* or *green oats* and cultivated grasses are all relished well.

4. It is interesting to note how sheep feed on hills. In a hill country where sheep are grazed in large numbers, the observer is sure to see along the hillside many sheep paths like little terraces

indicating that in grazing the sheep do not pass over the hill but rather gradually work along the side to the top. Possibly, the native abode of domesticated sheep was in the high treeless plateaus and mountains. Most sheep enjoy grazing on the high places in the pasture. Some of the modern breeds have been kept on low level lands, so long, that it is now doubtful whether they would take to the hills from choice.

5. Comparatively few studies have been made of grazing behaviour of sheep. Field observations in semi-arid and tropical wastelands indicate that tips of green leaves are searched out from the base of tussaks when the pasture is dry. Depending upon availability of grazing, sheep irregularly travel 4 to 5 km a day, but when the pasture is sparse they travel farther. Strong wethers have been observed going almost 10 km.

Sheep prefer to graze in the wind and cooler hours. They are disinclined to graze around the hot part of the day. They suspend grazing and move towards water as air temperature rises in the morning. If the pasture is adequate, sheep cease grazing between 2 to 3 hours after sunrise in the summer. However, when the pasture is inadequate in summer, sheep extend their day grazing time. Many a Bakerwali sheep flocks are in the habit of night or late evening–early morning grazing. There is a marked difference in grazing behaviour in temperate region and northern hemisphere from the subcortices. Sheep in the rich alpines of Himalayan states resort to grazing between 10 am to 1 pm and again from 4 to 5 pm. Rest of the time they rest and ruminate only.

In the tropical area and in hot sun of summers in subcortices, sheep prefer to be in the shelter or shade. It is not unusual for them to stand or lie about in-groups either near water or on the open place in shadeless areas. Like highland grazing during very cold or forbidding weather the sheep may not go out to graze before 10 am.

The sheep has a small mouth with which to gather approximately 1 to 1.4 kg of dry matter a day. A sheep may have to spend 3 to 4 or even up to 8 hours each day in grazing steadily to obtain its fill. Out of full grazing duration, there is a resting pause after every 2 to 3 hours grazing bout of chewing the cud. When left undisturbed the sheep go on ruminating and masticating in regular succession, sometimes in half sleepy state.

6. Intensity of grazing varies from maximum near shelter or watering points to a minimum at points remote from shed or water. Pasture and rangelands are the natural habitat of sheep. This herbivore possesses the unique ability to survive on natural vegetation and thrive under extreme climatic conditions and forage variations. Sheep avoid entering the pasture areas of tall vegetation. Usually nibble at tiny blades of vegetation, preferring small tender grasses. They chew forage more thoroughly than cattle. Liking and disliking of sheep to a particular type of pasturage in comparison to other animals indicate that no other animal has the ability to utilize pastures so efficiently (Table 4.1).

Suitability of pasture for different types of livestock more so for sheep is of paramount consideration for proper utilization of land to avoid damage to herbage.

7. Following heavy and continuous rains the grass grows rapidly and may provide such a dense cover that the sheep are unable to travel far from

Table 4.1: Percent intake choice of range plants of domestic livestock

S.No.	Vegetation	Horses	Cattle	Sheep	Goats
1.	Grass	90	70	60	20
2.	Weeds	04	20	30	20
3.	Browse (Bush and bramble)	06	10	10	60

Source: Bell, H.M. (1978)

water, thus many animals get confined in comparatively small area. This local 'over-stocking' may have two effects;

    a. The conditions favour a rapid increase in Haemonchus and allied worm burden, which frequently escapes the notice until mortality occurs.

    b. The composition of pasture changes. Many useful annual plants disappear in good season and bare ground occupies spaces between the perennials.

8. Sheep are able to exist without water longer than most domestic animals. This may be due to the reason that they have usually large salivary glands. It has often been thought that sheep don't need any excess water, but such an assumption is erroneous as even in cold weather it drinks 2 to 3 litre water daily. In water deficient environments or under high temperature above 40°C or under saline concentrations approaching 1%, the sheep become selective to pick up certain green grasses or pods that possess high water content and compensate the shortage of drinking water thereby. When water is available during summer, sheep may drink frequently during day.

BREEDING BEHAVIOUR

Sheep in general and by nature is a seasonal breeder. The wild types exhibit a well defined breeding season. In the high terrains of Ladakh these breed in late autumn/early winters and lamb at the end of prolonged winters. The domestic sheep too shows the same type of seasonal breeding activity, though a different rhythm in the two hemispheres. In the northern part of the globe the breeding season is witnessed mainly from late summer or early autumn to late autumn. Most of the sheep in India, particularly the northern zone breeds follow this pattern. Decreasing day length appears to govern the breeding behaviour. As an exception certain Deccan plateau sheep do also breed from February to April. So the lambing synchronises with the monsoons foliage flush. In the southern hemisphere the breeding season sets in the first half of the year instead of September-October. Merino and other breeds in the Ocaenia continent have their breeding season opposite to the northern hemisphere.

Under natural course, it is not possible to have lambs born at any time in a year. Most of the domestic breeds of sheep are mono-oestrous, very few animals revealing dioestrous tendency, which means ewes in majority come in heat in just one season and rare few in two seasons of the year.

It is however claimed that there are certain strains in India too, that can produce lambs in more than two seasons at the fancy of the breeder. Such a proposition of out of proper season lambing brings mixed fortunes. A high plane of feeding and availability of green fodder to the lambs and ewes if not provided can spell disaster.

During oestrous the ewe remains in heat for about two days. In young ewes, period is less but in old it is longer. If she is not bred or fails to conceive after service by a ram, the oestrous recurs in about 16 to 21 days. In case not bred, then she is likely to show heat recurrence for 2 to 3 months regularly. Because of such successive oestrus cycles at intervals, the sheep is classed as seasonally polyoestrous. The oestrus may pass off as 'silent heat' or with low intensity in older ewes.

Rams possess a natural instinct to detect heat by the very smell and movements of the ewe.

PROLIFIC NATURE

148 ± 3 days is the usual gestation period for ewes. Minor breed to breed variations exist in the length of period of pregnancy in exotic as well as Indian sheep breeds. But for certain breeds like Patanwadi, Lohi, etc. Indian sheep usually give birth to a single lamb. Twinning is just 2 to 3%. Occasionally an ewe might drop triplet or more. The crossbreds of Merino and its sister breeds have been found to give 5 to 6% twinning under our conditions. Since the ewe has but two teats, that function, she is not well prepared to take care of more than two lambs. Prolific breeds tend to throw two lambs in a higher percentage of ewes.

Genetic control on number of lambs born exhibits a correlated manifestation for higher milk potential in many prolific sheep breeds.

Though the heritability of twinning is relatively low, yet due to careful selection and breeding of proper stock of twinners it may be possible to improve prolificacy. Certain sheep breeds, viz. Romonov, Welsh Mountain, etc. have over 150 percent lambing rates.

PSYCHO-BEHAVIOURAL ENDOWMENTS

Folding habit

Sheep when allowed to choose between shelter and open prefer to sit or rest on raised or high places. Their liking for high well-drained and airy resting or sleeping ground appears inborn and very marked. Wild sheep even today can be seen roaming on the high exposed cliffs and mountain slopes. The domestic sheep too appears to have acquired such a behaviour and tendency from the ancestor sheep. This may not be true, however, of sheep that have been raised on barns. It is only in the severest winter weather that sheep abandon such spots for lower, wind-protected patches. After the lamb is few hours old it constantly seeks some eminence, such as its mother's back, a bale of hay, manger or a rock. Young sheep occupy elevated places more readily than do the older ones. Hoggets go higher up for grazing on a hillside than older ewes and rams.

The traditional sheep breeders in the temperate region and elsewhere are quite conscious of the nature of sheep. They generally accommodate sheep at night in open, raised and slopy ground. This keeps the flock neat, active and healthier.

Lamb recognition

Every human being and even sheep is known to possess a distinct smell. This has been attributed to pheromones. Sheep too have keen sense of smell. An ewe can recognize her newborn lamb by sniffing. But in a few days sheep can distinguish it at sight. In case of perplexity she almost realizes on her nose for recognition. Apparently the odour by which the ewe identifies her new born off spring is due to some thing coming from her, for in case she refuses to own her lamb, the expert professional shepherd rubs the lamb against the ewe to induce her to own the off spring. Some times he places some of her milk on its rump, the point where she usually sniffs at the lamb. At times a pinch of salt is sprinkled on the body of the lamb to make the ewe lick the lamb which ultimately helps in owning the lamb. Under congested conditions and in transportation early in life the peculiar smell of the lamb is lost. This results into large scale disowning of lambs by the mother ewes at times.

Gregariousness

The flocking instinct of sheep, i.e. the liking or the tendency to keep together, is gregariousness. This instinct is not so pronounced in some breeds as it is in others. But there is no breed that is known not to possess it. The Merinos and Ramboullet have the trait most strongly developed. On the other hand almost all the English mutton breeds are less inclined to stay close together while grazing. They normally spread out in the vast pasture while grazing. Yet any thing that frightens, like howl or growl of a jackal, barking of a dog or bursting of a cracker make the whole lot to flock together at once. The Indian sheep too express this behaviour, but marked among them are migratory and semi-migratory sheep of the temperate and arid zone.

The flocking instinct is so strongly ingrained in our sheep that when any individual sheep gets separated from the flock, it is an unusual happening. There is regular bleating by the sheep till it spots the flock again. Some times, the sheepman on finding an individual sheep alone considers the same ill or injured. Gregariousness is of particular advantage in Australia, New Zealand or USA where dogs are used to muster or collect the flock in the ranches and to shift from one paddock to another. In the alpine pastures and even Shivaliks one is amused to see sheep coming from all corners of the pasture at dusk to join the other flock members for a trek to the folding place. This avoids straying of animal. But where the flocking instinct is of low order, compact body or flock formation is not there and loss due to predators is more. In the extensive but unfenced pasturelands any herder can loose some of his sheep by straying.

Sheep follow a leader

Closely associated with the gregarious instinct of sheep is its tendency to follow a leader. As a pet individual, it follows the owner like a shadow. Goat being a very active and intelligent animal is often used to lead the sheep flock for grazing or returning back home. There is an old saying, "where one sheep goes, all others will follow". If the leader moves on, takes a long leap; passes through a narrow passage or even plunges into the water the rest of sheep flock or couple of animals after the leader behave the same way. About fifty years back an incident of this nature happened in Paddar area of Jammu. A gaddie sheep flock moving over a precipitous narrow path along river Chenab got frightened. The goat leader could not turn back and fell into the river. The sheep flock followed suit and in a couple of seconds a part of the flock jumped down and was lost in the river.

Nervousness

At the sight of wild animals sheep become so frightened that they run wildly here and there. Sudden barking of a dog or a shrill voice near the pen leads to stampede just by fear psychosis.

At the ranches when approached by strangers, they exhibit restlessness, fast running, dashing and even jumping over fences. A couple of imported Rambouillet sheep from American ranches (almost three decades back) suffered injuries, fractures and even physical breakdown at our farms in the process of handling, till getting familiar to new shepherds.

Snorting and bleating sounds are given out at times. Wild sheep in Marcelong and Gaya heights in Ladakh when sighted by the author started trumpeting fore foot as a signal by the leader to flock mates before hurriedly making off to deeper mountain ranges.

Timidity and Defencelessness

Sheep are known great timid domestic animals. They lack the ability to defend themselves against predators and other animals. Vultures and eagles take a good toll of newborn lambs. Worst enemies of sheep are the dogs, jackals, wolves, bear and panther in India. The dingo, a wild dog makes depredation on flocks in Australia. Wolf and the coyote particularly haunt sheep in the ranges of USA.

While any of these animals may kill the sheep, their attacks are almost as deadly, if they just chase or bite. In case they are bitten, death may result from the infection of wound.

Aggressiveness

Horned breeds of sheep are said to be less prone to predators than the hornless. Strong masculine breeds are aggressive and males less afraid than ewes. However, spirited ewes with lambs at foot have been observed to defend their young ones. Some rams attempt butting when approached by a stranger. Both ewes and rams in certain local breeds try to scare away the enemy by stamping the fore foot. In the wild as well as some local sheep, this behaviour is considered a forewarning to the other flock members of an approaching danger. Aggressiveness is much pronounced during ram infighting and mating. The hard butting and charging acts at 'ram fighting sport' often result into injuries and bleeding

NONRESISTANCE TO DISEASES

Sheep do not show much indication or evidence of illness until they are very sick. This is perhaps the reason for the statement that 'a sick sheep is a dead sheep'. A careful shepherd however picks up the sick sheep in time to save it. To be a successful sheep raiser, he must learn to discover at once that something is wrong with his sheep, before they are taken as good as dead. Twice inspection, i.e. while letting-out in the morning and letting-in, in the evening provide the best opportunity for the sheepman to appreciate any ailing sheep.

Certain breeds apparently resist disease better than others do. For instance the indigenous (Indian) sheep appear resistant and less fragile to parasitism than the crossbreds, the latter are lesser prone than the pure exotic breeds introduced in this country over the last couple of decades. Hence it seems probable that general hardiness may have been more or less disregarded in the development of some of the modern breeds.

Sheep express themselves differently than other dumb animals. It is only a keen eye, thorough observation and knowledge of sheep psyche that can help locate a real problem. Diagnosing a sheep ailment poses yet another puzzle. Instances may be cited here of sheep, disinterested in grazing, standing listless with suspended rumination and lowered head that was suspected for a digestive disorder. Symptoms and initial inference proved misleading and finally it turned out to a simple case of sternal sinus. Yet in a similar other case only a maggot infested wound in the vulvar region was the real cause of sickness which in fact was mistaken for a serious internal ailment to start with. *Per se* behaviour in fact evaded the conclusion initially. Suspicion in both the cases arose from the foul smell evinced around the animal and confirmation of actual disease came only after turning the animal topsy-turvy, during examination.

GENERAL BEHAVIOUR

By nature sheep is a neat and tidy animal. It discards low-lying, damp, humid, congested, less-airy and dirty dwelling and shelter. It is a simple observation that sheep maintained under such environment are unthrifty and remain disease infested all the time. Foot rot, respiratory disorders, mastitis, pizzle rot, etc. affect the flock quite often. Intensive housing may lead to infestation of lice, ticks, keds and mites. Flies torment the

sheep most. Not only do they make it restless, the nasal bot *(Oestrous ovis)* and skin bot *(Hypoderma lineatum)* are a source of disease, discomfort and low production.

Animals, which are used to outside grazing and drinking, particularly the adult sheep, would reject mouldy fodder, trampled hay or grazing in a field where other animal have moved about. To the unlike smell, they are so sensitive as to sniff out just in first attempt. Inexperienced shepherds try to offer the same rejected fodder repeatedly. Sheep normally keep away and it is only under starving conditions that unfit feed and fodder are consumed reluctantly. The outcome is invariably unfavourable.

Clear and running water is preferred over stagnant and still water. Quite often the sheep are made to drink water at the village ponds or to graze on the marshy lands and dewy grass, contrary to the liking of the flock. This often results into picking up of leach infestation and worminous load or gastro-intestinal problems. Mere peep into the behaviour of sheep shall make the sheepman follow management and rearing on scientific lines. Adjustment of management on natural lines avoiding much handling, least disturbance, congenial and comfortable main-tenance have been found to result in better thrivability, proliferation and productivity of sheep flocks.

BENEFACTOR QUALITIES

Beyond the main contributions of wool, mutton, fur, skins, milk, manure, etc. the docile sheep is serving the humanity yet in many other ways.

Eco-restorer

Because of close grazier nature the sheep possesses mowing habits. Thus, it trims the golf grounds, play fields and roadside grass/strips evenly. Sheep also consume away weeds, and other extraneous growth of the rangelands. The spread of unwanted vegetation like Parthenium and Cassia is thereby kept under check. Most of burrs like Jojra

(Nagoora), Hubla, Kithri get stuck to the fleece coat of sheep while grazing. Only a lesser number drops on the ground. Fleeces infested with the seeds of these burrs reach the grading centres and carbonizing plants, where picking, crushing and decay of the burrs reduces the intensity of dispersal of burrs and thistles. No doubt the undigested seeds that are passed by the sheep in the dropping do give rise to bumper germination at the folding sites quite often, but this simultaneously facilitates easy and enmass removal.

Remarkable advantage to the farmer and forester accrues from the movement of sheep flock in the forest area or enclosures. Mature grass seeds are dispersed either in the faeces or through body coat. These are gently dibbled in the soil through usual gentle trampling under feet. Passing of excreta, i.e. dung and urine in that grazing area at regular intervals leads to manuring as well. The sheep therefore returns much more to the pasture than what it gets out of the same soil. Eco-friendly nature of sheep has served as the best eco-restorer of the grazing areas at certain sheep farms, which were prone to degradation in face of exploitation. Surprisingly even the wild fauna like Ibex, antelopes and hare feel undisturbed among the merrily grazing sheep flocks in the alpines. The other carnivorous species of wolf, bear, leopard and the panther thrive well in the highlands and forest grazing lands at the cost of sheep.

As a laboratory animal

Young lambs and even adult sheep are commonly used in laboratory for testing of pharmacological actions of drugs. The sheep tissues and the animal too are utilized for growing micro organisms, isolation of infectious organisms and passages. In the field of biologicals, and vaccine production the importance of sheep is second to none.

Supplier of industrial raw material

Besides the supply of wool for making woollens in cottage as well as organised industry particularly carpets, tweeds and the worsteds, the sheep is in great demand for lamb and mutton supply. In certain sheep surplus states like Rajasthan, the live sheep sales and mutton exports add sizeably to the state revenue and farmers' economy.

Utility of sheep skins for fur and leather; endocrine glands for hormone preparation; hooves, horns, cartilages for gelatine manufacture, gut for catgut, sausages, and as reprocessed feed for small animals and fish, etc. hair for varied utility articles make the sheep an indispensable animal.

Sheep — a pack animal

In high mountain ranges in the temperate region of this country where other transport means are either lacking or the approach is inaccessible for the pack ponies, sheep is employed for transportation of essential commodities like grains, salt, etc. An adult ram or wether of 2 to 6 year age carries 8 to 10 kg load on its back in a specially prepared double haversack 'the shutt' made out of goat hair. The flock of pack sheep ascends the tough mountain terrains or passes like a cavalry. Where ever a plain plateau or halting stations comes, they spread out for grazing. The back load never slides as it is tied to neck and thigh wool.

Even today hundreds of Changthangi rams are seen transporting commodities in the interior of Changthang, i.e. to Kurzok, Kargyam, Chambur, Kharnak-Rupcho and Surchu valleys across high mountain passes and along the Silk route. This practice has been in vogue in extreme hilly region of Sikkim, UP and Himachal Pradesh particularly the districts of Kinnaur, Lahaul Spiti, Kulu and Chamba. Over 300 pack sheep belonging to a royal household of erstwhile Chamba state used to transport the winter requirements of land locked Pangi valley over the Saach pass till recent times. This flock would present a fascinating view of extraordinary utility of sheep to the tribals.

PHYSIOLOGICAL PARAMETERS

Parameter	Normal range
Body temperature	38 to 39°C
Respiratory rate at rest (adult sheep)	12 to 15/min.
Heart rate	70 to 89/min.
Ruminal movements	2 in 3 minutes
Breedable age (ewes)	15 to 20 months
Gestation period	148 $\pm$ 3 days
Oestrus cycle recurrence	After every 16 to 21 days during breeding season
Duration of Oestrus	12 to 36 hours
Postpartum heat	20 to 80 days (Generally within 40-50 days)
Body temperature of lamb at birth	Ewe's rectal temp. (C°) + 0.5°C
Scrotal temperature for efficient spermatogenesis	Ram's rectal temp. (C°) −2 to 3°C

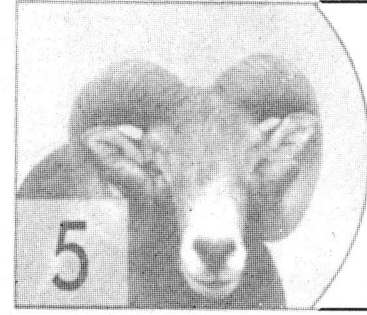

TRADITIONAL SHEEP HUSBANDRY

SOCIOECONOMIC BACKGROUND

Until mid twentieth century the practices of sheep husbandry followed in India were quite primitive ones. The reasons were obvious. Generally it were the nomadic tribals and poor rural communities who engaged themselves in sheep rearing. They passed on the inherited sheep property and the vocation as such from generation to generation. But for solitary instances, there was lack of attention towards their livestock improvement or their upliftment. Sheep rearing was neither an alluring job nor could it attract educated elite or affluent classes in the profession.

The returns provided meagre subsistence only and were not commensurate with the inputs of hard toil and discomforting life. The concept of extensive pasture ranches or big grazing holdings like Australia, New Zealand, USA, Russia or England did not exist in this country. The shepherding communities who were mostly landless or marginal farmers depended on pastures owned by others for feeding of their sheep.

Natural calamities and weather vagaries made the sheep vulnerable under the open sky. Insecure conditions, the ferocious wild animals and other predators took a heavy toll. The pests, which struck at times, proved disastrous in absence of proper disease control measures. Sheep were often exposed to forage competition with the large animals and the latter or even goat invariably found a preferential response.

Sheep byproducts were considered a material for family or local consumption only. Farming sections found the manure pellets more important than mutton or wool. No incentive market for wool existed in early days in the country. Only English market (at Liverpool and Manchester) offered a reasonable price for our valued carpet wool. Within the country there was hardly any organised centre for utilization of wool but for cottage industry and a few woollen mills. Not much scientific know how existed within the country. Marketing and commercial aspects were of least consequence to the sheep farmer. The shepherd however, continued to believe in the age old colloquial adage:

"Oontaan wale sada dwale,
Majhaan wale adhey,
Piddan wale sada sukhaley
Panwen muk jaan sabhe"

'The camel owners are invariably bankrupt and the buffalo rearers are half way; sheepmen are always comfortable even if there is a catastrophe'. The contribution of sheep in the rural and agricultural economy is well projected in the following Rajasthani couplet:

"Gabri sonadi tharee meengni sonari,
Thara daan dhan se para,
Ne oon sonara taar,
Dheena dhaya kraije ladli rani"

'O, beautiful sheep, your pellets are gold precious, the penning arena full of wealth and house holds with milk, your wool is a golden fibre; O dear, rani (queen)'

REARING SYSTEMS

Old testaments, dating back to 11th century AD and earlier bear reference to shepherding by ancient tribes in India. Nomadic people (like Bharwads, Kurbars, Dhangars, Gaddies, Baker wals, Chagpas, etc.) have been moving to and fro with their sheep and goat with the change of season for pasture lands. Others (viz. Raikas, Thoda, etc.) who settled and opted for agriculture herded their sheep alongwith other livestock at or around their dwellings. During grazing and water scarcity periods they too under took short distance sojourns from their habitations for brief periods. Thus there have existed three distinct patterns of sheep rearing since ages, i.e. the migratory, semi-migratory and the stationary.

Migratory system

In India bulk of sheep population possessed by nomads and tribals in northern temperate region of J&K, HP and UP hills is managed on migratory pattern. The flocks spend winters in warmer low altitude belt. With the onset of summer these shift by slow stages to hills and alpines. In certain cases the distance covered is 300 to 400 km and altitude ranges from 500 to 4500 m. To and fro migration by slow stages takes about two month each time. Three months are spent in high lands and rest almost five months in the bushy forests of the lower ranges. The movement is within the respective state only. Migratory flocks remain in the open the whole year round. Adequate pasturage is available to them in the hills during summer stay.

In Rajasthan almost twenty lakh sheep remain in a state of perpetual interstate migration to Madhya Pradesh, Uttar Pradesh, Haryana, and Gujarat. Most of these flocks spend the dry season in Chambal valley. Some of the flocks do not return to their homes, especially of Jodhpur division, whereas, about 70% spend 3 to 4 months in the home tract. Rainy season is spent in the forest and hill ranges within Rajasthan. Likewise tribals in Gujarat also undertake long migration to other districts and adjoining states. The prolonged outside stay of flocks of hot arid region of Rajasthan, Gujarat and other states is aimed at obtaining grazing and drinking water in the dry and lean period. Some of the flocks of northeastern Tamil Nadu and northern Karnataka are also migratory. The distance traversed by them is not extensive.

Semi-migratory system

Short distance movement within State/Division or District with the change of season in search of grazing grounds is quite common. In the temperate region of Jammu and Kashmir (particularly the Kashmir valley and Rajouri-Poonch districts) or in other states where sheep farmers have grazing and feeding resources for the sheep for winters around their village dwelling and for summers in closeby hills and river valleys, migration for short summer periods is practised. These farmers invariably have small or marginal land holdings. The intention is to keep the flocks away during crop cultivation period. Their home areas serve as halting station to receive lambing, conduct shearing and mating of flocks. Harvested crop residues, stubbles and fresh grassy growth serve a boon to these flocks at the owner's property. Manuring of fields for next crop is also possible during the stop over period.

Semi migration or temporary migration system is prevalent in Rajasthan where at least 2 to 3 lakh sheep return to their home villages at the start of monsoons and leave again before the onset of winters. In Haryana, Gujarat, southwestern UP., flocks also resort to restricted migration. Sheep of Maharashtra, Karnataka, Andhra Pradesh and Tamil Nadu in part are also semi-migratory. Flocks of eastern zone especially of the states of Sikkim, Arunachal Pradesh and southern Orissa undertake limited to moderate distance migration.

Problems of migratory system

In the modern times the migratory and unsettled life of a sheepman and shepherd is looked upon with curse. On one hand it is beset with innumerable problems and hazards to them and on the other the extension of scientific operations like artificial insemination, mechanical shearing, immunization or other breeding and health cover measures are difficult to accomplish satisfactorily while in transit and in far off pastures.

Since decades and centuries the migratory breeders and their flocks have followed some self ordained routes of travelling from their habitation to rich pastures. They have adopted certain halting sites enroute, depending upon availability of space, grazing, water source and weather protection. These areas stand encroached by and by. Shortage of pasture has lead the breeders to move to longer distances in search of grazing. Entry restrictions and heavier taxation further impede the intrastate movement. The remaining away of members in far off areas with flocks for long periods does not favour the settlement of families.

Some of the migratory routes fall along the national highways. The breeders are scared to follow the flocks on these heavy traffic roads. Public resents the movement and grazing of flocks along the village paths located enroute migratory tracks. Usual thefts of livestock and loss due to predators add to the anxieties of a transhument nomad under insecure transit situation. Protection of wild life and safety of fresh plantations appear running counter to shepherd's profession and health and security of sheep. Wide spread growth of obnoxious weeds/vegetation, creation of large wild life parks and sanctuaries, extension of irrigation, urbanization, deforestation, reclamation of pasture lands and slopes for crop cultivation all add to the difficulties of a shepherd and migratory sheep.

Sedentary system

Rearing of small number of sheep alongwith other livestock on stationary footing round the year by various farming house holds is not new in this country. In parts of Rajasthan, Gujarat, Deccan plateau, Haryana, Punjab and other states smaller size flocks are maintained around the village grazing lands, vacant holdings, forest area, etc. Around 80 percent of the flocks in Gujarat and Rajasthan are stationary in nature. Sheep strength

of such flocks is generally 40 to 70 animals per flock. On mixed farming system a couple of sheep are reared by small and marginal farmers and poor rural peasantry in almost all the states.

Invariably the sedentary flocks are of smaller size than the other two systems. An economic unit size in stationary conditions is 30 to 50 sheep. Depending upon the extent of feeding resources the strength at times is just 5 to 10 sheep. In the irrigated and agriculture areas, roadside, canal bank grazing, crop harvest residue, top feeding, sown fodder crops, etc. are made use of. With the squeezing of pasture lands and onslaughts over migratory sheep, the stationary sheep rearing is picking up in many states.

Mandya, Hassan, Bellary and other sheep of South India are the best examples of sedentary sheep. In Punjab, the border district sheep like Munjal and Nali are thriving very well. The plains of Jammu and orchards of Kashmir valley have offered good scope for such sheep.

Problems of high degree parasitism and disease, fly strike, wool yellowing, higher cost of feeding and maintenance are some of the handicaps of stationary sheep rearing. These sheep generally do not present an attractive look and give a dirty appearance because of intensive housing like wintered flocks of the cold region. The owners resort to regular or weekly bath to sedentary sheep, which improves look but spoils the quality and get-up of fleeces.

EXISTING MANAGEMENT PRACTICES

Feeding

The shepherd in India has from ages learnt the art of rearing and feeding of sheep. He appreciates the increasing forage needs of the flocks by way of growth, production, and lamb bearing and lamb rearing. Nutritionally less important dry periods applicable to dairy cattle do not hold good for sheep entirely. During the productive life of sheep the uninterrupted growth of wool and mutton place a continuous demand on the body reserves of the animal, which require replenishment. The maintenance feeding as such implies differently to the sheepman for the "ever producing" animal. Though oblivious of the scientific basis and feeding values of what he feeds, there is awareness about proper maintenance of sheep and additional requirements imposed by pregnancy lambing, drought, severe winters, convalescence and other unfavourable conditions.

At times the poor or deficient pastures fail to provide adequate nutrition. Energy utilised in search of grazing over long to and fro movements are not compensated by the available grazing. Changes in the pastures status and composition affect the condition of sheep. Shifting to the new pastures, providing increased hours of grazing, resorting to cooler hour pasturing, practice of *Dakwaan Charai** are followed by the traditional Gaddie shepherd. Supplementation of grazing with preserved hay, fodder, pala (dry *Beri* leaves) and top feeding (lopping of fodder tree leaves and twigs) is usual all over the country. Even the feeding of crop residues, brans, gram husk, millets and grains like maize, barley, horse gram, cotton seed, etc. are initiated, if breeding, pregnancy and lambing stresses, so demand. Where sheep farmers possess land holdings, small quantities of grown green fodders like berseem, lucerne, oats, cowpeas, field beans, etc. are also fed.

At the sheep farms, varied types of feed mixtures used to be compounded and fed during 1950 to 1970. One such mixture containing the locally available ingredients is given in Table 5.1.

This was allowed for almost 6 weeks before lambing and 8 weeks after lambing to the breedable ewes in addition to day's grazing.

Subsequently maize found an increasing scale with corresponding decrease in quantities of black grams and oil cakes when it was realised that for the growth of wool certain vital amino acids are met through maize feeding. When the black grams grew costlier, rice polishings and groundnut cakes were used as substitutes. Mineral mixtures to the extent of 1 to 2% were usually added to all such feed mixtures replacing salt.

Another improvement in the late sixties consisted in adding multivitamin preparations, antibiotic feeds, fish liver oils, Liv-52 and molasses, etc. to the lamb starters containing wheat bran and crushed maize. Because of nutritional and intrinsic factors, these starter feeds were found to augment lamb growth, production and survivability. The last three decades have witnessed further advancement in rational feeding of sheep and research in nutrition of livestock in general in India.

Watering

Water springs, running streams, and river banks are in fact the main places where flocks converge by noon to drink water after morning grazing. Sheep in the hills and alpines of northern region or those migrating from western arid zone and

Table 51: Composition of feed mixture

Sl.no.	Feed article	%	Remarks
1.	Wheat Bran	48	Fed in varying quantities
2.	Black gram (crushed)	15	from 100 to 500 g
3.	Maize (crushed)	20	per sheep, per day
4.	Oil cakes	15	from a lamb
5.	Salt	2	to an adult sheep

* Controlled grazing and browsing in circumscribed pasture area through restricted movement of flock, to provide equal grazing opportunity to all animals. The experienced shepherd regulates the movement of animals through whistling and sounds while standing/sitting at a prominent point in the pasture.

Deccan plateau to far off locations have a sole objective of grazing availability near or around water abundant river valleys.

In the plain rural countryside, the village ponds, rivulets or irrigation channels serve as water source for the sheep. Quite often a channel or a watering trough is prepared near a village well or a spring. At times the flock is driven to an oasis in the arid zones miles away for drinking. In the latter situation watering may be possible once a day or on alternate days only.

At organised sheep farms proper water supply is generally laid out, which extend to various paddocks, sheds and watering points in the pasture. Watering troughs are cleaned regularly. Contaminated and left over quantity if any in trough is drained and replaced by fresh one. Care is taken that the troughs are not so deep as to cause drowning of lambs.

Salt licks

Providing weekly or periodic salt licks is a common practice with sheep owners in India. Either a lump of rock salt or compact salt brick is used or crushed salt is spread by the shepherd on stones along or near the watering source on the day of offering licks. There is a belief among shepherds that fresh grazing in the alpines causes sourness of sheep teeth, which can be mitigated through salt licking. The animal exhibits better interest in grazing after a usual lick. It was observed in the migratory sheep that when salt licks were delayed or stopped, the sheep started licking belongings of the shepherd at the camp.

A sheep is fed 10 to 25 gm of crushed salt in the weekly lick. Salt is not given to young and suckling lambs. To the experienced sheepman the licks provide an indication of health of his flock. Some of the animals harbouring Fascioliasis are observed with mild bottle jaw condition the very next morning of the salting. A few others suspected for internal parasitism may develop watery transient faeces instead of normal pellets, a day or two after salt licks.

With the introduction of mineral mixtures and their addition to the compounded feed, there is hardly any need for the additional salt licks. The sodium requirements of the animals are met for normal body functions through salt licks in absence of concentrate feeding. The mineral mixtures are however a better source of various mineral elements than the salt licks.

Wool harvesting

The shepherd harvests the wool at right and appropriate periods to the best advantage of both the man and the sheep. This act of cutting and removal of the wool from the body of the sheep is termed "shearing". Process of shearing is generally accomplished with the help of hand shearing scissors by the traditional shepherd. Shearing is done twice or thrice in a year depending upon season and growth of fibres. Most of the southern zone sheep grow hairy coat so do not necessitate shearing. The fine wool merino and cross breds that possess a compact fleece coat do not shed and are shorn once a year only. Desired length of fleece coat and a measure of economy in labour engagement are achieved by resorting to single annual shearing.

This is a seasonal, labour and time consuming flock operation. Hand shearing being an outmoded practice is gradually getting replaced by machine shearing which has got multiple overriding advantages over the former.

Shelter

But for wintering of sheep at the time of lambing or shearing in extreme cold conditions, any elaborate housing of sheep is not advocated in U.S.A., Asia or even in Australia where only some shelters are provided in the ranches. The range sheep at times remain outside in the snow*

---

* Flocks maintained in open under snowfall conditions at Daksum (Kashmir) during 1972-73 showed least adverse effects (Kaul, M.L.-1974)

Transhument sheep rearing in India is attributed to nomadism and their flocks also remain under open skies.

Under permanent migrations the breeders provide no housing to the sheep excepting big bamboo baskets or temporary shelters made out of twigs and hay for the young lambs. Tarpaulin covers are also used at times. Winter protection is only ensured for the young lambs. The shepherd, or his family, in case of Bakerwal tribe, carry with them mobile equipment like tent or tarpaulin on a pony back. Changpas prepare their own woven shelter out of goat or yak hair. This is quite tough and withstands the severe chilly winds of Changthang (Fig. 39, PLATE 7). Underground sheds or bunker attached to the main houses are used to accommodate sheep in extreme winter conditions of Ladakh.

In the hills elsewhere, when winter is severe or snowy weather prevails, the flock is accommodated in kacha apartments adjacent to the owners habitation or on the ground floor. A lambing pen is usually attached to the flock shelter.

Under stationary flock rearing a thatched shed having mud masonry walls with an open enclosed space is the usual housing provision. This is generally made up of locally available cheaper, wooden or bamboo poles, kharkana (*S. sachharum*) sticks, thatch grass or polythene sheets (Fig. 5.1). This practice is common in almost all the warmer sheep rearing areas in the country. In the warmer areas of Rajasthan, Gujarat and southern states the flocks rest for the night in open fields. At times these are penned in proper enclosures erected near the dwellings or away from habitation.

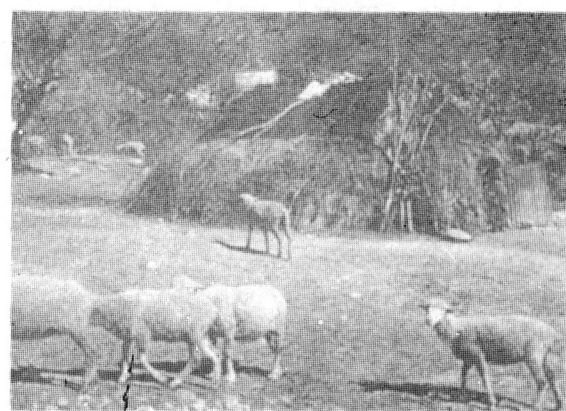

Fig. 5.1. Sheep enclosure with a thatched shelter.

the valuable stock well protected and scientifically managed. In Kashmir valley farms where prolonged wintering shelter is required, a baton flooring system was introduced. This helped in escape of droppings and urine and avoided damage to sheep and their fleeces. The long term effects have not been encouraging. The production of gases like ammonia, methane, and carbon dioxide in this system, prove more deleterious. In some of the well managed farms in hotter states and CSWRI. ventilation, exhaust and air circulation facilities have been created to minimize heat load. Even underground paddocks were provided at CSWRI. for the exotic sheep to reduce the effect of high environmental temperature and drift. Water spraying and use of khas-khas tatties is also practised to maintain the exotic costly sheep in fit condition.

Merits and demerits of housing

There are quite a few points for and against winter or summer housing of bigger flocks. Like in-wintering and lambing of sheep in cold European countries and northwestern U.S.A., farms in India are provided sheds. Shelter provision at the lambing time has its own advantage. Risk to old ewes, weak stock and young lambs is avoided under heavy rains and blizzard conditions. Both sheep and shepherd feel comfortable in severe

Housing of farm sheep

Though cheap housing is practised by and large, yet at certain stations pucca sheds with GI. or asbestos sheet roofing, elaborate manger, hay rack and watering and light facilities are provided. Open and attached chainlink closures are also constructed to serve as paddocks. Objective behind this expensive provision is to maintain winter. Feeding is facilitated. Other operations of sheep handling, lambing, marking and health cover can be accomplished conveniently. Rest to pasture is ensured. Inspection of lambs and ewes is easier inside. Incidence of internal parasitism is less in the housed sheep. In hot and arid zone, the covered underground paddocks save the fragile animals from summer heat and hot air draught. Where the breeder can afford a shed, it is preferred to have kacha floor and pucca walls up to half of the height and rest covered with pig iron or chain link mesh. The roof may be thatched one or made of asbestos or corrugated GI sheets (Fig. 5.2; Fig. 40, PLATE 7).

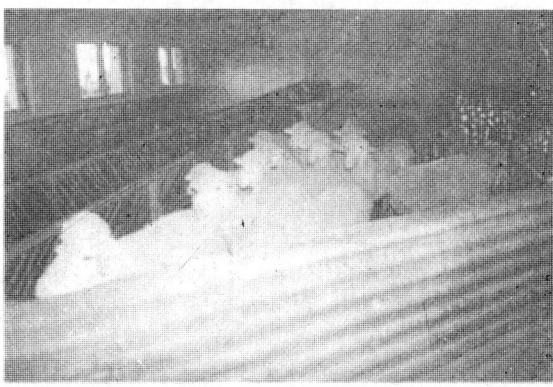

Fig. 5.2. Inside view of an improvisd pucca sheep shed.

The highly expensive sheds however make sheep rearing uneconomical. Intensive housing in winters makes the sheep dirty due to soiling. Wool tips degenerate under belly and in thigh regions. Ectoparasitism and mange in the housed sheep are more than those moving in open paddocks. Mastitis is higher in in-wintered ewes. Pizzle-rot is another malady commonly observed in inten-sively housed ram flocks. Gases that accumulate in imperfect ventilated sheds cause tremendous loss to the health of sheep. Though the warm environment of sheds promotes growth of lambs, but prolonged housing lowers their resistance to chill and atmospheric drifts. Deaths due to trampling, congestion, and accumulation of gases

in the housed sheep especially in humid conditions have been observed quite often.

As a matter of fact, housing of sheep needs to be discouraged unless warranted essentially. Then too, a cheap design, with proper ventilation and drained flooring is recommended. Shelters and sheds must permit entry of fresh air and light. There should not be any dampness or high humidity inside. Proper spacing is equally important.

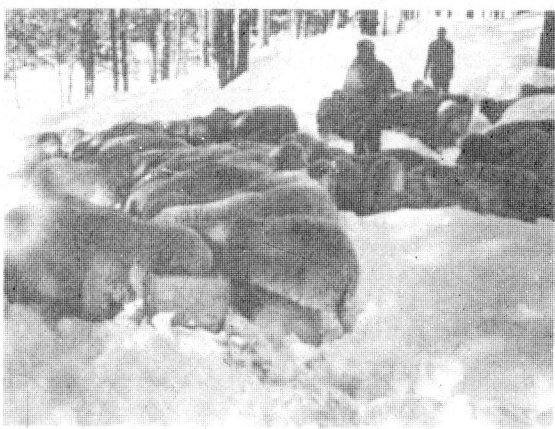

Fig. 5.3. Sheep feeding in open snow conditions at a Kashmir valley sheep farm

Sheep folding

In England, Australia and Texas (USA), 'sheep folding' is the usual practice of managing and rearing of sheep flock. It is the confinement of a flock on an area of a few hectares of fodder crop or pasture for feeding. The area is defined by using a suitable form of portable fencing, comprising poles and wire. It is so arranged as to circumscribe a flock within the forage area for a couple of days. Necessary watering point, a shelter for sheep and a light source are provided. At times a low voltage connection is also run through the fencing to deter animal crossing. When the fodder of the area is consumed, the hurdles are shifted so that the flock goes over to another stretch of fresh and unsoiled ranch.

Rearing flock on such a pattern saves energy of finding food by the animal. System is more suitable for mutton sheep rearing and development of sire herds as it ensures rapid growth and early maturity. The other advantage is the convenience of shepherding and labour economy. Property owner can inspect and follow improvement regularly while avoiding repeated interference and handling of flock. A make shift fencing and provision of shepherding dogs is the main necessity.

The sheep folding system connotes differently in India. Here land and pasture holding, at the command of shepherd are too small. It implies allowing the flock to sit and rest for the night in a limited area or corner of pasture or harvested (non-cropped) field. An acre of land may suffice a thousand sheep. The basic resting place or shelter for the night stay is quite erroneously termed as 'sheep night pen' or 'sheep fold' and named by the tribals, a "Bara", "Goth", "Dera" "Enylara", etc.

Space requirement

Migratory sheep mostly stay outside and do not attract much attention to spacing. Semi-migratory sheep like sedentary ones are housed during winters and at lambing period. Farm sheep too are accommodated in sheds. Any faulty provision of floor or air spaces can lead to huddling and result into serious consequences. Lacrymation observed in housed lambs and sheep in the morning is a sufficient indication of ill-spacing, ill ventilation and ill drainage. An experienced sheepman on entering a sheep shed would immediately perceive the presence of obnoxious gases like Methane and Ammonia just because of eye irritation. Therefore against traditional sheep housing, elaborate sheds planned on scientific lines are considered at various organised sheep farms.

The need for proper ground as well as air space deserves due emphasis (Table 5.2). Breed (to breed), sex (to sex), size and age group of animals, ambient temperature, humidity, wool coat condition and breeding status are some of the factors that determine the varying space requirement of sheep.

Thus a shed of 15 m × 10 m dimensions shall accommodate 120 to 150 ewes at lambing time exclusive of ground area occupied by feed mangers, hay racks, channels, etc. which account for almost one-fourth of the floor area assuming height of side walls at 2 metres and top (centre) truss points 3 to 3.5 metres high.

Table 5.2: Tentative space requirements for housed sheep

Sl. no.	Age category	Type	Floor area (m²)	Air space (m³)
1.	Lambs	Local and C.B.	0.2 to 0.3	0.5 to 0.7
2.	Weaners/Hoggets	–do–	0.3 to 0.5	0.7 to 1.2
3.	Yearlings	–do–	0.5 to 0.7	1.2 to 1.8
4.	Maiden ewes/Wethers	–do–	0.7 to 0.9	1.8 to 2.2
5.	Adult ewes	–do–	0.9 to 1.1	2.2 to 2.5
6.	Ewes with lambs (en-flock)	–do–	1.1 to 1.2	2.5 to 3.0
7.	Individual Lambing pen	–do–	1.2 to 1.3	3.0 to 3.4
8.	Rams	–do–	1.2 to 1.3	3.4 to 3.4
9.	Exotic ewes	Rambouillet Merino Corriedale	1.2 to 1.3	3.0 to 3.4
10.	Exotic Rams	–do–	1.3 to 1.5	3.4 to 3.7
11.	Exotic Studs (in individual pens)	–do–	1.6 to 2.0	3.7 to 4.2

Feeding troughs

In the shed, paddock or ranch, feeding troughs are provided for the flock to ensure hygienic feeding and to avoid wastage of feed and fodder. Varying with age, breed, size, sex, etc. the following dimensions for feeding troughs are adopted:

Length of trough or space per sheep	40 to 50 cm
Width of trough	20 to 30 cm
Height of trough	20 to 35 cm
Depth of trough	12 to 18 cm

Portable troughs are made of half curved GI sheets supported on angle iron stands. The channelled structure is held in position on the stands either by welding or through nuts and bolts. The fixed ones are usually pucca, made of cement and concrete. Additional racks made of angle iron and iron bars are provided for fodder feeding.

Compartmentalisation

At lambing time when the villagers house the sheep inside, an ordinary partition for the lambed ewe is made of wooden planks or bamboo strips or tree twigs/branches tied together. Suckling lamb once accepted by the ewe is at times separated by the shepherd and covered under a big bamboo basket or retained in the lamb pen while the ewe moves out for grazing. This practice is continued for a fortnight or so till the lamb accompanies the mother for grazing.

At farms temporary shed partitions or pen preparation is done by using galvanised steel sheets, framed chainlink or ordinary chain link rolls. Lambs are retained in the shed till 3 to 4 weeks age. By that time essential routine of marking, docking and feed starters are completed. Lambs grow young enough to accompany mother to nearby pastures or grazing fields. The age-wise pens maintained for them are then removed, allowing open space for their free movement and frolicking.

OTHER ASPECTS

Flock coverage

In most parts of northern India, major breeding takes place in September–October. An extended breeding season up to beginning January has been noticed in certain sheep flocks. Improved grazing conditions after rainy season and availability of crop residue facilitate a natural flushing. In temperate region the spring breeding is not much advocated for fear of lean grazing for young lambs and mother ewes during winters. In the southern region March–April breeding too yields equally good lambing percentage. In addition to primary autumn mating, the February–March breeding of sheep is also conducted at times in the western arid and semi-arid zone.

The sheepman is quite conscious in selecting a suitable breeding season for higher lambing, better survivability and growth of lambs. He is guided by the age-old experience in evaluating comparative merits of various mating seasons. Weightage to various parameters of successful lambing receive due consideration at his end. Some of the sheep breeders attempt to obtain 3 lambings in two years instead of one lambing in a year by exploiting the phenomenon of two breeding seasons in a year. Ram is run with the ewe flock in both the seasons and even round the year.

In smaller stationary flocks, ram is a regular component of flock and is hardly withdrawn. The lambing may also spread over a longer period. Number of receptive ewes in off breeding season is invariably less than 25%. Lambing received as a result of that is just 5 to 10%. This contributes towards marginally higher lambing rates in the stationary flocks than the migratory ones.

Sheepmen generally castrate the off type and inferior male lambs at an early age. Wethers are retained for fattening and sale at handsome price at a later period. The selected ram lambs are maintained separately as future breeding sires. Where sheep development schemes are operative, these ram lambs of the breeder may also be sold or exchanged away and a pedigreed sire replacement obtained. Properly managed rams are fit for breeding at one and a half-year age. Breeding performance is normally satisfactory till 6 to 7 year age.

Under the existing practices where the keeping of ram in the ewe flock in non-breeding season is considered imperative, the shepherd tries to tie an apron to body barrel anterior to prepuce. Ligation of prepucial sheath or tying of a forelimb used to be resorted by the shepherds to avoid untimely or illicit covering. Being cruelsome the practice is discouraged by the sheepmen now.

During breeding season, the selected rams are kept with the ewes' flock for 40 to 50 days so as to cover at least two heat cycles. One ram per 50 breedable ewes or so is allotted. For small and marginal farmer sheep units or under other State/ Centrally sponsored programmes, a provision of one ram for only 10 to 20 ewes is made.

Flock size

Sheep is hardly kept individually anywhere by the farmers. It is only on mixed farming and feed lot conditions or on reasons of ram fighting sport, fancy, ceremonial purposes, etc. that one comes across one or two sheep with a house hold.

Traditionally too, only flock rearing is considered a viable proposition. The size of flock may however vary depending on factors like manpower, shepherding expertise, feed and pasture resources, natural calamities, demand and supply and returns of marketing of sheep products, etc. The seasonal variations have bearing on the sheep holding. Size of the flock increases at lambing time and the number decreases before breeding when the sheep farmer disposes off the surplus or unfit animals. Conditions of disturbed environment may lead to distress disposal and fall in numbers. Mode of rearing also influences the flock strength.

There is dearth of range lands in India. Therefore big sheep properties do not exist. The flock size is gradually dwindling. Migratory flocks are invariably of bigger size. The range may be 50 to 500 sheep in various regions. Himachal Pradesh and Jammu and Kashmir states have

bestowed Bahak rights, i.e. grazing rights in highland pastures to the tribals. So a couple of families of a tribe move to a particular pasture jointly with their collective sheep holdings.

Semi-migratory flocks are usually of smaller size, varying from 20 to 200 sheep. Small farmers own lesser number. Two, three or even more sheep farmers collectively constitute a flock of 200 to 500 sheep or even bigger one. They pool their manpower while moving to a prospective pasture. This practice is quite popular in all the sheep rearing zones. Economy in shepherding and collective security are the prime advantages of pooling together. The Chopan system is another corollary of the semi-migratory pattern in Kashmir and elsewhere in temperate region. A chopan on the pattern of Raika community shepherd of Rajasthan collects the sheep of various households of a village and carries the same to the hilly meadows for summer months on terms of cash, wool or sheep as wages. The strength of individual villager's sheep may be just 10 to 20 only.

Stationary sheep rearing is predominantly a part of mixed farming in this country. A household may possess a small flock of five to ten sheep. A man of the family escorts these sheep to the common village grazing ground or nearby forest alongwith other livestock. The recent trend of developing viable sheep units has lead to raising of size from 30 to 50 sheep or more, thus affording a whole time job for a member of a family. In Deccan plateau particularly in Mandya and Hasssan sheep breed areas small flocks of 15 to 30 sheep are reared quite commonly. In plain belt of Punjab, Haryana, Jammu and parts of Gujarat the flock size increases even to 100 sheep or so.

Flock composition

The age and group wise make up of sheep flock is an important parameter to determine deterioration or progress of that flock. Higher number of healthy younger breedable sheep is a progressive sign. Composition depends on the lambing percentage, the survivability, and the pattern of selection, culling and disposals. A good breeder would like to retain as many fit breedable ewes as possible. In certain areas the ram lambs are sold just at hogget or yearling stage as observed in stationary flocks. Bakerwal sheep breeders castrate the male stock early and maintain as wethers or even as mature rams up to two year age or above. Disposal is made when they attain excellent fat condition in September–October after grazing in alpine pastures. To obtain extra crop out of old ewes, some breeders prefer to delay sale of old ewes, thus the number of female stock is high in those flocks at a particular point of time. Usually 2 to 3% selected ram lambs and 25 to 30% ewe lambs are retained as replacements.

The strength of male and female stock, young and adult ewes or that of breedable ewes and female hoggets also varies from season to season in a particular year. No hard and fast norms can be laid. Flock constitution as observed in general, over a number of progressive sheep holdings is presented in Table 5.3.

Tending (manpower) requirement

At various sheep farms in the country varying type of routines and flock operations are followed. Rearing systems differ so the labour requirements are also different. The duty hours are fixed in certain farms, and shepherds work on shift basis. In others a whole time work pattern exists, still in many other farms casual or part time engagement of manpower is resorted to.

Running of flocks on contract basis is also being tried. But out of all the systems, the traditional management (of whole time-shared responsibility) is considered satisfactory one. In this system one senior shepherd is made incharge and is assisted by two or more shepherds depending on the strength of flock. Besides the usual grazing, feeding, assistance in recording observations, upkeep and care of the flock is also vested in them. On an average one shepherd for 50 to 60 sheep is the criterion. Additional labour for lambing and flock breeding is provided when the number of sub-flocks increase.

In the private flocks one shepherd over 100 sheep is the tentative yardstick. Migrations, lambing, shearing and certain other flock operations increase the workload. Assistance of family members is often available. But that may not suffice all the time. At times expert shepherds are engaged or services hired/shared on mutual help basis.

Extent of engagement of tending persons in private flocks in India is in quite contrast to ranch flocks in Australia, New Zealand or USA. where just one or two persons look after a few thousand sheep in the paddocks assisted by shepherding dogs.

In Russia's commune sheep farms a sheepman is entrusted a flock of a thousand sheep or so. The size of the flock may reduce to even 200 heads. Family is often a source of extra labour as paid shepherds. Engagement of both male and female labour is a part of entire association of the family with the flock.

Table 5.3: Flock composition in two seasons

Sl. no.	Category of sheep	Period/Seasons	
		Post lambing (March-April) %	Post culling/ pre-breeding (Sept.-Oct.) %
1.	Breeding rams	1-2	2-4
2.	Adult ewes	40-45	45-50
3.	Maiden ewes and Female yearlings	12-15	8-10
4.	Young lambs	35-40	25-30
5.	Wether and male yearling	5-6	10-12

NEW PERCEPTIONS

At the advent of industrial revolution in Europe the invention of refrigeration facilitated the preservation and shipment of meat. The demand for the mutton and wool produced a global sheep boom in the early 20th century due to First World War. Sheep advanced countries like New Zealand and Australia took enterprising initiative and became the major source of lamb supply to Europe. International market for wool also improved.

This brought a realization in India as well about improved sheep production. Possible contribution of sheep in rural economy and upliftment of tribals began to be appreciated. A couple of dedicated sheepmen and veterinarians* took up the challenging task of sheep and wool development. Attention was primarily focussed on the improvement of poor producer local sheep germ plasm.

With the dawn of independence of the country the prevailing protracted approach and age old practices took a turn to a scientific thrust and introduction of scientific sheep breeding systems. New schemes were launched in various areas of the country. IVRI and ICAR played a vital role in the initial phase of sheep development. Scientific know-how and directions about better sheep health and breeding programme percolated down to the extension worker and even the sheep farmer, which led to a renewed awareness and interest in the profession of sheep rearing, soon after independence of the country.

---

* Rai Bahadur (Dr) P.N. Nanda, former Dir. Pb and A.H. Comm. to GOI; Dr. H.K. Lall (UP); Dr. D.N. Kaul (J&K); Dr. N.L. Narayana (Rajasthan); Dr. Gurbax Singh Mahal (Pb); Dr. V.Krishna Rao (AP); Mr. S.S. Khot (Maharashtra); Padam Shri Dr. G.A. Bandey (J&K); Dr. C. Krishna Rao (Former A.H. Comm. GOI); Dr. A. Ramamurthy (TN); Dr. K.C. Nayyar (HP); Dr. Guru Dutt (Pb); Dr. P. Bhattacharya (ICAR); Dr Ganeshan Kale (TN); Dr Krishnama Charulu (AP) and a galaxy of scientists of IVRI and other institutions of various states.

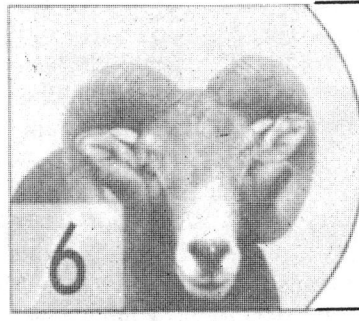

PRODUCTION SYSTEMS AND PASTURAGE

SHEEP SUSTENANCE

In addition to scientific breeding, proper housing and health cover the feeding management of livestock is of great importance. Inadequate nutrition is one of the main factors responsible for slow growth, low production, disease susceptibility and higher mortality in sheep in prenatal as well as postnatal stages. Poor condition of pastures, disturbed ecosystem, poverty of sheep farmers and ignorance about modern practices have all contributed to improper feeding of these animals.

The feed requirements of high yielding cattle and buffaloes are generally met through stall-feeding. Most of the cultivated fodder, dry fodder of meadows and available grain feeds are diverted for these dairy animals. Therefore, excepting pasturage little is left with the farmer to feed his sheep. The tremendous increase in human population has further resulted in feed and space resource competition with animals. The livestock number too has gradually increased over the years and made the forage situation complex and strained among various species of domestic animals (Table 6.1).

The sheep sustenance source, the grazing area, is fast shrinking. Permanent pasture and other grazing land in India was around 11.93 lac hectares and area under fodder crops was 7.94 lac hectares during 1984-85. These are estimated to have shown a decline to 11.84 lac and 6.82 lac hectares respectively by 1987-88. The density of livestock per unit of pasture has greatly increased. Consequently the share of forage availability per head has fallen appreciably in certain areas. The resultant non-availability of forage has in certain cases, made the livestock and its owners to migrate to neighbouring areas and states in search of feed.

LAND USE PATTERN

The land use pattern figures for 1975-76 (released by the Ministry of Agriculture and Coop., Goverment of India) are:

Table 6.1: Population of domestic ruminants in India

Sl.no	Type of livestock	Population (million)			
		1982	1987	1992	1997
1.	Cattle	192.45	197.70	205.43	209.08
2.	Buffaloes	67.78	73.90	84.49	92.19
3.	Goats	95.25	101.79	115.28	120.60
4.	Sheep	48.76	49.90	50.81	56.47

Source: (1) Livestock Census reports; (2) Statistical Abstract India (1997); and (3) Indian Agriculture-IEDRC (1999).

Total geographical area	3,287.78 thousand sq. km
Cropped area out of above	52%
Forests	20.2%
Permanent pastures	3.8%
Cultivable waste land	5.3%
Fallow land	6.7%
Miscellaneous under trees and groves	1.2%

After excluding forest areas the availability of land for grazing is left to the extent of 17% only. This is further squeezing due to extension of agronomic activities and irrigation, habitation and colonization, industrialization and creation of communication network, etc.

Arid and semi-arid areas of the country have the bulk of sheep population. The extent of arid areas is 3.2 lac sq. km of hot desert of Rajasthan, Gujarat, Haryana and parts of Southern Peninsula and 0.7 lac sq. km of cold desert of Ladakh which together constitute almost 11.8% of the area (Patnayak and Singh, 1985).

The semi arid area is 9.86 lac sq. km (about 29.6%) spread over various states, viz.

1.	Maharashtra	19%
2.	Karnataka	15%
3.	Andhra Pradesh	15%
4.	Rajasthan	13%
5.	Tamil Nadu	10%
6.	Gujarat	9%
7.	UP	7%
8.	MP	0.6%
9.	Punjab and Haryana	3%

The availability of grazing land in the temperate zone states of Jammu and Kashmir, Himachal Pradesh, Uttaranchal, Sikkim and Arunachal Pradesh too is precarious, notwithstanding the vast stretch of alpine pastures in the Himalayan ranges (Table 6.2).

The Shivaliks, Pir Panjal, the inner Himalayas and ranges in Central and Western India have suffered deforestation, unprecedented pasture reclamations for crop husbandry, denudation and ecological degradation. Creation of large scale closures, sanctuaries and wild life parks have further curtailed the movement of pastoral flocks. Unscrupulous exploitation of alpine pastures and corals is discernible. The vegetative destruction ensuing there from can hardly make the sheep to have a mouthful fodder. On a low and deficient plane of nutrition from the pasture, the sheep production per head is not expected to improve.

The recent attempts to develop drought prone areas and waste land with improved types of grasses, legumes, fodder trees and shrubs for increasing their carrying capacity is expected to provide some relief, yet the fodder shortage of 36 percent existing in eighties of last century in the country is predicted to rise to 41 percent by the beginning of current century.

FORAGE AVAILABILITY

The availability of forage for sheep varies from zone to zone, area to area and season to season. Acharya (1982) has enlisted the various types of grasses, edible shrubs and fodder trees existing in different regions (see Table 6.3).

Temperate zone

Winter pasture

In Uttaranchal, Himachal Pradesh and Jammu and Kashmir, the migratory sheep either stay around

Table 6.2: Extent of grazing area availability in various regions (Acharya 1982)

Sl.No.	Region	Natural grazing area (m.hec)
1.	North temperate region	7.68
2.	Eastern region	30.48
3.	Southern Paninsular region	34.90
4.	Northwestern Arid and semi-arid region	45.63

Table 6.3: Livestock population (1992) and forage resource position (1987-88)

Sl. No.	States/U.Ts	Total livestock (000)	Sheep population (000)	Permanent pastures and other grazing lands (000 hec.)	Area under crops (000 hec.)	Fodder seed production farms
1.	Andhra Pradesh	32911	7787	881	133	4
2.	Arunachal Pradesh	842	30	–	–	2
3.	Assam	16062	150	184	3	1
4.	Bihar	47930	1690	137	12	4
5.	Goa	243	–	1	–	4
6.	Gujarat	18598	2027	846	857	3
7.	Haryana	9143	1044	30	510	1
8.	Himachal Pradesh	5106	1079	1216	8	3
9.	Jammu and Kashmir	8703	2947	125	34	3
10.	Karnataka	29568	5432	1135	78	17
11.	Kerala	5834	29	3	2	2
12.	Madhya Pradesh	46744	836	2790	878	4
13.	Maharashtra	36404	3074	1381	810	1
14.	Manipur	1290	14	–	–	1
15.	Meghalaya	1182	23	17	–	3
16.	Mizoram	203	01	4	–	1
17.	Nagaland	1074	03	–	–	2
18.	Orissa	22742	1840	711	–	4
19.	Punjab	10222	526	4	924	3
20.	Rajasthan	48441	12497	1817	1438	5
21.	Sikkim	385	16	69	–	7
22.	Tamil Nadu	25007	5849	134	200	8
23.	Tripura	1591	05	–	–	3
24.	Uttar Pradesh + Uttaranchal	64799	2404	349	923	13
25.	West Bengal	35090	1490	7	3	12

Source: Live stock Census Reports; Malik C.L. (1990); Directorate of Economics and Statistics, Min. of Agri. (G.O.I.).

Shivaliks or in adjacent plains during winters. Stationary ones are housed on a semi-intensive pattern. Forage in the former case comprise of:

1. A variety of grasses ranging from poor quality *Heteropogan, Themeda, Aristida* to medium quality *Iseilema* and good quality *Cyanodon, Bothriochloa, Dicanthium, Sehima, Trifolium* species and other local medics.

2. Bush-bramble browsing, consisting of *Carissa spinarum* (Garna) *Adhatoda vasaka* (Brahkar, Basuti) *Zizyphus* (Jharberi), *Morraya* (Drankdu, Curry patta), *Cassia* species (Hadwan), etc.

3. A variety of creepers and wild vetches.

4. Top feeding of tree leaves particularly that of *Grevia sps.* (Dhaman), *Albezia sps.* (Siris, Sareen), *Leucaenia* leucocephala (Su-Babul), Sesbenia (Cu-Babul), *Zizyphus sps.* (Ber), *Acacia sps.* (Kikar, Phalai, Kher varieties), *Olea sps.* (Olive, Kohu), *Azadirachta sps.* (Neem), *Morus alba* (Mulberry Toot), *Bauhinia* (Kachnar), etc.

5. Crop stubbles and farm residues.

6. Unusual plants, viz. weeds like *Lantana, Parthenium, etc.* in varying quantities.

7. Cultivated fodders and grasses, viz., Berseem, Barley, Oats, Lucerne, Cenchrus, etc.

Besides the availability of some of the above fodder, the stationary or indoor confined sheep of the colder region derive their forage from:

1. Preserved *Chrysopogon, Narcissus* (Kahe-Krisham, Iris) and clover hay.
2. *Salix* (willow, bisa), *Ulmus* (elm, bren) and *Rubinea* (hilly kikar) tree leaves.
3. Still in extreme winter conditions of Ladakh and Lahaul-Spiti Artemisia plants and local *Lucerene* (oal) hay, etc. are the main fodder source for the prolonged winter housed sheep.

Summer pastures

In the lower ranges *Cyanodon* (Khabbal-Dub, Bermuda grass), *Chrysopogan, Bothriochloa,* wild ferns, vetches, Trifolium and local Medicago varieties provide grazing. Browsing on shrubs and top feeding of *Rubinea, Quercus* and wild Rhododendron trees is also available. However, during migrations the sheep hardly get maintenance fodder on the transit routes. The quality of forage is of no consideration and main concern of the shepherd is to arrange grazing or fodder for the flock. The movement is solely at the cost of body reserves of the animal. Some zealous and feed conscious sheepmen on the other hand arrange grazing area from a private or government owned sources even on exorbitant price.

On arrival in the sub-alpine and then alpine ranges of the Himalayas, these sheep have access to rich pastures growing *Poa, Festuca, Bothriochloa, Lolium, Dactylis* species and a variety of clovers of excellent nutritional value, containing 12 percent or more protein. Since crude protein and crude fibre ratios are quite favourable in the mixture of these grasses, the intake is less and rapid body weight gains are attained in limited hours of grazing in the limited period of alpine stay.

North western arid zone

This forms the vast stretch of sheep rearing in India. The number of sheep is commensurately quite large as compared to other regions and the population is steadily on the increase. The natural pastures are in a degraded state due to over grazing, erratic rains, burning and erosion. Grazing areas in this drought prone region are in bad shape. Pasture vegetation consist mostly of poor quality grasses like *Heteropogon, Themeda, Aristida,* etc. A sparse cover of legumes also exists in certain tracts. Availability of forage is hardly sufficient for 3 months in a year. For the remaining part the average carrying capacity of the poor rangelands of the arid region is only 2 to 3 sheep per hectare. Even though the pasture contains almost 15 percent crude protein in some instances, the energy supply from the pasture is very low to promote weight gain. Better grasslands of arid region consist of *Dichanthium, Cenchrus, Lasiurus* species. On the sown pastures of *Cenchrus ciliaris, C. settigerus* and *Penicum antidotale,* the capacity improves up to 8 sheep per hectare. Proper protection of pastures through fencing and controlled grazing practices at Central Arid Zone Research Institute Jodhpur improved forage yield of poor, fair and good rangelands by 148, 92 and 116 percent respectively.

Most of the grasslands are deficient in nitrogen and phosphorus. Application of 40 kg N_2 + 20 kg P_2O_5 per hectare increased yield and protein of the sown grass species of *Cenchrus* and *Sehima.* The high costs of nitrogen fertilizers is curtailed through introduction of legumes like *Delichos, Stylosanthus, Siratro, Atylosia, Clitoria,* etc. These legumes are a good nitrogen source to range lands also. The natural legumes of these pastures are *Rhyncosia, Indigofera* and *Tribulus.*

Fodder tree leaves are an important source of nutritious forage for sheep in the arid and semi-arid region. *Zizyphus numularia* (beri) leaves are preserved in dry state (Pala) in Rajasthan, Gujarat, Haryana and Madhya Pradesh for winter feeding of sheep and lambs. *Prosopis cinararia* (Khejri) *Ailanthus excelsa* (Ardu), *Albezzia* species (Siras), etc. are some invaluable top feeding source. Loppings are also available from fodder trees like: *Gymnosporia spinosa* (Kandera); *Acacia species* (Babool); *Bauhinia variegata* (Kachnar); *Su-*

Babool (Agasti); *Zizyphus mauritiana ingadulcis* (Ber); *Colophospermum mopane* (Mopane); *Azadirachta sps.* (Neem), etc.

The crude protein, dry matter and crude fibre in various tree leaves of this zone ranges from 9 to 20 percent, 20 to 40 percent and 7 to 27 percent respectively. Land use pattern reveals that permanent pastures in these tracts is just about 1 percent, thus negligible.

Gangetic plains

The extent of fallow and cultivable wasteland is more in Bihar because of coal fields and undulating hilly terrain. The scope of maintaining flock on extensive system of grazing are least. Weather is hot and humid and rainfall around 100 cm. This holds true for eastern districts of Uttar Pradesh and parts of Orissa and West Bengal adjoining Bihar.

Only tall and coarse grasses grow, which are not suitable for sheep. These are less nutritious. Sheep and goat can graze on their stubbles only, left after cutting. Sheep population as such is too less in the Gangetic belt of UP, Bihar, West Bengal and even in northern Orissa. Position of forage availability and sheep population in the north eastern states is identical except Arunachal Pradesh and Sikkim. Hilly terrains of the latter states have a cover of good quality grasses, which can support a sizeable sheep population.

Southern peninsular and coastal areas

In the southern peninsular region of Maharashtra, Karnataka, Andhra Pradesh and Tamil Nadu bountiful surface grazing and even shrub browsing is available in many parts. *Cyanodon* (Dub), *Chrysopogon, Dicanthium, Penicum, Ischaemum, Andropogon, Themeda, Aristida, Saccharum* species of good to inferior grasses are a few to be found in the pastures mixed with medium types. Many of the tropical grasses grow in the natural pastures. The nutritive value of these grasses varies widely with season and advancement of maturity. Early grazing provides required nutrition. But in late stage high fibre content and crude protein deficiency result in lowering of nutritive value.

Such poor pastures hardly provide maintenance to sheep. Some of the established pastures in the drought prone areas and fodder belts have *Cenchrus* species and legumes like cowpeas, field beans *Stylo, Siratro* or *Atylosia* species. In the Bannur breed area of Malavalli Taluka, horse gram (Kulthi) cultivation is a valuable source of fodder and grain ration for sheep.

This region is next to the north western arid zone in sheep strength. Due to availability of grazing around the villages, the flocks are stationary. They invariably remain within the district. Less than 20 percent sheep undertake short distance migration. Uncultivated fields, farm back yards, village kahcharai, forest lands and road side grazing help in maintenance of sheep. Crop residues and stubbles are utilized to the best advantage. Groundnut or horse gram husk is at times used to supplement feeding in late pregnancy and post lambing.

In the coastal belt there is high rainfall and tall grasses grow. The high humidity and temperature are unfavourable for sheep. As a result of hostile environment and varied land use pattern, sheep concentration is negligible along the eastern and western coasts and in Kerala.

REARING MANAGEMENT

Sheep ranching is least practised in India. Land and pasture holdings are small with individual farmer. The tribals or nomads who mostly rear sheep are invariably landless or have limited land resources. The usual tendency is to not invest anything on the development of pasture holding belonging to others. The investments made if any by the sheepman to augment feed resources makes his rearing profession quite uneconomical. Under migratory rearing the flocks spend most of the time of the year in to and fro movement between the two distantly located summer and winter pastures. Majority of flocks in the temperate region and a sizeable sheep population of the northwestern arid zone undertake long migrations.

Partial migratory rearing is prevalent in hills where tribals and farmers have their hearth and homes and own their land and grazing area. For a short period during summers their sheep move to nearby pastures where grazing and water availability is assured one. The distance of up and down movement is not long. Generally the two pastures are within the same district or in the adjoining districts.

Stationary flocks rearing is lesser practised in temperate zone but predominantly followed in western and southern regions of the country. Owners possess limited sheep strength only. A suitable sheep germ plasm which is adapted to the regions of high summer temperatures, humidity and scarcity of foliage and water is the main factor for successful sedentary sheep rearing. In the states like Punjab, Haryana and eastern Rajasthan where round the year fodder availability exist, this system finds favour. In Karnataka, Andhra Pradesh and parts of Maharashtra where beside assured grazing, acclimatized indigenous sheep germ plasm exists the stationary sheep rearing is doing fairly well.

Production pattern

Within aforesaid systems production pattern may be:

Subsistence type: The subsistence rearing is maintaining the animals on grazing/browsing or stall feeding or both. The practices may be followed according to the circumstances and feed fodder resource availability with the farmers.

Extensive type: The extensive rearing method involves a minimum amount of labour and expenses. The grazing of sheep is resorted to in the village common lands, i.e. gochars or shamlats, ravines, vacant road or canal side strips, uneven waste lands and non-agricultural lands, etc. for maximum number of hours.

Intensive type: In the intensive rearing there is no chance for grazing. The animals are completely stall fed. Shelter is essential for maintenance purposes. Though protection of animals from weather vagaries and deleterious effects of pastures vegetation is ensured, this system has least applicability in sheep and is suitable for dairy goat production only.

Semi-Intensive: Pattern is a combination of extensive management and zero grazing. It involves controlled grazing in fenced or reserved pastures alongwith supplementary ration feeding. It is practiced when sufficient grazing or browsing is not available. Top feeding is quite relevant under semi-intensive rearing. Feed lot sheep farming in Punjab, Haryana and plain belt of Jammu and Kashmir and rearing at most of the sheep farms in this country is on this very pattern.

GRAZING MANAGEMENT OF PASTURE LANDS

Grass cover is the best soil binder. Open soils bereft of surface cover of grass, creepers and shrubs are more prone to erosion. The one with a tree canopy having a cover of trees, shrubs and grasses are less exposed to soil leaching and serves the livestock better. The grasslands with a better utility for livestock have thus a better status of soil conservation. There is realization now, of not interfering with the life cycle of annual species and growth of perennial one's in the pasturelands so as to allow ample chance for seed maturation and dispersal. Controlling the number of animals grazing per unit of pastureland, i.e. controlled grazing with respect to number and grazing time is important. Exceeding the carrying capacity of the grazing area is to expose the same to overgrazing and depletion of natural flora. Various grazing systems followed are:

Rotational grazing: This is a system where pasture lands by compartmentalization are provided alternating period of grazing and rest. The extensive pastures are divided into paddocks through fencing. The sheep flocks are let loose there by turns and withdrawn. The rest period provides for fertilization, irrigation and regeneration in the cropped paddocks. In natural pastures, during off grazing season, the seed formation and dispersal helps in the continuity of flush growth. Such a system is commonly practiced in Australia, New Zealand, USA, UK and some other sheep advanced countries. The limitation of vastness of pastures in India *vis a vis* the livestock population do not afford rotational practices of grazing, but for at some well organised farms.

Strip grazing: It is a type of controlled grazing, where movement is restricted within a paddock through electric fence. This improves utilization of pasture and prevents selective grazing.

Creep grazing: Like creep feeding in the sheds, provision is made in the fenced paddocks for the lambs to move ahead of the ewes in an effort that the lambs get fresh grazing on a flush growth. The chances of lamb growth acceleration on such a system are much better.

Deferred grazing: Instead of paddock maintenance it is generally the common or reserved pasture that is allowed for livestock. The system is to delay or defer grazing till seed maturity and permit sufficient growth and content of foliage. This is in fact what a forester, ecologist or a sheepman prefers, i.e. to take care of seed formation and avoid elimination of valuable grass species.

Alpine pasture is getting grazed as soon as grasses sprout soon after snow melting. The seed formation stage is rarely approached. This evidently results into sparseness and depletion of pasture flora. Attention is therefore needed to delay entry of livestock by a month or so in certain portions of the pasture for protection, growth and vigour attainment of plants and possible seed formation. The only disadvantage of delayed entry of flocks is the problem of prolonged retention of animals in the lower ranges and lowered palatability of forage of deferred areas, approaching maturity. Deferred grazing poses a similar situation in other regions also during bumper growth in monsoon period. The delayed entry of sheep helps in the maturation of seed.

Altnernate grazing: To provide rest to the pasture it is left ungrazed in a season or a year. On one hand it helps in the recovery of dying varieties of grass and herbage and on the other regeneration is facilitated. However, in a well-grown pasture

incidents of fire take place. To avoid the same, grazing restrictions and cooperation of sheepmen, and vigil by all concerned is essential.

Differing stocking intensity system: The forage status of pasture varies from time to time in a year. The seasonal condition of pastures determines the stocking rate. The flock may be maintained over the area, but when the growth is luxuriant as in monsoon, the stocking rate may be higher. The number is however brought down at times of low growth of vegetation, or as soon as drought or scarcity conditions appear.

Regulated flock movement*: It is a unique grazing method practiced by traditional and experienced Gaddie shepherds. While sitting at one corner the shepherd makes the flock to move in a circumscribed unfenced patch of a bushy pasture by the sound of whistle only. There is no impinging upon the adjacent pasture area. The hush-hush movement of the flock is avoided. The system is helpful in providing fair grazing opportunities to healthy and weak, adult and young animals alike. Once the foliage is consumed the flock is moved on to the next area.

Cut and carry system: No entry of stock in the pasture is allowed. The forage, i.e. grasses, bushes, leaves, etc. are cut and carried for feeding to livestock. Under the social forestry scheme, this method is advocated to avoid animal interference with the closures. The system though good for the pastures under forestation, is suitable for dairy cattle, dairy goat or feed-lot sheep but runs counter to natural grazing instinct and economic rearing of a larger flock.

Controlled grazing: What ever system of grazing may be adopted, the application of scientific criteria of optimum grazing, carrying capacity and rest to pasture, the periodicity of grazing in a particular area (which constitute controlled grazing) is the right approach for the health of pasture. Controlled grazing keeps the pasture as perpetual source of nutrition. While assessing the farm strength, i.e. the livestock

---

* Dealt as 'Dakwan Charai' in the earlier chapter.

number to be maintained and farm economy, the carrying capacity of its pastures under controlled grazing system is the surest way of avoiding bad effects of grazing on the pasture vegetation.

PASTURE EVALUATION AND CARRYING CAPACITY

Sheep and goat can thrive well on the available natural forage alone, i.e. grasses, edible creepers, shrubs, fodder tree leaves and weeds, etc. existing in the usual pastures. Much attention in India has not been paid to nutritional components and the evaluation of pastures. The important aspect of correct assessment of the quantity and quality of the pasturage consumed by these animals is over looked. Their nutritional requirements are met by a wide variety of pasture vegetation. It is invariably difficult to obtain a representative sample of the type of forage consumed.

The heterogeneity of the vegetative intake is influenced by the period of year, season, rainfall, nature of flora, terrain, number and category of livestock stocked in the pasture, etc. Early stages of growth, mature condition of grasses or even the draught situation influence the composition of the pasture and consequently the sheep pick.

Where extensive system is practised in the village common lands and grazing for maximum hours is allowed, a carrying capacity of 8 to 10 sheep/hectare is possible. Under semi-intensive management conditions where adequate supplementary ration feeding is provided for, even 10 to 15 sheep are accommodated. In semi-arid region the natural pastures may carry 2 to 3 sheep per hectare. A gradual gain from October to November and in January-February may be noticeable.

The average grazing capacity of reserve pastures (adaaks) is generally around 6 to 7 sheep/hectare on the basis of 70% utilization. On the poor grassland which need improvement, the grazing capacity for maintenance purposes is suggested as 2 to 5 sheep/hectare per year by Dabadghao (1959). However, in the migratory rearing pattern and under three tier silvi-pastoral foliage

conditions, the reasonable carrying capacity is around 8 sheep/hec. In the degraded state of Kandi-Krewas and Shivalik pastures or in the semi-arid region a stocking rate of more than 3 to 5 sheep/hectare is not permissible.

Composition and nature of available fodder from the pasture helps to determine the carrying capacity and the type of livestock it can sustain preferentially. This aspect is of importance from intake and digestibility basis. A good grass cover is suitable for sheep and cattle. Presence of edible bushes is liked by the goat and even sheep. A combination of these with tree loppings and fodder crops is useful for the livestock in general. The existence of weeds renders it partly unfit for animals other than the small ruminants.

INGREDIENTS OF RATIONAL SHEEP GRAZING POLICY

Sheep and goat are selective in their grazing and browsing. In cut and carry system the animals do not have any choice of selection. One has, therefore, to be more careful in feeding these animals than the usual practice adopted in large animal rearing. A good pasture is all that sheep needs.

Three tier silvipastoral system of vegetation, i.e. surface cover of grasses, a lower canopy of edible bushes and shrubs and higher one of fodder trees is an ideal situation. Medium to good quality grasses are relished. Coarser and poor quality grasses are a last resort. Edible bushes are too valuable. These provide almost 2 to 3 times more forage matter than the grassy area matching their canopy. The bush and tree loppings are a good source of vital nutrients. Their fodder leaves are not so vulnerable to wither under drought conditions and serve the best during lean periods.

Complete reliance on top feed source like Leucaena and Sesbenia can be harmful. Due to presence of 'Mimosine' the prolonged and ad-lib feeding of such like tree leaves is known to cause loss of fleece, abortions, infertility, itching, fall in milk secretion, etc. An intake of 25 to 30 percent of such leaves of the total forage at some sheep farms in Jammu and Kashmir was observed to develop shedding of wool.

In seasonal fodder scarcity areas or where the quality of forage is inferior, the fortification of grasses with leguminous fodder crops, urea, etc. and with molasses improves acceptability, palatability and nutritive value of poor quality fodder. Such chaffed, treated and ensilaged forage material can be fed up to 2 kg per 50 kg body weight for providing proper roughage.

Policy approach: Concerted and permanent measures for pasture improvement and forage production are called for. It should lay a simultaneous emphasis on conservation, propagation and regeneration of indigenous varieties of grasses and top feeding plantation. Faulty grazing and mismanagement of grass lands has to be avoided. Exploitation of pasture vegetation for fuel, hedge, charcoal preparation, etc. and overgrazing are responsible for denudation and damage to surface cover and existing flora. Scientific research backup and proper grazing methodology need priority attention.

Emphasis is also needed to develop degraded range lands and marginal lands, not suitable for crop production, into pastures. Indiscriminate crop cultivation on steeper slopes, reclamation and noutods of hilly pastures of 25–30° or above gradient has resulted into soil erosion and serious damage to grazing potential.

Least interference with the life history and seed production of pasture flora is essential. This implies controlled grazing, i.e. fixation of number of animals of a particular species with due consideration to season, period of grazing and carrying capacity of the grazing area. Controlled grazing on protected reserved range lands is the best method of utilizing the natural range lands.

To sum up, the conservation of natural flora of pastures, reseeding, avoiding overgrazing, practising controlled and delayed rotational grazing, introducing better quality perennial grasses, encouraging suitable three tier pasture forage resources and augmenting fodder cultivation constitute the elements of a rational grazing and forage development strategy. The education of graziers, their involvement and cooperation in the pasture and fodder resource related problems is of great importance. This in turn demands an integrated approach and coordinated effort of the involved agencies. In depth study and research on the much neglected edible forages and to develop better varieties for sheep consumption need priority attention. Further damage to edible natural flora and their extinction has to be checked. Nutritive evaluation of pastures of various zones is required.

EXTRANEOUS PASTURE FLORA

Pasturelands in India, have two types of extraneous vegetation, the toxic plants and the burr weeds. The former is consumed by the sheep under fodder scarcity and drought conditions resulting into adverse effects and even fatal poisoning at times. The latter category is of some of the weeds that produce bristly or hooked burrs. When the sheep move about for grazing in the weed prevalent pastures, the burrs get attached to the fleece coat causing discomfort to the animal and the handler. Occasionally damage to vital organs and even deaths are caused by them by piercing the skin and then the vital organs. Burry wools fetch low price. Common poisonous and burr plants in pasture lands are:

1. Lantana camara: (Punj phulli, Bara phulnoo, Ramphool)

This is a shrub of medium height, growing up to 2 to 3 meters at times. The flowers are of at least five different coloration. English people introduced it in this country as a hedge and ornamental plant around 1942. Now it is found in almost all the regions and at elevation up to 1000 m. The Shivaliks have a profuse cover of Lantana. The grazing and all barren lands have been usurped by this plant in many parts of the country. This weed is poisonous for the livestock, particularly the young cattle, sheep and goats. The active toxicant is lantadane-A. It causes hepatic damage and interference in the secretion of bile (Raina and Raina, 1997), leading to impeding of bile flow and severe constipation.

The bile stasis and engorgement produce jaundice, photosensitization like conditions, toxaemia and eventual death. The young ones, which are not used to such vegetation, suffer severely, death rate varying from 70 to 80 percent. In adults, however, the effects of intake are not so fatal. New stock entry into lantana infested pastures is always risk prone.

The adult goats and local sheep are casually consuming the leafy growth. The after effects are not favourable. There is sudden fall in milk production in lactating ones. The suckling young ones of lantana consuming mothers show unthriftiness, depraved appetite and anaemia. Varying type of treatment like glucose saline or Cal. gluconate infusion, anti-histaminics and liver correctives and laxatives are tried. The flock owners generally practice citrus fruit juice drenching. Water milk or milk whey are considered good fluids for GI tract and as calcium supplements in Lantana poisoning. In untreated cases of poisoning death may ensue in a couple of hours to 2 to 3 days. Recovered animals show prolonged weakness, drying, peeling and scarification of skin and shedding of wool. The spread of weed in fields and pasturelands has resulted into tremendous loss to grazing and fodder availability.

Control: The plants find use as poor man's fire wood, for charcoal preparation, as hedge material and for lawn decoration. Further utility of it as raw material in paper industry, light furniture and insect repellent have all made it to sustain and grow profusely in certain areas. The weedicides used so far have not been successful in enmass eradication. Biological controls being tried at various institutions have yielded partial results. The use of an insect/beetle in Almora region in Uttaranchal to control this obnoxious plant has proved quite successful. The other plausible eradication measure appears manual removal, though uprooting also involves lot of labour and soil disturbance due to deep rooted nature of the plant.

2. *Ipomoea carnea*: Commonly known as Akk locally, is being used in the countryside in India as a popular hedge plant. The wide spread growth in barren areas, fields, pastures and road side strips has led to its becoming another menace for agriculture and pasturing. The dried twigs are used as cheap firewood by the rural poor and labour classes.

The unaccustomed and yearling sheep at various stations and even the imported sheep were found to consume the leaves of Ipomoea voraciously leading to a typical type of addiction. Such animals subsequently did not relish any other fodder or feed and craved only for the Ipomoea plant, leaves. Strangely the sheep and goat affected with Ipomoea poisoning when kept in an open area having varied good quality fodders opted only for the leaves of Ipomoea. At occasions even forced starvation of addict sheep did not alter this tendency.

Toxicity: The ingestion of this plant is reported to result in salivation, diarrhoea, weakness, anaemia, staring eyes, lack of interest in surroundings, aloofness, anorexia, staggering gait, incoordination and subsequent paralysis and death. Patnayak and Singh (1972) and Christopher (1990) found that the plant toxins cause haemolysis of RBCs of sheep and degeneration of liver and central nervous system. On postmortem, general oedema, pale spots in the liver and cerebral changes are observed. Akk poisoning or addiction is rarely a flock problem as only individual animals may take up eating of Ipomoea leaves under drought or starved conditions. In a lone instance however, six out of fourteen imported Rambouillet stud rams stationed at Chingus (Rajouri, J&K) developed marked Ipomoea poisoning in 1987 winters. Recovery ensued on shifting and prolonged treatment. Control or eradication of the weed has hardly been attempted anywhere.

Treatment of affected cases consists of:

- Clearing the GI Tract with saline purgatives.
- Restricting movement of the animal to areas having accessible leafy growth of this plant.
- Atropine sulphate i/m or s/c @ 0.25 mg/kg body weight TID.
- Glucose, normal saline parenteral administration.

☞ Liver extracts, other liver protectives and correctives, tonics and vitamin preparations if administered, may also help.

3. Ageratum connyzoides: Nillijari, Nilphulia, Chhota phulnoo.

Like many other weeds this plant has found its entry in India alongwith the imported food grains. The deep green leaves with sky blue flowers make it another beautiful ornamental plant. Profuse flowering and light nature of seed help fast dispersal and spread to cultivable fields, damp lands and even shady areas and avenues. It invades and over powers the indigenous grass cover and other surface growth of the pastures with which it grows in close association and proximity. Nilphulia weed grows up to 800 m (MSL) altitude.

Toxicity: It is equally fatal to the young sheep and goat that forage on the weed. The animal may remain ill and dull, off feed for a day or two before collapsing.

Eradication: Some weedicides are reported effective but the subsequent damage to indigenous vegetation makes their use with utmost caution. Twice flowering seen in certain areas poses another problem for manual picking. The areas where uprooting was accomplished completely in one season, developed a fresh bumper growth in the next season.

4. Parthenium hystero-phorus: Known as 'Congress grass, China weed, Pandhari phool, or carrot grass in many parts of the country and 'safed phulli' by the tribals. It is yet another obnoxious weed imported with food grains from American continent in late fifties. After appearance in Maharashtra, Karnataka and some other states, this weed has spread like a wild fire to other regions. Rarely has any weed established itself so menacingly in the cultivated lands, pastures, vacant plots, roadside strips, railway tracks, residential premises or even roof tops as Parthenium. Seed germination and plant growth start in early spring even under dry conditions. Second flush and flower bearing occurs in May-June, followed by third one in August-September. Flowering is terminal but profuse. Seed is too light and fluffy. Leaves are highly, incised like that of carrot, hence called as 'carrot grass'. The Parthenium shrub is 1 to 1½ metre in height and well branched.

Toxicity: It is an environmental as well as health hazard. Flowers, leaves and other parts cause severe irritation of mucosa and dermatitis. Allergic reaction in human being is visible on the face, lips, around eyes, etc. within minutes of handling or touching a plant. Sheep frequently move about in the thick stand of this weed. The adult animals develop a mild reaction but in young lambs and kids the allergy may be well pronounced. Scratching of face, swelling of face, lips, ears, eyelids, reddening and ulceration of commissures or rashes over the bare skin areas are often seen. Eczema like condition develops at times. Coughing and bronchial asthma like problems as observed in human beings also appear in tender animals, terminating fatally in certain lambs.

Parthenium browsing: Adult sheep and goats do consume the plant especially in October-November. The extent of this unusual browsing is up to one-fourth of total daily intake and depends on the availability of normal forage in the pasture. Better the forage availability, lesser the consumption of weed.

Control and Biological effects: Pasture after pasture has been depleted of grazing by this weed due to partial or complete suppression of growth of pastoral herbage. Contrary to this the remarkable feature is the reduction of Nagoora burr (*Xanthium strumarium*) in the parthenium infested pastures. Bumper parthenium growth takes place in early monsoons forming a canopy. The tough Nagoora seeds germinate later. But once the seedling comes up, it degenerates under the compact canopy of parthenium, failing to receive sunlight. The jojra burr which once appeared invincible to control has been eradicated naturally to almost 50 to 60 percent in weed competition and subjugation by parthenium.

Following control measures are advised.

Mechanical:

1. Manual uprooting before flowering. Use of hand gloves and masks is essential. Mass

participation of all the involved agencies is desirable in the eradication programme.

2. Cutting before flowering, stacking and burning.

3. Suppression through ploughing, hoeing, smothering, flooding or turning of the land soil, etc.

Chemical: Various weedicides have been tried at Karnataka Agricuture University, Bangalore, and PAU, Ludhiana, including Atrazine spray at 1–1½ kg per acre in 200–250 litres of water before flowering. But the use of all such herbicides has to be viewed with caution on account of anticipated damage to useful grasses and fear of residual effect of repeated use in the soil.

Biological: So far effective biological control measures are not much practiced. Pine tree plantations along the roads are reported to reduce weed growth. Competitive fodders and grasses also contain the spread and growth of parthenium. Many plant pathogens are considered as potential and cost effective means of weed control. A beetle, *Zygograma bicolorata* introduced recently in the weed infested pastures has proved partially successful in localised eradication (Sharma, 2003). No myco-herbicide fungus has so far been found suitable for this weed.

An instance of natural control based on field observations, is cited here. Cassia spp. (Hedwan) once usurped the inner Shivalik pastures. Severe Gastro-intestinal and hepatic disorders usually ensued in sheep on consumption in November-December. The spread of *Xanthium strumarium* (Nagoora/Jojra) from 1950 onwards gradually suppressed the growth of Cassia spp. The incidence of toxicity by eating of such plant by sheep has gradually come down, but Nagoora burr then fast emerged as a most vexing problem for sheep and their owners during seventies and eighties of 20th century. The spread of parthenium has overtaken the former burr/weed with the passage of time, thereby lessened burry wool production in early nineties. Parthenium weed now reigns supreme in all corners. A competition among the flora for survival further reveals that *Cannabis indica* (Bhang) growth subdues the flush of carrot grass in the main growth period of rainy

season. Where parthenium existed in abundance in previous years and cannabis got introduced advertently or inadvertently, only the latter had a luxuriant growth and parthenium almost got eliminated in turn. Further observation and research in such a natural biological phenomenon might provide an effective means of control of parthenium in the years to come.

5. Abrus precatorius: Commonly known as Ratti, is a pod bearing wild climber found in the subcortical parts in this country. The seeds are typically demarcated into red and black colour areas. It is not eaten normally by any kind of livestock. Sheep may however browse on Ratti pods and leaves, during the pasturage scarcity periods in the months of May and June.

Poisoning: The plant as well seeds contribute towards hydrocyanic acid production. Thus the consumption of leaves and particularly the pods proves fatal. The hydrocyanic acid content of the pods varies with the season. It has been found to be 12.5 percent in March and increases to 26.5 percent in May on fresh basis. Since the Ratti plant is less common, the cases of Ratti (HCN) poisoning are also rare.

Treatment: Consists of administering lavages for stomach wash or in inducing vomission, but is not of much utility. Sodium thiosulphate serves the purpose of nullifying the action of cyanide group and is prescribed in all such cases.

6. Aconite poisoning: Aconite species plants exist in abundance, scattered in the alpine pastures of northern temperate region of India, growing amidst the Rhododendron and other shrubby growth. At times a sprinkling of the plants may also be found in aconite notorious alpine pastures at an altitude of 3000 to 4000 m. The height of the plant may go up to three-fourth of a meter. The goats out of their browsing habits and daring attempts to sneak in thick shrubs fall an easy prey to aconite eating and poisoning. Incidence of aconite plant eating in sheep is lesser but is of fatal severity invariably.

All the parts of the plant are poisonous. Leaves and flowers are commonly consumed and result in fast appearance of poison symptoms. Roots are too toxic. The gaddie shepherds collect, dry and preserve the aconite roots. These are powdered and in very small quantities fed to sheep flocks mixed with powdered salt licks during winters. This as per them makes their sheep less vulnerable to poisonous effects of Aconite during summers on entry into infested pastures.

Symptoms and remedy: Goats in many cases show nauseating symptoms and attempt at vomition. Any success in vomiting out brightens the survival chances. Sheep do not exhibit marked nausea. Hence are found dead soon, before administration of any treatment. The usual approach in aconite poisoning cases is to administer 5 percent solution of $CuSO_4$ to induce vomiting.

Since aconite is cardiac depressant so alcohol is given orally to stimulate. Digitalis is also tried to improve cardiac function. Gastric lavage may not be much effective due to multichamber condition of stomach and much larger size of rumen. As a precaution the experienced shepherds pick up and destroy the aconite plants prior to the entry of flock in the aconite known highlands.

7. Rhododendron poisoning: One of the rhododendron varieties growing as a shrub in the alpine pastures of Pir Panjal and Dhauladhars produces toxicity when eaten by sheep. The thick leaves are less relished and do not cause any serious problem. But the flowers are invariably consumed by the goats and even sheep producing serious poisonous symptoms.

Generally the symptoms and suspicion arise when the animals grazing in Rhododendron infested pastures attempt at an unusual act of vomiting and belching out. If the animal is successful in ejecting out the ingesta, the poisonous effects get allayed. Otherwise the condition aggravates and death may ensue within two to three hours in untreated cases. Invariably the poisonous rhododendron consumed sheep are found dead only in the pasture or in the pen.

Prevention: Shepherds avoid moving of flocks to rhododendron shrub growing patches especially during flowering period. In certain pastures the intensity of the shrub growth has come down due to its utility as fuel by the migratory nomads and tribals. The curative aspect consists of symptomatic treatment and other measures as resorted to in other cases of vegetation poisoning.

8. Heteropogon grass: This poor quality sub tropical area grass poses a big problem for the young animals. *Heteropogon contortus* (Seriala or spears or lumb grass) produce spear like bristly seeds in bunches. These get attached to fleece, face, legs and other parts of the body of sheep. The presence of hair/scale like growth on the seed of this grass helps in the progressive movements of the bristles towards the skin. Ultimately it pierces the skin causing irritation, discomfort and dermatitis. Further penetration inside the skin and gradual passage towards vital organs results into tissue damage, abscess formation, haemorrhages, etc. Orchitis is one major problem in rams moving about in speargrass infested pastures. Hepatic damage and traumatic pericarditis are the common conditions caused due to *Heteropogon controtus* bristles. Flocks of the farms that are fed a mixed meadow hay containing Heteropogon grass often develop abscess in the buccal cavity, throat, and salivary gland region or neck particularly in lambs, due to piercing and lodging of bristles.

Grazing or harvesting of spear grass pastures and meadows in the pre-flowering stage lessens Seriala problem.

9. Xanthium strumarium: Nagoora burr—Commonly known as Bathurst burr in New Zealand and Australia and Nagoora or Jojra burr in India. It is the most obnoxious weed and burr as far as sheep and wool are concerned. It did not exist on this soil half a century back. After entry, it has spread menacingly to all parts of the country. The seed is tough with hooked prickles. It is highly viable due to laden food reserves with ability to germinate under adverse situation, soil and climatic conditions. The plant is not eaten by cattle and is not relished by even sheep and goats. Rapid growth gives it the advantage to compete well with other vegetation. Rather it propagates at the cost of other herbage and by suppressing the same.

Seed survivability is almost cent per cent even after a dormancy of a year. Once it invades an area it has the capacity to hold on to the terrain. The structural and morphological characters enable its dispersal through the agencies of wind, water, animal, man and all other means of transport or carriage.

Losses: Since last three decades it has been an enemy number one for woolly sheep and the sheep man. The capability and the tendency of the Xanthium seed to stick fastly to the wool coat and least possibility of the burr getting removed, damages the wool absolutely. Prickly bristles irritate the delicate skin of the sheep to the extent of rashes, bruises, orchitis and damage to external body parts. The profuse sticking of Nagoora burr makes the animal restless and the sheepman's handling difficult. The jojra infested sheep loose physically. There is thus a multifold loss of wool, mutton and sheep health. Thick growth of Xanthium not only eliminates the under cover of grasses and other forage, but also impedes the sheep movement in Nagoora habitat.

Eradication: Manual removal in pre-flowering monsoon season has been found quite result oriented.

The use of weedicides like 2, 4-D and MCP-A (2 methyl, 4 chlorophenoxy acetic acid 450 g per acre) in crops and established pastures or MCPB application (2 methyl, 4 chlorophenox butyric acid) has been found useful upto flowering stage.

Though biotic factors, bacteria or fungi have not been able to check this plant, the spread of parthenium has to a great extent overpowered the Nagoora growth in early stage and thus eliminated the same from certain Parthenium encroached pastures.

Chicorium intybust (Hubla, Kasni)

It is a deep rooted seasonal plant growing in the hills and especially at sheep penning sites profusely. Leaves are green and broad like spinach. There are two distinct varieties which grow in a range varying from 500 to 3000 m in the temperate region.

Growth starts on the arrival of summer rains in hills in May or soon after snow melts. Sheep, goat and even cattle relish the leaves. Another leafy flush takes place in July-August. On the long flowery pedestal are born the seed which are with multiple small hooks. When the sheep move about for grazing these burrs get stuck to the fleece on the forehead neck, britch region and on the sides of the body. Sticking can occur in green stage, but get shed later on. On ripening the burrs turn brown and are not shed so soon. In certain cases fleece burr content may be even 3 to 5% which looks dull brown otherwise.

After October the plant parts overground wilt and further growth ceases to regenerate in next March-April.

Removal of burr sticking to fleece is affected through the use of curry combs. In doing so some finest fibres of the fleece are also combed out with the burr. The fleece cannot be de-burred completely. Such wools fetch lower price. Because of bruises caused by combing, such a practice prior shearing is discouraged now.

Carthamus oxycantha (Kanyari, Kandyari)

It is a wild growing thistle plant with wide ranged habitat. The leaves of this shrubby plant as well as the stem itself possess the bristles which prick and irritate the skin of the animal and man coming in contact. Lambs are scared to take the leaves but the goats relish the forage.

The flower heads appear at the terminal ends in the form of corium full of thistles. When the seed is ripe the thistles get attached to the fleece of the sheep that try to browse and move about in the Kanyari plant infested pastures. These add to the vegetable or burr content of the wool. The handling of the animals becomes problematical. At times the needle like thistles reach the skin and penetrate causing trauma and damage to the vital and delicate organs.

Rumex sps. (*R. nepalensis*—Albal, Kulayee) and burr clover (Sareedee) are usual pasture forages which produce burry seeds. These burrs also damage wool and torment the sheep, but are not as injurious as Nagoora burr. Local vegetation named Pakhreh (*Tribulus terrestrus*, land caltrops), Kithri-Lendha (*Rupalia lappacea*-producing sticky jojree), Kashmiri thistle (*Circium falconeri*), Parkanda, Chhoti jojri, etc. are other burr producing plants of rangelands in certain areas that stick to the sheep coat inseparably.

Some of the field vegetation that the agronomist considers as crop weeds is in fact a good sheep forage from a sheepman's angle. *Avena fatua* (Jungli javi), *Medicago denticulata* (Menna), *Melilotus indica* (Senji) and *Chenopodium alum* (Bathu) are a few such examples. Whereas wild growths like *Fumaria parviflora* (Papra, Gajri) are of no use to either of them.

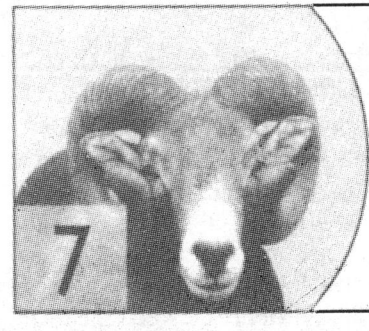

SHEEP NUTRITION AND FEEDING

7

APPROACH TO FEEDING MANAGEMENT

A know how about the nutritional requirements at various stages of life cycle of animal and knowledge of what to feed, how much to feed and the feed values of the material to be fed constitutes judicious feeding. This obviates wastage of nutrients, ensures palatability and economy in livestock feeding. Rational feeding involves scientific estimation of requirement of nutrients, viz. proteins, carbohydrates, fats, vitamins, minerals, water, etc. and takes care of breed, sex, age, body weight, season factors in tune with time to time demands of breeding, pregnancy, lactation, growth, fattening, wool-meat production and extent of movements, etc. A uniformly static feeding schedule does not work. Proper feeding necessitates adjustments in feed fodder demand and supply under varying situations.

Sheep possess a unique ability to survive on natural grasses, shrubs and farm waste products like crop residue. Pastures and ranges are the natural habitats of the sheep and they thrive on them under extremely wide climatic conditions and utilize most adverse types of vegetations.

Some of the important points in successful flock management include:

1. Abdundance of good pastures throughout the growing season.
2. Proper feed and care of the ewes before and after lambing.

3. Control of parasites.
4. Lamb production type—market demand and supply.

A well planned and economic nutritional management is of pivotal importance as feed accounts for about 55 to 60 percent of the total cost of rearing the sheep.

Poor grazing lands or the ones deteriorated due to overstocking can not ensure adequate availability of feed and nutrition to the pastoral sheep. This poses a serious hindrance to efficient sheep production where main stay is the pasture alone. The challenge at hand for sheep industry is to devise ways and means to solve nutritional problems. Steps other than the conservation of pastures, improving top feed resources, fodder conservation and processing, etc. are also called for and include supplementation with cheaper, surplus grains, agro-industrial byproducts and other useful, edible wastes.

EFFECT OF NUTRITION

Pre-breeding and conception stage

Research made in India and abroad reveals that adequate feeding of hogget ewes leads to better development of reproductive tract. The yearlings and maiden ewes fed roughages and grains tend to develop puberty earlier and produce larger graafian follicles than the control group fed on

Chief Contributor: Dr. R.K. Sharma (Ph.D) Assoc. Professor, (Ani.Nut.) SKUAST-J.

roughage alone as found on slaughter of treated ewes. Maturity and puberty are breed linked traits. The low feed group Rambouillet crossbred ewes of sheep farm, Billawar (J&K) showed a delayed growth. First successful conception took place around 2 to 2½ years age instead of 1½ year (Gupta, 1972). Fertility rate in ewes of higher fed group has been found higher though not significant. The horns of pregnant and nonpregnant uterus of well fed ewes were larger than the poor fed group.

To improve ovulation rate the practice of increasing the nutrient intake and utilization to improve body condition before breeding is referred to as flushing. This is accomplished by moving ewes to better pastures, deworming and feeding supplements. The flushing period starts 4–6 weeks prior breeding and continues for a week during the breeding season. Underfeeding usually does not delay the onset of breeding season, though at times the breeding season may pass off as silent heat in younger ewes maintained on maintenance feed only. For securing fertilization the number of services or inseminations in poor fed group is more. The reproduction function quickly regains with the improvement of feeding. The ewes flushed but not to the extent of fatness, i.e. lean or thin ones, shed more ova from the ovaries, though this may not be reflected in simultaneous improvement in lamb crops. Twinning rate has been found considerably higher in the flushed group of ewes at some of the farms and plain area sedentary flocks. Appropriate flushing limits barrenness of flocks. Moving the ewes to fresh good pastures, a fortnight prior to ram joining, reduces the proportion of dry ewes and avoids spread of major lambing beyond six weeks.

Developing foetus

The nutritional requirements of the foetus are met in a number of ways. The ovum contains sufficient reserves for its early division. Later the *uterine milk* supplies nutrients to the embryo. The formation of placenta provides the channel where by nutrients from the mother blood stream flow to the foetus.

There is a very close contact between the blood vessels in the cotyledons attached to the lining of the uterus and those of the placenta. In the cotyledons, gases such as oxygen and nutrients like carbohydrates, proteins, fats, minerals, vitamins and water partake from mother to the lamb placenta.

The most interesting features of this transfer is the distribution of the nutrients between the ewe and her lamb and the transfusion of nutrients across the villi in the cotyledons. This distribution of nutrients however, depends on the metabolic rate of foetal tissues. When the foetus in early age is small, its total demands of nutrients are small. As it grows, its metabolic rate declines and there is a shift in the basis of its competition with its mother. As pregnancy advances, the developing foetus competes against the ewe's liver, muscles, and reserves of fat suggesting that it can exercise an independent demand on nutrients' circulation in the blood of mother.

The growth of foetus is uniform during first 15 to 16 weeks of gestation irrespective of how well the ewe is fed. In under nourished ewes, however, the foetal losses may be higher during early pregnancy especially when body weight declines by one-fourth or so in about two months. During the later part of last six weeks of gestation, growth and body weight differences are influenced greatly by the plane of nutrition. Better fed same age group pregnant Rambouillet ewes at sheep farm, Reasi dropped more viable lambs with birth weight average of 3.6 kg against the lower nutritional group of ewes where lambs at birth averaged 3.2 kg in weight. Well fed ewes themselves gained 5 to 8 kg more weight during the last two months of pregnancy. The requirement of digestible proteins/nutrients in this period increase by 40% and that of Ca and P more than 100%. A provision of 300 g or more of concentrate having 25% DCP and 75% TDN is advised. Feeding extra to meet heavy demands of unborn lamb is known as *steaming up*.

Noticeable reductions are found in the fat reserves and liver of lambs born to poorly fed ewes. The alimentary tract, the bones, the heart, pancreas, and nervous tissues suffer least reduction, while the blood vessels, muscles and lungs encounter immediate reduction in weight. It is thus clear that the way the ewes are fed during the last weeks of pregnancy may affect the birth weight of foetus and its survivability.

Oxygen is essential to the tissues and the demand of the foetus depends on its stage of development. Large well formed lambs have a higher oxygen consumption. Haemoglobin content in blood is the carrier of oxygen. Its affinity for oxygen increases as pregnancy advances. Oxygen requirements increase enormously and rapidly during the last 6 to 8 weeks of gestation. Unless the blood haemoglobin level is adequate at this stage foetal loss may ensue.

As parturition approaches the attachments between the foetus and maternal cotyledons start snapping. The foetus must either escape from the uterus to obtain enough oxygen by breathing or die.

Carbohydrates: Glycogen, glucose and fructose are important carbohydrates for the nourishment of foetus. Glycogen occurs in the foetal and maternal placenta and in the uterine milk of the ewes though the amount is not large.

Foetal blood fructose has a higher sugar level than that of the blood of adult ewes, but glucose level is about the same as in the mothers blood. This is probably because fructose can not cross the placental barrier while glucose can. The normal range of glucose in sheep blood is cited between 40-65 mg per 100 ml blood. In some laboratories in India the mean blood sugar values for non-pregnant ewes on maintenance feeding showed a normal range of 30-50 mg/100 ml.

Proteins: Many nitrogenous substances cross the placenta from the maternal to the foetal circulation. Some antibodies circulating in the ewe blood may pass unchanged to the foetal blood, there by protecting the new born lamb from disease. The vaccination of ewes in advance pregnancy with single, bivalent or multi-Clostridial vaccine has the sole objective of achieving active immunity in new born lambs particularly against Lamb dysentery, Entero-

toxaemia, etc. It is probable that the foetus obtains free acids from the maternal blood stream and those are re-synthesized into proteins by the foetus.

The nitrogen requirements of foetus appear higher. The rate of nitrogen uptake by a goat foetus rises from 0.75 g/day at 100th day age to 2.0 g/day at 120th day and 5.50 g/day at 140th day, respectively.

Fats: The lipid levels in the blood of sheep foetus rise and fall with variations in lipid levels of ewe's blood. In foetal blood lipids probably reflect changes in the balance between fat synthesis and fat break down, i.e. lipids in foetal blood should be high when the ewe is under nourished and she is mobilising her fat reserves.

Minerals: Na and Cl occur in foetal blood at par with their concentration in the maternal blood.

Iron: The iron content of the foetus increases rapidly after about 80th day of gestation. The amount of iron stored in the liver of the lamb is not readily influenced by the amount of iron in the ewe's diet.

Copper: Content of the lamb liver rises during the last 50 days of gestation and it is influenced by the amount of copper in the diet of the ewe. It may be lower than that of the mother. Lambs born to ewes suffering from copper deficiency may suffer incomplete development of spinal cord leading to the 'Sway back' condition in the early life of the lamb. The Cu content of the liver of effected lambs may be as low as 8 parts per million on dry matter basis.

Ca and P: These are essential for the development of skeleton and bones of lambs. Foetal blood levels of Ca and P are higher than those of pregnant ewes. This means Ca and P are passed across the placenta against the concentration gradient, may be through process of active selection. The demand of lamb for the two elements is so great that ewes maintained on a low Ca diet may even draw on the reserves in their own bones in order to meet the demands of foetus they carry.

Vitamins: are essential for the healthy growth of foetus and for this purpose supplementation of at least essential vitamins in the diet of mother ewe deserves attention.

Birth and newborn

Variations in the nutrition level of pregnant ewes may influence the length of gestation though not very markedly. Fat ewes are said to experience greater difficulty during lambing than ewes in stores or forward store condition*. Assistance is needed more frequently at lambing in certain ewes. But this may be more of a breed to breed difference and matter of management. Some pastures may predispose ewes to dystocia and serious lamb losses occur. Clover rich pastures produce estrogenic effect and peculiar kind of infertility, lowered conception rate, parturition problems and prolapse of uterus.

Effects of plane of nutrition on birth weight, growth and survival are appreciable. The poor fed ewes rarely deliver healthy, viable and sound growing lambs. As a safeguard, urgent attention towards feeding of pregnant ewes, is needed once reduction in their body weight is imminent. On this account supplementary feeding is advised for last 40 to 50 days of pregnancy.

The prenatal and postnatal feeding of ewes are equally important. The mothering ability, besides other aspects rests partly on the nutrition of the mother ewe. To maintain an average increase of 100 g lamb weight per day, lamb is required to consume half a litre of milk. The Rambouillet cross bred lambs having birth weight around 3 kg, attain 9 to 11 kg weight at one month age and 15 to 16 kg by the end of second month. The daily gain in weight is around 200 to 250 gm/day in the first month. In exceptional well fed cases the lamb weight of 18 to 20 kg may be achieved in two months.

The drain on the ewe in the first month is heavy. Tentative intake of at least 1.5 to 2.0 kg total digestible nutrients (feed units) containing 10% digestible proteins is the requirement of the ewe. The average daily weight gain gradually declines. Mothering effect and dependence on mother's milk also decreases once the lamb is switched over to starter feeding. To allow for the initial growth of lambs it is always desirable to allow additional feeding of lambed ewes for at least 8 weeks. Pasturage is invariably deficient in India to meet the required nutrients particularly the digestible proteins, Ca and P. Thus supplementary grain feeding of ewes becomes all the more important for foetal growth and to meet suckling needs of lamb, aggregating to 100 to 120 days in all.

Suckling lambs: Ewe's first milk after parturition called colostrum, is a rich source of nutrients and immuno-globulins which protect the lamb against diseases. Colostrum should essentially be fed to the lamb as being laxative as well, it clears the gut of muconium. 50 to 100 ml of colostrum shall suffice. When larger quantities are suckled, a temporary diarrhoea may ensue.

The lambs depend only on mother's milk for first 3 to 4 weeks. After about a fortnight they start to consume small quantities of fine supplemented feeds, the starters. Foster feeding may be necessitated at times, due to death of mother ewe, disowning or early drying of the mother. Bottle or nipple feeding of warm milk replacers is often tried, but does not yield as good results.

Creep feeds: Suckling lambs are initiated with supplemented succulent fodder and creep mixtures, known as creep grazing or creep feeding respectively. This enjoins the establishment of a creep feeder which is an area where lambs nibble or consume feed without competition from their mother ewes. The amount of creep mixture consumed by the lambs are inversely proportional to the amount of milk available from the dams.

However, after 6 to 8 weeks age, most of the lambs consume significant amount of creep feed in addition to mother's milk unless they have access to high pasture. The composition of such creep mixtures is presented in Table 7.1.

---

* good or very good condition but not fat.

Table 7.1: Composition of creep mixture
(Verma, 1995)

Ingredients	Percent		
	I	*II*	*III*
1. Maize crushed	67	50	30
2. Barley crushed	–	17	37
3. Groundnut cake	10	10	10
4. Wheat bran	10	10	10
5. Fish meal	10	10	10
6. Common salt	1	1	1
7. Mineral mixture	2	2	2

Creep ration should be well balanced, palatable and clean.

Growing lambs

After the rumen is developed, good quality leguminous fodder/hays should be provided. The requirements of nutrients are different for replacement ewes and lambs in comparison to finishing lambs. Finishing lambs are required to gain weight rapidly, however, replacement lambs are intended for breeding and weight gain is secondary. Lambs can be grown and finished on high quality pasture, on pasture plus supplementation or in dry feed-lot systems. The type of system depends on desired marketing time (faster gains can be made in a dry lot), type of lambs to be sold (lean versus more fat cover), available feed resources and economics. Rapid growing animals are required to be given concentrate mixture in addition to grazing, while on low quality grazing pastures. The concentrate mixture supplying 20 percent CP and 70% TDN can be prepared from maize 25%; wheat bran 32%; pulse chuni 26%; GNC 15%; mineral mixture 1% and salt 1%. The concentrate mixture to be given depends upon body weight and quality of grazing material (Table 7.2).

To produce leaner lamb carcasses, dry lot feeding may not be required. Dry lot feeding systems are designed for rapid lamb growth and usually involve two to three diet changes through the finishing period (Ely, 1991). Lambs are usually adjusted from pasture-based feeding to concentrates by feeding ground hay (30 to 50%), mixed with grains maize, oats, barley, (50 to 60%), molasses (19% to improve palatability and reduce dust) and possibly an antibiotic premix (1%). Ammonium sulphate may be added to reduce problems of urinary calculi. Various appropriate feed mixtures suggested by Ely (1991) serve as examples of diets for growing lambs (Table 7.3).

Table 7.3: Compounding concentrate feed mixtures for growing lambs

Diet	Lambs weight range		
	30 (kg) (%)	30 to 40 kg (%)	40 kg to market (%)
Diet 1			
Cracked maize	48.0	58.0	68.0
Chopped hay	33.0	23.0	13.0
Soybean meal, 44% CP	11.5	11.5	11.5
Liquid molasses	5.0	5.0	5.0
Di-calcium phosphate	1.0	1.0	1.0
Trace mineral salt and Se	1.0	1.0	1.0
Ammonium sulphate	0.5	0.5	0.5
Diet 2			
Ground ear corn	60.0	30.0	–
Cracked corn (maize)	–	30.0	60.0
Chopped alfa-alfa hay	27.5	27.5	27.5
Soybean meal, 44% CP	6.0	6.0	6.0
Liquid molasses	5.0	5.0	5.0
Trace mineral salt	1.0	1.0	1.0
Ammonium sulphate	0.5	0.5	0.5

Table 7.2: Feed and fodder requirement of growing lambs (Ranjan,1997)

Body weight kg.	Concentrate mixture g/day	Roughage oat hay g/day	Remarks
12-15	200	400	8 hours grazing can be
16-25	250	600	substituted in place of oat hay
26-35	300	700	

Replacement stock

Replacement ewes are generally identified at 3 to 4 months of age and fed in such a way that they lamb at 1½ year of age. Fat should not be given to replacement ewe lambs, as this can decrease milk production potential. Replacement rams should be allowed free access to pasture and supplemented so as to achieve a growth of 150-200 g/day. Once mature, grazing alone can meet the maintenance requirements.

Feeding for wool production

Since the wool is rich in sulphur containing amino acids, cystine and methionine, the diets for wool producing sheep should be planned in such a way that they supply adequate amounts of these amino-acids. Low level of protein in the diet hampers fibre growth affecting staple length adversely. A break in wool fibre is usual in sheep maintained on unsatisfactory nutritional plane. Fibre strength,

length and even diameter get reduced during periods of stress caused by changes in temperature, pregnancy, lactation, etc. besides nutritional deficiencies. Minerals such as selenium, copper, cobalt, iodine, iron, etc. play important role in wool production.

MAINTENANCE AND GROWTH

Pasture is the main source of sustenance of sheep in India. But for northern alpine grazing lands and developed or reserve pastures elsewhere in the country, the grazing areas are in a vegetatively degraded state. Carrying capacity is hardly 1 to 2 sheep/per hec. Extent of pasture lands is shrinking and livestock number is on the increase. Thereby the number of animals per hectare of available pastures has also risen. Most of the pastures are hardly efficient to provide maintenance to a flock for a limited season only. Growth may be satisfactory in certain months but stagnant and reversed in others (Fig. 7.1).

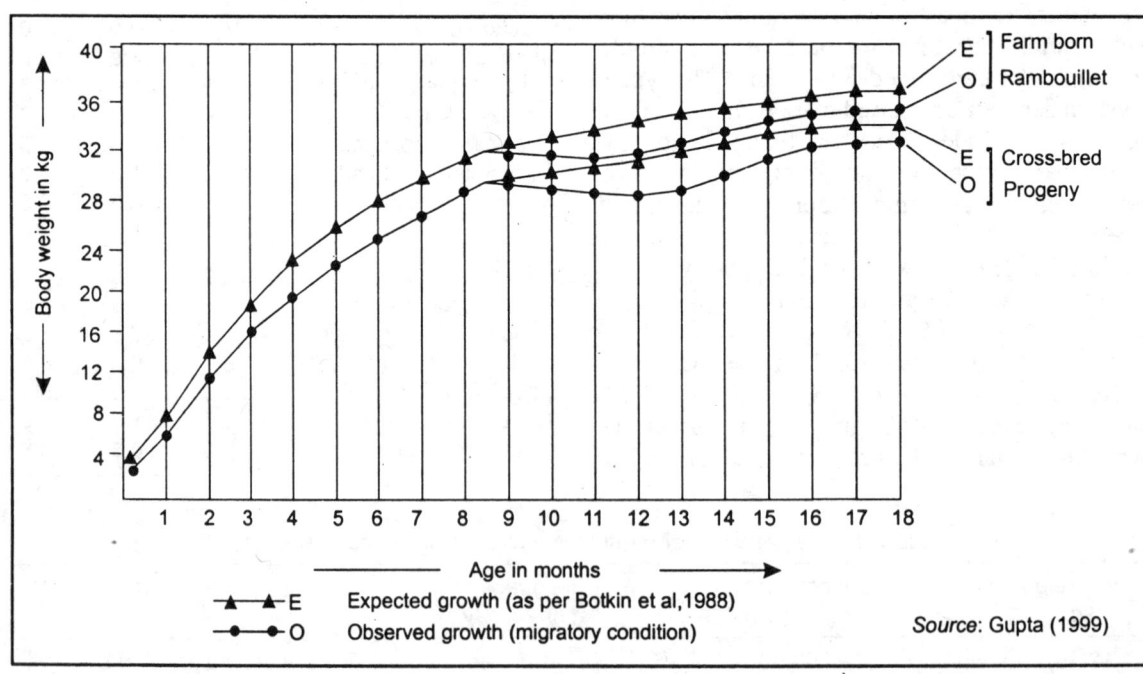

Fig. 7.1.   Growth studies of farm born sheep (Rambouillet block and cross breeds–J&K) in relation to pasture status.

In the Northern Temperate region the gain in weight of lambs is uniform and gradual from Feb-March to September-October. Ceasing in gain takes place in November and there is general loss in weight from December to February. Besides winter stress, this downward trend in weight is attributable to a reduction in forage availability. Studies into pasture feeding *vs.* growth of sheep over 8 years at one farm and for six years at another revealed a marked fall in sheep weight during lean pasturage from December to February (Gupta, 1999). Loss so suffered could partly be made good in the next favourable season only. In northwestern arid and semi arid zone. Sheep weight gains are reported from June to December. A loss in weight is invariably imminent in February due to significant reduction in the vegetation.

NUTRIENT REQUIREMENTS OF SHEEP

Physiological state of health, age, production and reproduction status (as discussed earlier) and environmental factors are the key to determine feed requirements. The latter vary depending upon environmental temperature, wind velocity, humidity, stress factor, wool length distance travelled while grazing, intensity and extent of mutton gain. Inadequacy of nutrients in the sheep diet can cause poor fertility, lower milk production, reduction in lactation period, lower wool production and increased susceptibility to diseases.

Various scientific authorities, viz. ARC (1980), NRC, (1985), Sheep Council of Australia (1990) and CSWRI, too have published nutrient requirements for sheep which are an ample guide for planning balanced rations.

Dry matter (DM)

Stall fed sheep can consume 2.5 to 3.5 kg of dry matter per head per day from quality roughages. Sheep may consume 15 per cent more DM on pasture than when stall-fed with the same feeds, which is especially true when pasture is succulent. With inferior quality pasture the total intake may be considerably lower, thereby affecting the nutrients supply.

Energy

Generally the energy is the most limiting nutrient in ewe and doe nutrition. The major source of energy are pasture (forage, range and browse), hays, silage, byproducts, feeds and grains. However, a good quality pasture, hay, silage or byproducts usually meet the energy requirement most economically. The high moisture content of some feeds such as silage/pasture may reduce the animal's intake and thereby necessitate provisions of supplemental energy through grains. Supplemental energy is also necessary for rapid growth, rapid foetal development or lactation to meet high energy demands. Energy deficiencies may result due to shortage of feeds, drought, low dry matter content of pastures, over mature feeds or snow covered pastures. Outcome is retarded growth or weight loss, reproductive failure, low milk and fibre production and high mortality rates. The total digestible nutrients (TDN) requirements for maintenance of mature sheep for energy is 0.027 $w^{0.75}$ kg/day.

Protein

Sheep being ruminant, depend on the microbes of rumen to manufacture most of the amino acids required for desired production. As with other ruminants, quantity of protein in the diet is more important than quality of protein. Young suckling lambs require high quality protein in the diet, as their rumen is not fully developed. Rumen microbial population are able to utilize nitrogen from proteins of feed origin and also nitrogen from nonprotein source to synthesise amino acids, however, some of the amino acids such as methionine, lysine and threonine may be limiting. Wool fibre being composed almost entirely of protein, necessitates to have greater proportion of protein in the sheep diets. Feeds high in protein are usually expensive and therefore sheep diets often contain urea, a cheaper source of nitrogen. Guidelines for using urea (Sheep Industry Development, 1992) in sheep diets are as follows:

- Urea can be used up to 1% of total diet or 3% of the concentrate portion, but should never exceed one-third of the total nitrogen in the diet.

🐏 Urea should be introduced into the diet gradually to allow for adaptation by rumen microbes and full adaptation takes 2-3 weeks.

🐏 Urea should be thoroughly mixed into the diet to allow uniform intake and prevent high levels of intakes.

🐏 Urea should not be used in the diets of young lambs.

Pastures in vegetative stage or browse generally meet the protein requirement of sheep. Low protein feeds such as hays, silage and byproducts are required to be supplemented with protein to achieve the desired production. The oil cakes such as soyabean, cotton seed, peanuts, etc. though expensive, are the most common protein source used in sheep diets. Recently protein blocks (20-200 kg) containing natural and NPN source of nitrogen are often being suggested for animals on pastures for protein supplementation. The total protein requirements of sheep may be calculated from the digestible protein values using the regression equation given below:

$$Y = 0.929\ X - 3.48 \text{ where } Y = \text{Digestible protein}$$
$$X = \text{Crude protein}$$

An animal weighing 30 kg needs about 400 g TDN and 40 g DCP per day for optimum wool production within its genetic potential. A level of 10% protein in the ration has been found adequate for wool production, since feeding beyond this level has no beneficial effect on wool yield.

Recent concepts about protein requirements

For many years the basic unit for estimating the protein requirements of ruminants was digestible crude protein. Total protein and DCP were the units adopted by NRC (1985) in estimating the nutrient requirements of sheep. However, progress in understanding and quantifying the processes of digestion and synthesis of protein in the rumen in the last couple of decades has led to the realization of the inadequacies of the DCP system. The major short coming of DCP system for calculating the nitrogen requirements of ruminants arise from:

1. the extensive degradation of dietary protein in the rumen and its incorporation into microbial protein.

2. the presence of undigested microbial protein arising from rumen and the hind gut.

3. the inability to differentiate between the absorption of amino acid nitrogen, ammonia nitrogen or other forms of non-amino acid nitrogen.

4. the inability to account for differences in animal response according to the form of dietary nitrogen and

5. the failure to relate nitrogen requirements directly to energy intake and energy concentration in the diet N_2. In the past 10-15 years many countries have introduced new systems (British RDP/UDP system, the French PDI system, the Swiss API system, the Nordic AAT-PBV system and US-NRC AP system) based on predicting the supply of microbial and feed protein to the intestine, the digestion of protein and absorption of amino acids from the intestines and the efficiency of utilization of absorbed amino acids for maintenance and production. Although all these systems are similar in concept, they differ in details and continue to be subject to review and improvement.

Minerals

Mineral requirement of sheep are dependent on many factors such as age, sex, breed, growth rate, physiological status, amounts and chemical form of ingested minerals and interaction with other nutrients and minerals in the diet. (Sheep Industry Development, 1992). The mineral requirements and toxicities are well established for sheep (NRC, 1985). The important macro-mineral requirements of sheep include Na, Cl, K, Ca, P, S and Mg whereas common micro-mineral requirements include I, Cu, Co, Fe, Mn, Mo, Se, Zn (Pond, et al, 1995).

Salt, the most common, cheapest and highly palatable form of Na and Cl should be provided free choice. The salt should be provided in loose form as compared to blocks, because sheep at times tend to bite the block thereby damaging their teeth.

Most forages contain adequate amounts of potassium (K), however, its supplementation may be required when animals are on high grain diets or mature or drought stressed pastures or stressed by transport and are on new concentrate based diets.

Calcium and phosphorus are closely associated and are required for normal development of teeth, bone and skeleton. Lactating animals have higher requirements of Ca and P and their deficiency may affect milk production. In general, deficiency of Ca or P or their inadequate ratio (< 1-2:1) can reduce growth and may cause metabolic disorders like milk fever, etc. Sheep and goat efficiently reuse P by recycling it through saliva, however, sometimes sheep recycle more P per day through the parotid salivary gland than is required in the diet. Their utilization is dependent on vitamin D and hormones. As long as Ca is not given in excess it is always absorbed with a reasonably constant and high efficiency (ARC, 1980).

Magnesium deficiency (Grass tetany) most commonly occurs in sheep and goats grazing lush, fast growing pastures in the spring which are generally rich in Na and K and poor in Mg. Sheep consuming such pastures may fall to ground, froth at mouth and may rigidly extend and relax the legs. Untreated animals may even die. This can be prevented by provision of adequate levels of Mg in diet and can be treated by intravenous administration of Ca and Mg in the gluconate form.

Sulphur is essential for live weight gain, wool and hair growth as it functions in the synthesis of amino acids such as methionine and cysteine, the former being the most limiting amino acid for fibre production. Routine feeds usually contain adequate amounts of S but may be deficient in mature hays or drought hit stressed pastures. A ratio of dietary N to S should be 10:1 especially when NPN is component of ration because rumen microbes need a source of S and N at the same time to synthesize methionine and cysteine.

Copper has the narrowest range between what is required and what is potentially toxic. Sheep are most susceptible to Cu toxicity than cattle or goats, however, the actual threshold value of dietary Cu varies with factors such as presence of dietary antagonists and length of time of feeding (ARC, 1980). Copper levels in sheep diet should never exceed 25 ppm. Cu and Mo have antagonistic relationship thereby causing Cu deficiency in animals consuming feed with adequate or low level of Cu and high level of Mo. Provision of Mo to the sheep diet can also reduce the toxicity of Cu.

Selenium is a relatively toxic element and the tolerance level of 3 mg Se/kg diet DM suggested by ARC (1980) for ruminants should be regarded as a maximum value. Se has a synergistic relationship with vitamin E. Growing or pregnant sheep require minimum of 10-15 mg vitamin E/kg DM, as a general rule. Higher levels may be needed if Se intakes are low or marginal. 'Stiff lamb' disease (White Muscle Disease) may occur in sheep due to deficiency of Se. Its deficiency can also effect reproductive performance. Toxicity may occur due to prolonged intake of Se rich plants or Se accumulating plants, which is a problem in some range areas.

Iron is generally adequate in most feeds and deficiency symptoms are rare in healthy sheep. Blood loss due to internal parasites can cause anaemia. Anaemic condition is very common in young lambs because of low body stores of Fe and low Fe content of milk. Iron status of the animal can be improved by 1/m injection of Fe, and management or regular treatment to reduce internal parasites. As with other ruminants, excessive intakes of Fe should be avoided to reduce the risk of interference in the metabolism of other inorganic elements.

Iodine: In the absence of goitrogens, ARC (1980) recommended that a dietary Iodine (I) level of 0.5 mg/kg DM should be adequate for pregnant and lactating cattle and sheep. However, in the presence of goitrogens dietary iodine concentrations should be increased to 2 mg/kg DM. Iodine is usually adequate in most feeds and its deficiency is generally exhibited in newborn by an enlarged thyroid gland clearly visible on the neck (goitre). Severely deficient lambs may be stillborn without wool. Iodised salt is the most common and cheapest supplement.

Zinc: In practice, up to 150 mg Zn/kg DM appears to be well tolerated by ruminants (ARC, 1980) and even higher levels often do not have observable adverse effects. The evidence that development of the reproductive organs require relatively high Zn intakes (Chhabra and Arora, 1985), the possible presence of interacting dietary components and low Zn body storage, requires high and continuous supply of dietary Zn. Deficiencies are rare but can result in reduced fertility, stiffness of joints, reduced weight gain, parakeratosis, impaired testicular growth and ceasation of spermatogenesis.

Manganese (Mn) requirements have not been clearly established for any ruminant species and they vary considerably according to dietary considerations. The Mn content of most forages is greater than 50 ppm and of most grains is from 15-40 ppm, so deficiencies are rare. Deficiency signs include difficult walking, skeletal abnormalities and lower reproductive efficiency.

Cobalt: Is needed by the microbes in the rumen to synthesize Vit. B_{12} but is usually adequate in most feed-stuffs. ARC (1980) and IDWP (1984) suggested that a Cobalt level in cattle and sheep diets of 0.11 mg Co/kg DM should usually meet Co requirements, however, high concentrate diets should contain 0.2 mg Co/kg DM.*

Vitamins

Sheep with fully developed rumen can synthesize amounts of the vitamin B complex, vitamin C and vitamin K, but they require dietary sources of vitamins A, D and E. Young lambs require vitamin B complex in the diet until their rumen develops. Sheep generally obtain vitamins or vitamin precursors in adequate amounts through grazing but supplementation may be necessary in stall fed or high producing animals. Vitamin A occurs in forages as its precursor carotene and approximately 1 mg of carotene is equivalent to 400 I.U. of vitamin A. In sheep and goats, vitamin A is stored in the body to meet the requirement for 3 to 6 months after removal of animals from pastures. Vitamin A deficiency is rare. Deficiency symptoms include night blindness, poor reproductive performance, keratinization of epithelium tissues and decreased resistance to infections. Vitamin A deficiency can be corrected by provision of vitamin A in the diet, or by injections of vitamin A or by feeding vitamin A rich feeds (green grass/legume hay).

Sun cured hays and green forages generally contain adequate amounts of vitamin D. Sunlight exposed animals obtain sufficient vitamin D to meet their requirements. Supplementation is necessary in confined animals with heavy fleece or dark pigmented skin. Deficiency symptoms include development of rickets or osteomalacia, which can be corrected by provision of vitamin D in the diet, or through injections or by exposing the confined animals to sunlight.

Vitamin E, a biological *antioxidant* is important to prevent white muscle disease and increases the shelf life of milk. It is not stored in the body in large quantities and is often included in the supplement for fast growing lambs and for lactating sheep and goats.

Sufficient amounts of B Complex vitamins are synthesised by the rumen microbes, however, they are required continuously as being not stored in the body in large amounts. Thiamin deficiency can cause *Polio-encephalomalacia* in sheep. Vitamin C is synthesised in the body of sheep as per requirements.

Water intake

In addition to drinking from watering source, sheep obtain water from feeds, snow, dew and oxidation of nutrients. Like other livestock the water intake of sheep depends on season weather condition, environmental temperature, type of feed and fodder offered, sheep movement, terrain where maintained, sex, age, breed, body weight and physiological state of health of animal.

---

* Deficient and unbalanced feeding of copper and cobalt in diet results in faulty growth of wool fibre.

In summers, dry weather, wind blasts, long journeys, dry forage or concentrate feeding, lambed and in-milk conditions increase water requirement. During winter and rainy season, succulent or green fodder consumption reduce water intake. Drier the feed, higher the water intake. The requirement may be as low as one litre per day in smaller sheep and rises to 3 to 4 litres for a good size sheep in hotter season. Pregnant sheep, lambed ewes, lambs, breeding rams and ailing sheep are adversely affected due to shortage of drinking water. Sheep of arid zone that are used to water scarcity conditions are less prone to immediate effects of deficient watering than temperate area sheep, the cross breeds or the exotic sheep.

Water intake expressed as kg per kg of DM intake for sheep in various physiological states and at different environmental temperatures is presented in Table 7.4.

In India, sheep are generally provided water *ad-lib*. It has however been observed that certain arid zone sheep can thrive on limited watering and show no untoward effect without water for 1 to 2 days. Experiments at Central Arid Zone Research Institute, Jodhpur, showed that both the ambient temperature and humidity caused change in water intake. Sheep with low blood potassium level (6 μg per lit) drank sufficiently less water than those having high potassium level (23 μg per lit). Heat balance in Bikaneri sheep was maintained under climatic stress by increasing heat loss through more of water intake. The depot fat (as found in Dumba sheep) and multi-chamber stomach help serve as water storage and temporarily sustain animals from water inadequacy.

FEEDING STANDARDS: RESEARCH IN INDIA

Scientific work in livestock nutrition in India was initiated by the Imperial Research Institute Pusa (Bihar) more than seven decades back and then carried out at Bangalore. Emphasis was more on large animal feeding. Sheep nutrition received little attention. IVRI made certain early head ways after independence of the country. Since seventies C.S.W.R.I. Avikanagar (Rajasthan) has organised specific research and investigation in sheep nutrition.

Feeding standards adopted by NRC (National Research Council of USA and Canada) and ARC (Agri. Research Council of UK) based on total digestible nutrients (TDN) and starch equivalent (SE) systems respectively have been in use in India. On very many accounts these are inadequate to answer the requirements of not so well fed animals, viz. sheep grazing on poor pasturages. Secondly, the rearing systems, the type of feeds, agro-climatic conditions and management in India differ widely. Thirdly, the NRC standards cover a higher weight group lambs (above 27 kg), where as Indian sheep are of smaller body weight than English breeds. Further the significance of volatile fatty acids (VFA's) came to be appreciated later. Therefore, instead of applying these standards in toto, the sheep nutritionists have undertaken

Table 7.4: Desired water intake (kg water/kg DM consumed) of sheep in different physiological states and at different environmental temperatures (Jarriage, 1989)

Sl. no.	Physiological state		Daily water intake (kg) at environmental temperature (°C)			
			15	20	25	30
1.	Lambs, growing or finishing		2.0	2.6	3.0	4.0
2.	Ewes, nonpregnant or early pregnant		2.0-2.5	2.6-3.3	3.0-3.75	4-5
3.	Ewes, late pregnancy with single lamb		3.0-3.5	3.9-4.6	4.5-5.3	6-7
		with twin	3.5-4.5	4.6-5.9	5.3-6.8	7-9
4.	Ewes lactating	First month	4.0-4.5	5.2-5.9	6.0-6.8	8-9
		Later months	3.0-4.0	3.9-5.2	4.5-6.0	6-8

redefining the requirement of Indian sheep quite recently. Sufficient data of experiments on sheep feeding has generated after 1970 and suggestions advanced by CSWRI about the nutrient needs of Indian sheep.

Dry matter: Dry matter consumption is important in livestock feeding. Srivastava and Chaturvedi (1971) found the dry matter consumption from pasture grazing sheep to vary from 800 to 1200 g per day. The growing lambs require 3 to 5% dry matter of body weight. Higher the DM intake, satisfactory is the growth. Adult sheep, particularly the ewes consume 2.5 to 3% of their body weight for maintenance. The intake however depends on the type of feed, age, body weight, growth and production status.

Energy and protein needs: Nutrient requirements are often not met through sufficient dry matter alone. The energy and protein requirements are as much essential ingredients of feed nutrients. The systems of total digestible nutrients (TDN) and metabolizable energy (ME) are employed to arrive at the energy and protein

needs. TDN consumption is used as an indicator by various workers to represent energy intake.

Research observations at IVRI, CSWRI and other stations suggest that average consumption requirement of DM, TDN and DCP (digestible crude protein) of the ewes is 1105, 681 and 118 g/day respectively. Ram weighing 32 kg can be maintained on 397 g of TDN and 34 g of DCP per day. DM intake per 100 kg live weight is 3.35 kg, whereas TDN requirement is recommended at 1.3 kg/100 kg body weight. The results of trials of various levels of plane of nutrition on the performance of ewes and lambs (Patnayak and Singh, 1972) for major traits are as under (Table 7.5).

A high level of dietary protein in association with low energy plane does not produce satisfactory performance. Energy and protein in the diet should be in right proportion for optimum utilization and production.

A review made on research in India on nutrient requirement of sheep by Patnayak (1981) indicates that in adult non-producing animals TDN

Table 7.5: Performance of sheep at various levels of energy and protein consumption

Particulars	Plane of nutrition			
	High energy high protein	High energy low protein	Low energy high protein	Low energy low protein
A. Ewe performance				
Dry matter consumption (kg)	3.36	3.10	2.38	2.23
Lambing % (Av. of 6 reproductive cycles)	85.42	66.60	29.25	21.60
Mortality %	20.00	50.00	78	100.00
Wool production (kg) Av. of 3 years	1.90	1.70	0.9	0.7
B. Lamb performance				
Birth weight (kg)	3.25	2.47	2.54	2.23
Weight gain (kg)				
6 months	15.75	14.24	8.57	7.65
12 months	22.99	20.36	12.57	15.27
C. Dressing percentage				
6 months	45.9	44.1	44.0	38.3
12 months	50.4	49.9	44.3	45.0

Source: Patnayak and Singh (1972).

consumption varied from 340 to 450 g/day depending upon body weight and season in case of grazing animals. 10 g of TDN per kg live weight is enough for maintenance of sheep. To achieve growth rate of 100 g per day in lambs, approximately 25 g of TDN per kg live weight is required to be fed. The enhanced scale of 35 g TDN per kg live weight can bring about a growth of about 150 g (Table 7.6).

Table 7.6: Digestible crude protein requirement (g/day) for maintenance and growth of lambs (Patnayak, 1981)

Body wt. (kg)	Maintenance (g)	Weight gain (g)			
		50	100	150	200
5	10	15	20	25	30
10	16	20	25	30	35
15	21	23	34	40	47
20	26	34	42	50	58
25	31	41	50	59	69
30	36	47	57	68	79
35	40	52	64	76	89
40	44	58	71	84	98

Maintenance requirement of DCP are almost 1 g per kg live weight. In growing lambs 3 g of DCP per kg live weight is suggested. The suitable level of DCP to TDN ratio is 1:9. Lamb feed should have 13% crude protein. For adult animals a 10% level of CP is optimum (Table 7.7).

Table 7.7: Total digestible nutrient requirement (g/day) for maintenance and growth of lambs (Patnayak, 1981)

Body wt. (kg)	Maintenance (g)	Weight gain(g)			
		50	100	150	200
5	120	150	210	250	300
10	168	211	254	296	339
15	222	279	335	391	447
20	271	340	408	477	546
25	330	414	497	581	664
30	374	469	564	658	753
35	425	476	640	747	855
40	474	594	714	834	954

In general however, at twice the maintenance level of nutrients, the growth of 70 to 90 g is observed. Good growth is possible at thrice the maintenance requirements. These studies have provided a broad outline of energy—protein requirements of native sheep in our conditions.

Exhaustive studies about nutrient requirement for growth of lamb, gestation-cum-lactation and prime lamb development are called for.

Minerals and vitamins

The research work done in India has been reviewed by Patnayak (1981) and recommended maintenance levels are presented in Table 7.8.

Table 7.8: Requirement of different nutrients, minerals and vitamins for maintenance of an adult sheep weighing 35 kg/day

Nutrient/ mineral	Requirement per day	Mineral/vitamin/ nutrient	Requirement per day
Total feed	900 g	Co	0.2 mg
TDN	450 g	Zn	75 mg
DCP	45 g	Fe	60 mg
Ca	2.4 g	Mn	30 mg
P	2.0 g	1	0.1 mg
Mg	1.2 g	Mb	1.5 mg
NaCl	5.0 g	Se	0.15 mg
K	4.5 g	Carotene	1.5 mg
S	1.5 g	Vitamin A	750 IU
Cu	80 mg	Vitamin D	200 IU

COMMON FEED STUFFS—THEIR NUTRITIVE VALUES

Sheep consume forage including range land grasses, hay, bushes, top feeds, silage, etc. They utilize agro-industrial byproducts and feeds not appropriate for monogastrics. Sheep throughout the country depend on meagre range vegetation and natural pasture grasses and crop residues on cropped lands. These natural range and common grazing lands have generally been over-exploited and are dominated by extremely poor and generally annual grasses and shrubby vegetation.

These rangelands and natural pastures can hardly carry 1 sheep per hectare when unprotected and 2 sheep per hectare when protected. There is great prospect of improving these pastures through reseeding with more productive and nutritious perennial grasses and legumes and introducing fodder trees and shrubs. The nutrient content of roughages, concentrates and crop residues are presented in Table 7.9.

The tree leaves, referred to as emergency fodders for livestock form integral part of the feed for sheep. They serve as potential source of feed during December to March extending up to June when grazing material becomes scarce in arid and semi-arid regions and grazing lands are covered with snow in hilly areas. The nutritive value of important tree leaves is presented in Table 7.10.

Tree leaves contain anti-nutritive substances, i.e. tannins, which interfere with utilization of nutrients in feeds and fodders by complexing with various macromolecules, thereby making them inert to the action of digestive enzymes (Sharma and Samantha, 2003). The main anti-nutritional effects of tannins include reduction in voluntary feed intake, decreased digestibility of nutrients, adverse effects on rumen metabolism and toxicity. The total hydrolysable and condensed tannin contents of some common tree-leaves is presented in Table 7.11 Condensed tannins (CT) unlike hydrolysable tannins are not toxic to ruminants and when their concentration is below 4% of DM, they improve the nutritive value of herbage by binding to plant proteins and protecting them from excessive degradation in the rumen, besides preventing the establishment of parasitic nema- todes (Sahoo et al 2002; Sharma et al 2002, Min et al 2003). In addition bloat does not occur in ruminants fed forages containing condensed tannins (Singh and Bhat, 2001).

Table 7.9: Nutrient contents of common roughages, concentrates and crop residues (in per cent)

Feeds	DM	DCP	TDN	Ca	P
Dry roughages					
Pea straw	90	1.5	40.00	1.00	0.26
Arhar bhusa	90	4.0	45.8	1.4	0.06
Lucerne hay	85	11.0	50.0	1.42	0.22
Berseem hay	85	9.0	58.8	1.30	0.20
Cowpea hay	85	9.5	45.0	1.7	0.30
Masoor bhusa	90	4.0	44.0	1.3	0.05
Wheat bhusa	90	0	40.0	0.26	0.10
Paddy straw	90	0	45.0	0.14	0.05
Oat straw	90	0.8	41.0	0.30	0.09
Oat hay	85	4.8	45.0	0.33	0.17
Barley bhusa	90	0.8	44.0	0.30	0.08
Dry doob	85	4.5	40.0	0.36	0.10
Jowar Karbi	90	2.8	40.0	0.33	0.05
Green roughages					
Berseem	15	2.5	12.0	1.5	0.16
Guar	20	1.4	10.00	1.3	0.05
Lucerne	18	3.2	12.0	1.4	0.25
Cowpea	18	3.5	10.6	1.4	0.14
Pea	15	2.5	12.5	1.0	0.30

Table 7.9: Nutrient contents of common roughages, concentrates and crop residues (in per cent) *(Contd.)*

Feeds	DM	DCP	TDN	Ca	P
Sorghum/Jowar	25	1.0	16.0	0.50	0.10
Bajra	25	1.2	15.0	0.12	0.40
Maize	25	1.2	16.5	0.65	0.14
Guinnea grass	25	1.1	12.6	0.35	0.06
Napier	25	1.5	15.5	0.50	0.40
Maize silage	30	1.1	18.0	0.7	0.15
Para grass	25	1.5	11.5	0.4	0.10
Oat	25	2.6	16.5	1.4	0.21
Jowar silage	30	1.0	18.0	0.55	0.14
Concentrates/Grains					
Wheat	90	–	40.0	0.05	0.39
Barley	90	7.5	77.0	0.08	0.38
Oat	90	7.0	71.0	0.09	0.39
Maize	90	7.5	84.0	0.02	0.26
Gram	90	12.8	75.0	0.45	0.36
Arhar	90	13.0	68.0	0.35	0.38
Bajra	90	6.5	58.0	0.12	0.38
Jowar	90	7.0	68.0	0.03	0.30
Oilseeds and cakes					
Cotton seed	90	8.0	87.0	0.30	1.28
Cotton seed cake	90	18.0	72.0	0.28	1.25
Linseed cake	90	30.0	65.0	0.37	0.80
Groundnut cake	90	41.0	74.0	0.12	0.50
Sesame cake	90	38.0	78.0	2.0	1.60
Mustard cake	90	26.0	80.5	0.80	1.15
Linseed	90	7.5	85.0	0.50	1.00
Soybean meal	90	40.0	75.0	0.25	0.65
Animal byproducts					
Bone meal	90	21.0	69.0	29.00	14.00
Fish meal	90	45.0	65.0	5.00	3.30
Blood meal	90	89.0	90.0	0.30	0.25
Meat meal	90	50.0	65.0	9.80	4.50
Cereal byproducts					
Wheat bran	90	11.0	67.0	0.14	0.85
Rice bran	90	7.0	60.0	–	–
Pulse Chuni	90	12.0	68.0	0.40	0.35
Gram husk	90	0.3	54.0	0.22	0.20
Rice polish	90	12.0	67.0	0.24	0.50

Source: Prasad, J. (1996).

Table 7.10: Nutritive values of common fodder tree leaves (DM basis)

Trees	DCP (kg)	TDN (kg)	DE (Mcal per kg)	ME (Mcal per kg)
Ardu (A.grandis)	13.0	63.0	–	–
Banj (Quercus incania/glauca	5.7	43.7	1.92	1.58
Beri (Ziziphus jujuba)	3.1	30.7	1.35	1.10
Bamboo (Dendrocalamus strictus)	9.3	48.8	2.15	1.76
Bahera (Belesia)	16.7	54.6	2.40	1.97
Dhaman/Biul (Grewia oppositi folia)	16.7	54.6	2.40	1.97
Bel (Aegle marmelos)	10.8	56.7	2.40	2.04
Bargad (Ficus benghalensis)	0.81	17.8	0.78	0.64
Gauj (Millettia auriculata)	15.5	44.9	1.98	1.62
Jamun (Syzygium cumini)	0.02	17.5	0.77	0.63
Pakar (Ficus infectora)	1.61	18.3	0.81	0.66
Jharberi (Ziziphus nummularia)	5.5	51.1	2.26	1.84
Kachnar (Bauhinia variegata)	9.2	55.5	2.45	2.00
Khair (Acacia catechu)	2.9	46.3	2.04	1.67
Lasora (Cordia obliquoa)	5.4	26.9	1.18	0.97
Neem (Azadirachta indica)	8.4	53.3	2.34	1.92
Pipal (Ficus religiosa)	7.0	38.3	1.68	1.38
Sirin (Albizia lebbek)	10.5	49.3	2.17	1.61
Tilonj (Quercus dilatata)	4.2	43.2	1.92	1.58

Source: Ranjan et al (1959).

Table 7.11: Total tannin, hydrolysable and condensed tannin contents of common tree leaves (in per cent)

Sl. no.	Tree leave	Total tannin (%)	Hydrolysable tannin (%)	Condensed tannin (%)
1.	Bauhinia variegata	5.41	1.21	4.20
2.	Butea monosperma	1.05	0.75	0.30
3.	Grewia optiva	1.33	1.26	0.07
4.	Ficus religiosa	1.63	1.17	0.46
5.	Morus alba (shah toot)	0.75	0.69	0.06
6.	Quercus dilatata	4.65	3.87	0.78
7.	Quercus leucotricophora (Banj)	2.97	1.99	0.98
8.	Salix alba	0.80	0.71	0.09
9.	Melia azedarach (Drank)	1.30	1.18	0.12
10.	Olea ferruginea Indian olive, kohu	1.21	1.15	0.06
11.	Carissa spinarum	4.90	0.37	4.53

Source: Sharma et al (2000).

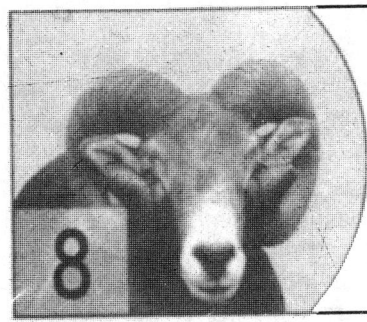

RUMINAL DEVELOPMENT AND SHEEP DIGESTION

ANATOMY OF RUMINANT STOMACH

The stomach in ruminants is very large and occupies nearly three-fourths of the abdominal cavity. It almost fills the left half of the cavity and extends considerably over the median plane into the right half. It consists of rumen, reticulum, omasum and abomasum. The division is indicated externally by grooves. The first three parts are often regarded as proventriculi or oesophageal sacculations, since they are lined, with a mucous membrane which is covered with stratified *squamous* epithelium and is non-glandular. The abomasum has a glandular mucous-membrane and is known as *true stomach*. The oesophagus opens into the stomach as a sort of dome, the *atrium ventriculi*. The abomasum joins the intestines.

Development of rumen in a young animal

At birth the true stomach, the abomasum, constitutes about 50% of the total stomach in sheep and other ruminants. In the subsequent weeks the position alters in the proportional development of various chambers of stomach. The initiation of starter ration helps in transition (Table 8.1).

At four months the rumen and reticulum are about twice as large as the omasum and abomasum together, but are collapsed and functionless.

Exterior of rumen has two surfaces, the parietal is convex and related to diaphragm. Visceral is irregular and related to omasum, abomasum, liver and spleen. Two curvatures are dorsal and ventral. Dorsal is related to roof of abdominal cavity and ventral to its corresponding floor. Extremities are anterior and posterior or pelvic. Posterior extremity has got ventral blind sacs. Interior of rumen is partially divided into dorsal and ventral sacs by the pillars which are folds of wall with additional muscular fibres. Anterior pillar projects backward and continues on either side as relatively narrow right and left pillars. Posterior pillar is nearly horizontal. It separates large dorsal and ventral posterior blind sacs and branches into dorsal and ventral coronary bands. Rumino-reticular fold corresponds to rumino-reticular groove and is opposite to 7th–8th ribs. Its dorsal

Table 8.1: The relative size of compartments of ruminant stomach at different ages

Name of compartments	Age in weeks						
	0	4	8	12	16	20–26	34–38
	Size as % space occupied						
1. Rumen and reticulum	38	52	60	64	67	64	64
2. Omasum	13	12	13	14	18	22	25
3. Abomasum	49	36	27	22	15	14	11

edge is concave and forms margin of rumino-reticular orifice.

The mucous membrane is brown except on margins of pillars where it is pale and studded with papillae approximately 10 to 12 mm long. Three types of papillae are mostly found in rumen.

Figure 8.1 shows the development of ruminant stomach.

1. Folliate—longest in size.
2. Filiform—medium, and
3. Club shaped or conical

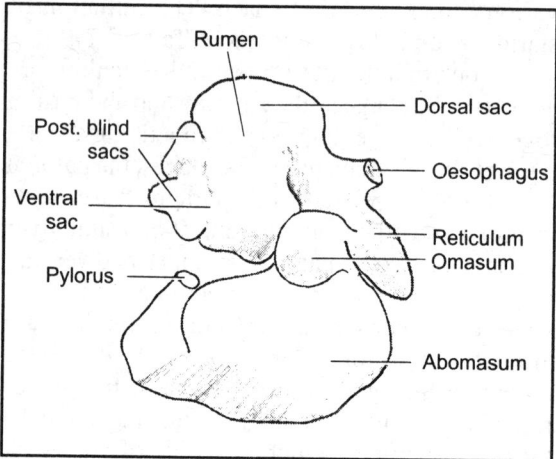

Stomach of adult ruminant

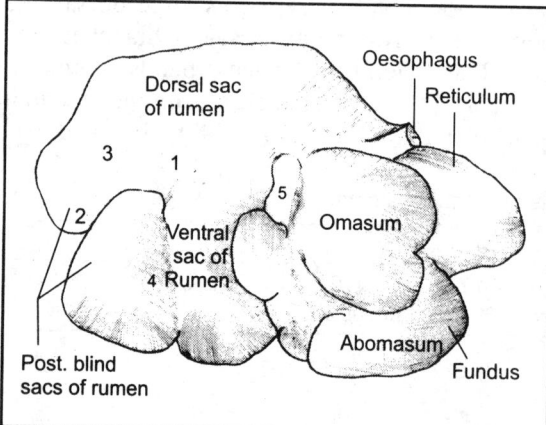

Fig. 8.1. Development of ruminant stomach.

Oesophageal groove: It begins at the cardiac end and passes ventrally on the medial wall and ends in reticulo-omasal orifice, which lies ventral to the 8th or 9th rib. Its length is 16 to 20 cm.

Reticulum: It is generally honeycombed. The mucous membranae is raised into folds about 10–12 mm high enclosing 4, 5, 6 sided cells. These folds are again subdivided by smaller folds and in the bottom studded with horny and pointed papillae.

Omasum: It is occupied by about 100 longitudinal folds—the *laminae omasii*. In cross section there are shorter laminae or still shorter of 3rd and 4th order. These are series of very low folds.

Sulcus omasii: It is a groove extending from reticulo-omasal opening to the omaso-abomasal opening and is 10 cm long. In the neck of omasum, the laminae change into thick folds, bear unguli form papillae. Omaso-abomasal orifice is oval, long and bound by thick muscular pillars-omasal pillars.

Abomasum: Consists of two parts—fundic and pyloric. The organ is divided into areas by constriction. First with many spiral folds and second resembles with that of horse stomach. Pyloric orifice is small and rounded. The fundus part of abomasum is adherent to rumen. It has got two surfaces, two curvatures and two extremities. Parietal surface is in contact mainly with abdomen floor and visceral surface for the most part related to rumen and omasum.

PHYSIOLOGY AND RUMINAL DIGESTION

The rumen is a storage chamber where the sheep keeps the ingesta. After grazing the animal retires to a shady and comfortable place to chew the cud, thereby, making a large amount of fermentation to take place in the ruminal storage. If left undisturbed the regurgitation of the ruminal contents takes place at almost a regular sequence. The churning movements of the rumen can be observed at a frequency of two in three minutes or so. Different types of micro organisms found in the rumen are bacteria, protozoa and fungi. These include:

Rumen bacteria

Cellulose degrading rumen bacteria

1. *Bacteroides succinogenes*
2. *Ruminococcus flavefaciens*
3. *Ruminococcus albus*
4. *Clostridium loccheadii*
5. *Eubacterium cellulosolvens*

Hemicellulose degrading rumen bacteria

1. *Butyrivibrio fibrisolvens*
2. *Eubacterium uniforme*
3. *Eubacterium xylanophilum*
4. *Coprococcus entactus*

Starch degrading rumen bacteria

1. *Streptococcus bovis*
2. *Ruminobacter amylophilus*
3. *Ruminobacter ruminicola*
4. *Succinomonas amylolytica*
5. *Succiniovibrio dextrinosolvens*

Sugar fermenting rumen bacteria

1. *Lactobacillus ruminis*
2. *Lactobacillus vitulinus*

Protein degrading rumen bacteria

1. *Bacteroides ruminicola*
2. *Bacteroides amylophilus*
3. *Butyrivibrio fibrisolvens*

Xylan degrading rumen bacteria

1. *Butyrivibrio fibrisolvens*
2. *Selenomonas ruminantium*
3. *Streptococcus bovis*
4. *Bacteroides ruminicola*

Acid utilizing rumen bacteria

1. *Megasphaera elsdenii*
2. *Veillonela parvula*
3. *Wolinella succinogenes*
4. *Oxalobacter formigenes*

Lipid degrading rumen bacteria

1. *Anaerovibrio lipolytica*

Methane generating rumen bacteria

1. *Methanobrevibacter ruminantium*
2. *Methanosarcina barkeri*

Urea hydrolysing rumen bacteria

1. *Streptococcus species*
2. *Staphylococcus species*
3. *Micrococcus species*
4. *Propionibacterium species*

Rumen protozoa

Cellulose utilizing rumen protozoa

1. *Eudiplodinium maggi*
2. *Epidinium ecaudatum*
3. *Diploplastron affine*

Hemicellulose and pectin utilizing rumen protozoa

1. *Epidinium ecaudatum*
2. *Eudiplodinium maggi*
3. *Polyplastron multivesculatum*

Starch utilising protozoa

1. *Entodinium caudatum*
2. *Entodinium bursa*
3. *Polyplastron multivesculatum*

Protein utilising rumen protozoa

1. *Entodinium caudatum*
2. *Entodinium simplex*

Rumen fungi

1. *Neocallimastix frontalis*
2. *Piromonas communis*

Production of volatile fatty acids

As a result of fermentation of complex carbohydrates the most important fatty acids produced

are acetic, propionic and butyric acid. The concentration of these fatty acids in the rumen content increases after feeding. Concentration of VFAs depend on the nature of diet. Foods with a high content of soluble sugars produce a rapid rise in fatty acids concentration. Starchy foods such as cereals and grains produce a slower rise, i.e. maintained over a still longer periods. The concentration of fatty acids in the rumen gives no accurate idea of the rate of production which is merely a measure of balance between production, absorption and passage from the rumen to the omasum as the food passes down the gastro-intestinal (GI) tract. The concentration of VFAs in the rumen may be as high as 12% of the dry matter.

The fatty acids are absorbed into the blood directly from the rumen and also from the omasum. Hence their level in the omasum is lower than in the rumen. It is still lower in the abomasum where it may be almost negligible. Finally large concentration of fatty acids also occur in the caecum where the fermentation similar to that in the rumen occurs.

VFAs after absorption enter the blood stream and are taken to the liver where propionic acid is converted rapidly to glucose. The rapidity of this conversion is clearly demonstrated by the effects of injecting sodium propionate, a salt of propionic acid, into normal sheep. 5 minutes after injection of 0.15 g of propionic acid per kg of body weight the blood sugar increases from a normal level of 40 mg/100 ml to approximately 80 mg/100 ml. This conversion has also been studied in sheep with very low blood glucose level following insulin treatment. Blood glucose rose from 4 mg/100 ml to 19 mg/100 ml blood in 8 minutes and to 31 mg/100 ml after 20 minutes. By 8th minute all the symptoms of hypoglycaemia disappeared.

Energy is derived from the VFAs which are the end products of carbohydrate digestion and to some extent from amino acids. Energy from these sources reaches the tissues largely in the form of glucose and acetic acid. Very little glucose is absorbed from the gastro intestinal tract of sheep. Therefore, the value of a pasture or of a ration may depend largely on the amounts of acetic, propionic and butyric acids produced from it and on its protein content.

Deficiency of feeds from which glucose can be formed is the main cause of energy deficiency in the diet of pregnant ewes. The effects of glucose deficiency are seen in those tissues that specifically require glucose, e.g. central nervous system in the ewes and of the developing foetus. Supply of energy or of glucose to these tissues depends largely on the level of glucose in the circulating blood.

Effect of nature of diet

The fibrous nature of pasture forage governs the rate of passage of ingesta through the alimentary tract. It also determines the amount of VFAs formed in the rumen and their rate of absorption. The diet also influences the amount of ammonia formed. To make an accurate evaluation of a pasture to sheep is difficult until all the aforesaid variables are examined precisely in relation to the energy requirements of sheep during pregnancy or otherwise.

The concentration of rumen microflora are in fluctuating state. Even within the sacchrolytic group the change in pasture, foliage or feed, result in a gradual increase or decrease of fermenting microflora depending upon the type and complexity of carbohydrates in the diet.

The proportion of VFAs in the rumen have been found to change after the penned sheep have eaten different diets. On all roughage diet the acetic acid accounts for about 75% of the total VFAs. If wheat, grain lucerne and maize was added to diet the total VFA content included about 63 to 65% acetic acid, 18 to 20% propionic acid and 16 to 18% butyric acid. When sheep are fed rations rich in starch, large quantities of lactic acid are produced and increase the acidity of rumen to a pH level around 5.0 and depress the production of propionic acid. The amount of saliva and ammonia formation during fermentation may also alter the relationship between VFAs content and the pH of rumen.

Sheep are predominantly graziers, but most of the study and research findings are based on stall fed cattle. The physiological differences that exist in sheep particularly are that:

1. the proportional growth of ovine foetus is rapid and it is extremely demanding. The foetus increases quickly as gestation advances.
2. The ewe body has comparatively smaller reserves of energy and the ability of pasture to meet the energy needs of breeding/pregnant ewes are often debatable, many ewes remain undernourished during late pregnancy.

Thus, the likely changes in the rumen of grazing sheep are more difficult to assess because feed intake is spread over a longer period of each day and the VFAs get constantly absorbed through the rumen wall. To measure the VFA production of such sheep (on grazing or ration) it is necessary to know:

- The amount of VFAs in the rumen itself.
- The rate at which the blood flows from the ruminal wall.
- The amount of fatty acids flowing from rumen into blood.

RUMINAL ABSORPTION

Ruminal digestion is a continuous process and volatile fatty acids are constantly being absorbed. Either these are used by certain tissues or are converted into glucose by the liver. Anything that interferes with grazing may interfere with the supply of energy and eventually lower the blood glucose level.

This process of anabolism and catabolism is controlled by the hormones secreted by adrenal cortex and anterior pituitary. Cortisol (ACTH) produced by the former stimulates the formation of glycogen in liver, muscles and transformation of proteins into blood sugar. The hormones of anterior pituitary and pancreas (insulin) influence the regulation of any fall in blood level if the demand for nutrients outstrips the supply. This break down of glycogen, fats and other body reserves depends on the rate at which some byproducts of catabolism as ketones can be disposed off by the liver.

The blood ketone level of a healthy nonpregnant ewe is usually 2 to 3 mg/100 ml of blood. When the liver is unable to dispose off the ketone bodies due to increased breakdown of reserves, the blood level may rise rapidly to exceed 20 mg/100 ml blood.

Blood glucose and ketone level analysis serve as useful indicators of nutrition and state of the pregnant ewe. Ewe flock on a falling body condition in advanced pregnancy period provides evidence of under nutrition if 10% of ewes have blood glucose around 25 mg per 100 ml coupled with ketone level of 10 mg/100 ml or more.

Control of blood glucose status

The amount of blood sugar in the ewe depends on:

- The rate at which propionic acid and amino acids are absorbed from the rumen and small intestines respectively and converted into glucose in the liver.
- The rate at which glucose is removed from the blood stream by the maternal tissues.
- The rate at which glucose is utilised by the developing foetus as such or for production of fructose.
- The rate at which glucose is mobilised from body stores of glycogen and tissue proteins.

The rate at which the volatile fatty acids are absorbed depends largely on the rate at which they are formed. This in turn is governed by the quantity and quality of pasture and the rate of food passage through the alimentary tract. Fibrous feed passes slowly through the rumen, thus depresses daily feed intake and reduces the amount of nutrient availability to the sheep.

As gestation advances the volume of uterus increases, pressure on ruminal volume ensues. Thus it is generally preferred to offer the ewe, feed frequently but at smaller intervals to maintain better feed intake levels.

COMMON NUTRITION RELATED DISORDERS

The common nutrition related disorders in sheep are:

Urinary calculi: is a problem associated with males, wethers and symptoms include difficult urination, straining, kicking at belly, bladder rupture (if stone lodged in the urethra) and finally death. It results due to accumulation of mineral stones. This can be prevented by management of dietary Ca: P ratios of greater than 2:1 and provision of ammonium sulphate (0.5%) in the diet (Church, et al, 1995) Stud rams maintained on high rations are prone to urolithiasis. The sigmoid flexure in the urethra complicates the expulsion of calculi or easing of retention of urine.

Enterotoxaemia type D (over eating disease): Is a very common nutritional problem occurring in animals on high quality (usually grain) diets. Incidence is further increased when the new stock enters fresh clover rich pastures. Symptoms include depression, abdominal pain and grinding of teeth. Sudden deaths may ensue. In per-acute cases young sheep die in the pasture without giving any chance for treatment. It is caused by *Clostridium perfringens* type D and can be prevented by timely vaccination.

Stiff lamb disease (white muscle disease): It is a nutritional muscular dystrophy, usually seen in animals of 6 to 8 weeks age and caused by deficiency of Se, vitamin E or both. The symptoms include low growth rate, difficult movements, stiff legs and finally death. Provision of adequate dietary Se and vitamin E prevents its occurrence.

Ketosis (pregnancy toxaemia, lambing paralysis): It occurs usually in poor condition animals (with twins or triplets) towards the end of gestation and is associated with the high demand of carbohydrates. The high demand for carbohydrates results in the depletion of body reserves, leading to higher levels of ketone bodies in the blood and urine. The symptoms include laboured breathing, staggering, impaired vision, breath and urine smell sweet. Specific dietary deficiencies of cobalt and possibly phosphorus may also lead to high incidence of ketosis, which may occur due to low intake of total digestible nutrients. But in cobalt associated deficiency the essential defect is failure to metabolize propionic acid into the TCA cycle (Radostits et al; 1995). Fat ewes experience a voluntary fall in feed intake in late pregnancy due to the reduction of the rumen volume by the pressure of intra-abdominal fat and the developing foetus. The disease can be prevented by adequate dietary carbohydrate sources during late gestation and can be treated by provision of propylene glycol or corn syrup by drench two to five times a day until the dam recovers. It is also recommended to increase the carbohydrate content of the ration for remaining gestation period.

'Sway back' post natal or young lamb lumbar paralysis: Appears within two to three week stage due to copper-cobalt deficiency. The salient development is dragging of hind limbs and 'dog sitting posture' of the lamb. Adequate levels of these elements in the diet of pregnant ewe brings down the incidence of 'Sway back'.

Some other nutrition disorders may result due to consumption of toxic or poisonous plants and feeds. Toxic or poisonous plants include those that are cyanogenic, contain alkaloids, or are photodynamic and may produce mechanical injury.

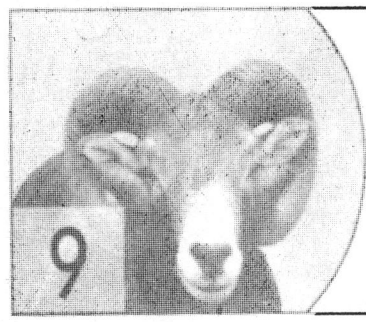

PRE-BREEDING MANAGEMENT OF FLOCK

PROCESS OF REPRODUCTION

In flock breeding the contribution of ram and ewe is at par. It is ultimately a single germ cell shared by each sex that normally unites to produce a lamb. Though the participation of ram is brief, yet it is attached a spatial breeding status. Only a limited 2 to 4 percent breeding males are maintained and cared for against every 100 or odd number of ewes. However, in the reproductive process or lamb bearing ewe is the sole participant. Right from the shedding of scarcer ovum, showing receptability and ram acceptability; efficient sperm transport, fertilization of ovum; implantation of embryo to carriage of pregnancy till viable lamb delivery is a body function of the ewe. Rearing of the lamb too, exclusively rests on the ewe.

Organs of reproduction

Ewe: The reproduction organs of the ewe consist of the vagina, uterus (os, uterine body and the uterine horns), the Fallopian tubes and the ovaries (Table 9.1). The nonpregnant uterus is hollow muscular organ, 7–8 cm long. Its body is short divided into two horns and swept into larger curves. Each horn communicates with the body cavity through the uterine or Fallopian tubes. The junction of each tube with its respective horn is known as uterotubal junction. At the other end uterus continues as a narrow canal of the cervix (os uterus) into the vagina which in turn terminates externally at the vulval lips.

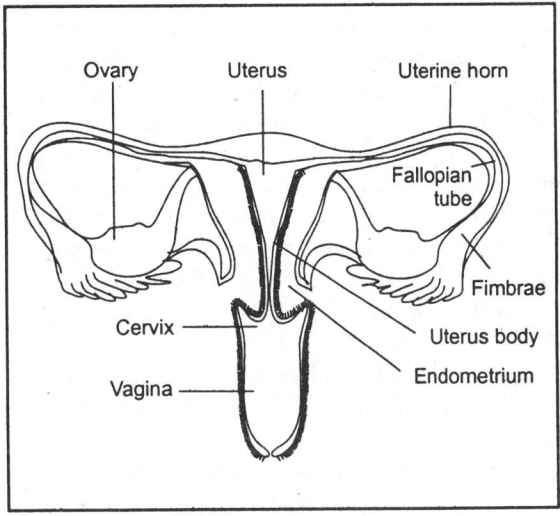

Fig. 9.1. Reproductive organs of ewe

The cervix of the ewe is thick muscular small lumen structure, with numerous folds lined with mucous membrane. The narrow tight passage forbids easy entry of insemination tube or probe into uterus. The walls of the uterus are about 1/2 to 3/4 cm thick and are mainly composed of smooth muscle fibres. There is enough elastic tissue particularly in the cervix region. This enables stretching and great expansion which is necessary at parturition time.

The mucous membrane lining the uterus is known as endometrium. It is in close contact with the deeper muscle layers of the uterine wall. Its thick deep cells are simple tubular and glandular in nature. On the internal lining of the uterus there exist numerous specialised areas known as cotyledons, the seats of attachment of foetal membranes. In a nonpregnant ewe these are small and slightly raised structures. During pregnancy they become greatly enlarged to provide sound attachment of membranes.

The cells lining the upper part of Fallopian tubes possess thin hairy ciliary growths which tend to move the ovum (when shed) down the tube through wave like motions. The vagina is lined with numerous layers of flat cells.

Ovaries are somewhat oval bodies about 1.5 cm in size and are covered by a special layer of cells known as germinal epithelium. The ovaries are formed during the early phase of foetal development, when groups of cells grow down from the germinal epithelium to form small nests known as primordial follicles. At birth each ovary contains many thousands of these follicles. When the young ewe attains sexual maturity they commence to develop successively. Cells in each follicle enlarge to form an ovum. As the follicle begins to mature it gets filled with a clear fluid which gives it a blister like appearance. Ovulation occurs when the follicle bursts and the ovum escapes (surrounded by a number of cells known as the cumulus).

The space left in the ovary by the ruptured follicle is soon filled with clotted blood. Later this is replaced by larger cells containing a yellow pigment. Therefrom develops the corpus luteum which is reddish brown in colour in case of ewe, rather than the yellow body in cattle.

Ram: The reproductive organs of a male sheep comprise the following.

1. a pair of testicles (testes) contained in the scrotal sac and separated by a septum. The scrotal sac hangs down externally. These glandular structures are solid mass of cells with germinal epithelial layers of cell on the inner most zone.

2. Epididymis: Is distinctly divided into three zones, head, body and tail and is the seat of maturation of sperms and passage from the testes to the exterior as seminal discharge through the vas deference, 'the spermatic cord'.

3. Spermatic cord proceeds from the posterior to the anterior along with urethra to open at the penile orifice externally for the discharge of seminal fluid, the semen containing sperms.

Endocrine control

The reproduction activity is regulated by pituitary *(hypophysis cerebri)* the mastergland located at the base of brain. The diverse external stimuli of light, heat, sound, smell, scenics, etc. originating from environment are received by the hypothalamus through the nerve cells. These are transmitted via neurons to the pituitary. The hypothalamus-hypophyseal mechanism is further linked with the whole endocrine system (Fig. 9.2).

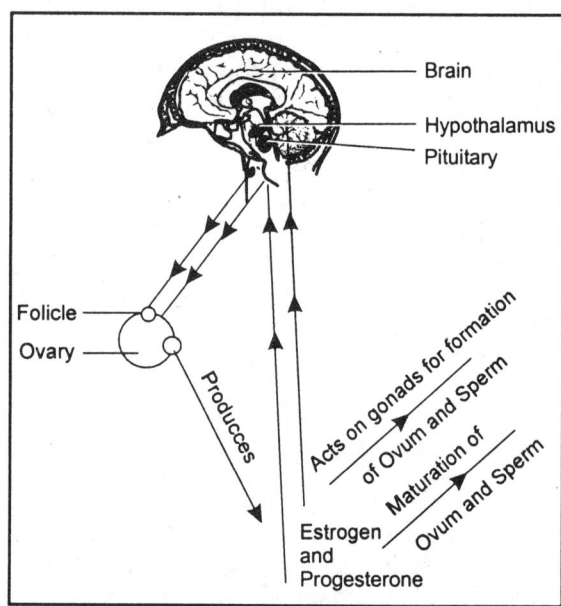

Fig. 9.2. Hypothalamus-pituitary-gonadal hormone complex

HYPOTHALAMUS-PITUITARY-GONADAL HORMONE COMPLEX

The hypothalamus produces gonadotropin geleasing factor (GnRH), which initiate the release of gonadotropin hormones from the pituitary, viz. luteinizing hormone (LH) and follicle stimulating hormone (FSH). Action of LH and FSH in both sexes is almost similar on the respective germ cells, but the levels in female is cyclic and vary at different phases of reproductive cell development and release.

Ovary produces a primary steroid hormone the oestrogen. Female puberty-maturity including development of udder tissue is mainly attributed to this hormone. Besides, it is responsible for the preparation of sex organs like vagina, cervix, uterus, etc. for male acceptability and covering. Its action causes shedding of ovum from the ovary.

Corpus luteum formed after the release of egg, produces another steroid hormone the progesterone, also named as pregnancy hormone. This takes care of the fertilized egg right from embryo implantation and foetal development till successful termination of pregnancy. Thus it is hypothalamic–pituitary–gonadal complex which controls the reproduction process.

Male sex hormones, the androgens, are also steroid in nature and produced by the testes. Like oestrogen in the female, the testosterone is the major most androgen of male, responsible for sperm production, male puberty, libido and masculinity; and development of allied characteristics.

Fertilization

Ovary produces egg cells (ova). All the ovarian follicles that start developing in the ovary do not reach final maturation and shedding stage together. At the end of oestrus one or a couple of eggs may be shed due to rising blood level of gonadotrophic hormones. Fimbrae or the finger like projections of the fallopian tubes pick up the ovum after shedding. The ovum further slips through the oviduct, being slimy, to reach the uterine horn. The slimy cover, the *zona pellucida,* acts as a barrier for entry of sperms other than of the same specie in the egg wall.

The male gonads of ram, the testes, like males of other mammalians have millions of primordial cells which give rise to spermatocytes. These develop into sperms. On releasing from testes these propel to epididymis. Maturation into a mobile cellular structure having clear head, mid piece and tail takes place in the epididymis. Genetic material is contained in the cytoplasm of the head covered by 'acrosome'. Secretions of accessory glands provide requisite floating material 'the seminal discharge'. While the tail portion imparts motility to the sperm, mid portion provides energy and enzyme hyalurinidase in the acrosome serves to dissolve the zona pellucida of the egg wall on coming in contact.

Out of millions of sperms in the ejaculate only a single sperm succeeds in penetrating the egg wall and fusing together of the DNA material (nuclei) of both cells takes place. The egg cell wall then becomes refractive to the penetration of other sperms, which ultimately perish.

The sperm count in a healthy ram ejaculate is almost a thousand million per millilitre. On insemination of semen or depositing into ewe's vagina on mating with the ram, the sperms move first through the cervix into the uterus and fertilization of the ovum normally occurs in the horns of the uterus. The fertilized egg, the embryo, starts dividing into 2,4,8 and 16 cell mass called the 'morula'. With further division embryo is a mass of cells with a fluid filled cavity. The 'blastocyst' (as named at this stage) descends to uterus body for implantation in the uterine endometrium.

Reproductive planning

The reproduction management of sheep is quite complex, particularly in enflock breeding and under varying rearing systems. Thus proper know how of conditions, the nature of animal, physio-environmental aspects and allied activities is desirable.

Though the ram is half of the flock and demands utmost care and minutest scrutiny the selection and preparation of breedable flock mothers too can in no way be neglected. The sound planning of all operations is a part of successful pre-breeding management. The flock owner or the incharge farm has to ensure the mating ewes in ready to breed condition at appropriate season and time simultaneous to sound maintenance and feeding. A detailed checkup of rams and ewes for reproductive health is an important routine. Fitness should be ascertained by individual handling and examination a couple of weeks in advance.

BREEDING ASPECTS

Breeding age

Maturity and puberty in sheep though related, are not synonymous. The former implies attainment of physical growth of body, bone and muscles and the latter is the development of genitalia and hormonal system, i.e. sexual maturity or breeding fitness in other words, prerequisite to normal reproduction. The native sheep show an early maturity preceding puberty. A Deccani, Nali, Gaddie ewe or any other sheep breed of Indian origin is fit to receive the ram and bear a lamb around 1½ year age. Instances are common where female sheep kept in association of rams in stationary and well fed conditions mothered a lamb at just 14 to 15 month age.

Gupta and Chopra (1974) reported that Rambouillet crossbreds of Gaddie and Poonchi sheep and even graded ones continued gaining size and weight up to 2½ year age irrespective of their genetic group variations. Various sheep farms postpone first joining of rams in the maiden ewes at 1½ year age as they are unable to nurture the lamb well. Even the Rambouillet ewes which attained breeding capability at 15 to 18 months in the home country failed to show off the tendency at the same age in their Indian born progeny. Their breeding is generally delayed till 1½ to 2 year age. At Govt. Sheep Farms in Jammu and Kashmir state just 15 to 20% of maiden Rambouillet ewes attained desired growth and mammary gland development by 1½ year age for viable rearing of an off spring. Capacity for early breeding is no doubt advantageous but underdeveloped udder condition exposes the lambs to starvation and increased losses (Figs 9.3 and 9.4).

The fitness of a male sheep for tupping is invariably considered at 1½ year age and above. However, at very many occasions ram lambs of 5 to 6 months age, running with the flocks of shepherds are noticed covering the ewes and producing inbred progenies.

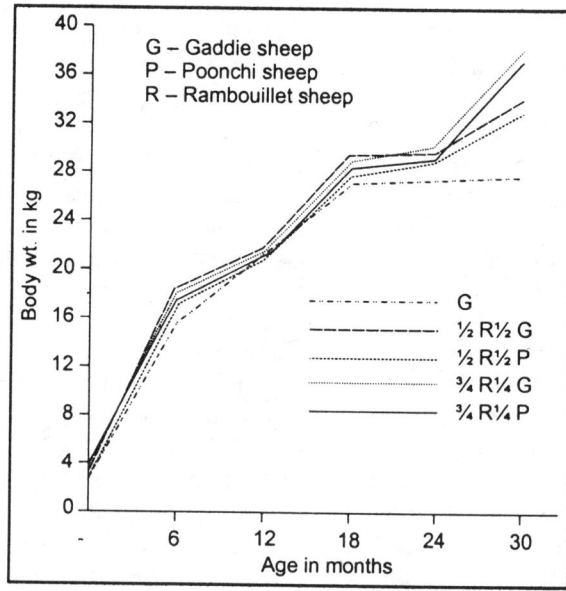

Fig. 9.3. Graph showing trend in body weight gains of various genetic groups of sheep at a J&K Farm (Gupta and Chopra, 1974).

Breeding season

In this context pattern of breeding season, factors controlling the breeding season and basic information for the development of suitable systems and practices of husbandry invite our attention. Many breeds of sheep exhibit a definite breeding season which restrict them to the production of one crop of lambs in a year. Merinos and some other breeds have an extended breeding season and are capable of breeding three times in two years.

There is a common trend in sexual activity of all the indigenous flocks irrespective of breed or location. Western area and Deccan plateau ewes generally come in heat regularly during spring. Deccani sheep, too breed through out the year but have three peaks. North temperate region sheep exhibit oestrus twice annually but of distinct intensity, short and mild in spring and longer and intense in autumn.

There is a variation in the occurrence of oestrus in the same ewe from year to year. Differences are also observed between the incidence and onset of oestrus amongst ewes of the same breed of

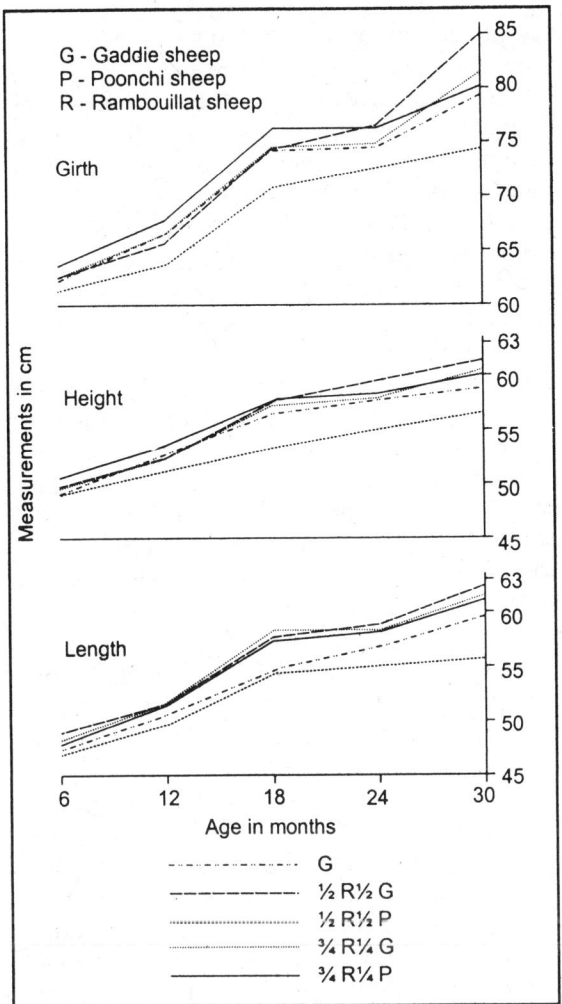

G - Gaddie sheep
P - Poonchi sheep
R - Rambouillat sheep

Girth

Height

Length

Measurements in cm

Age in months

```
------------- G
------------- ½ R ½ G
............. ½ R ¼ P
............. ¾ R ¼ G
------------- ¾ R ¼ P
```

Fig. 9.4. Graph showing trend in body size (measurement) gains of various genetic groups of sheep at a J&K sheep farm (Gupta and Chopra, 1975).

different ages and between ewes of same age but of different breeds. The sheep in north temperate region are by and large bred from September to November. However, the stray entry of a ram in an ewes flock during May to July often results in producing unplanned progeny in early winter.

Gradual decrease in day length (light hours) during change from summer to autumn and thence to winter is known to influence the breeding season. Fertility of sheep is related to the changes

in day length that occur between the longest and shortest days in the two hemispheres. The August to November is the main breeding season in the sheep of Northern hemisphere and February to April in the Southern hemisphere.

The decreasing day length or light hours set in motion the oestrus in most of the sheep flocks. The common physiological explanation advanced for this change in breeding season with changing light is that:

1. The light or photo-stimulus received by eye and the temporal region stimulates the anterior pituitary. An increased release of FSH takes place which in turn stimulates the ripening of the ovarian follicle and the secretion of oestrogen.
2. Light is concerned only so far as it provides the means of keeping the animal awake and that stimulation of the pituitary is affected by consequent changes in metabolism.

During breeding season when the ewes are run with a teaser/vasectomised ram it brings in sudden association of sexes and provides stimulus that usually occurs at normal joining. The breeding season is considered to have commenced when oestrus recurs regularly in the majority of ewes in a flock. At the beginning of season there may be considerable variation in the length of oestrus cycle. The occurrence of oestrus, stimulus and consequent sexual activity when the rams are joined with ewes are important from conception and fertility aspects. About 80% of the ewes in north temperate flocks show oestrus within the first 17 to 20 days after joining in early September. There after, the majority of non-conceived ewes come in heat every 16 to 17 days. This interval increases as the breeding season progresses.

The non-breeding season is the period when after joining of rams the majority of ewes are likely to be anoestrus. Wide variations in the incidence and onset of oestrus may be observed in the non-breeding season. Changes in ovarian activity associated with oestrus occur in vaginal contents of some ewes during greater part of non-breeding season, where as some other ewes fail to exhibit typical vaginal changes during oestrus in the normal breeding season. At the beginning and towards the end of each breeding season some ewes experience the so-called 'silent heat'. They shed an ovum without showing signs of heat.

Other observations

Variations are observed in other physiological changes associated with oestrus. These influence the result of mating. For instance the time between the onset of heat and shedding of ovum decreases as the breeding season advances. Likewise the length of oestrus and the number of twin ovulation gradually increase to maximum by the middle of breeding season. The net result is that if the rams are fertile, the proportion of fertile mating increases to reach its maximum at the middle of breeding season.

The duration of heat in sheep generally ranges between 16 to 36 hours. Ovulation takes place between 1 to 2 days after the start of heat. The postpartum heat occurs from almost three weeks to three months. Majority of the lactating ewes have a postpartum interval of 40 to 60 days.

On these observation it is based that at least some sheep of Indian breeds can be exploited to obtain two crops of lambs in a year, though in practice, the feasibility of more than one lambing per ewe per year appears remote. However, by modifying the management suitably the proposition of obtaining of three lamb crops in two years is advocated for good dividends.

Indigenous sheep do breed under usual environmental temperatures in the arid and semi-arid regions. The temperate zone sheep, the exotic cross breds and the pure exotic sheep need a lower temperature and cooler environment. The length of oestrus duration is not materially affected on a low or a high plane of nutrition in the native sheep.

Trends in breeding season

Limited information and only a few reports in this direction are available on Indian sheep. In Maharashtra the ewes mated at the major farms during May are reported tupped no doubt, but majority did not carry a lamb. At some of the sheep farms in temperate region where even teasers were not run prior breeding, the peak oestrus was observed in September–October, declined in November–December and was least in subsequent winter months. Interestingly the late August period is the one when the migratory ewes in northern temperate region show initiation of oestrus. Excellent receptability of these flocks in the highlands may be due to flushing, favourable temperature and other factors. But the sheep farmers do not prefer early season breeding and defer ram joining to mid September or even later. Like English breeds, the sheep in the temperate region in India experience a restricted breeding season which extends over autumn and winter months. During late spring and early summer few ewes come in heat, and thus the lambing seldom takes place during autumn and early winters. The Rajasthan sheep breed well during September–October and March–April. In the arid and semi-arid zones the early summer mating is advantageous as the lambs are benefitted by the bumper pasturage of post rainy period.

Comparative evaluation of progeny of Deccani sheep and its crossbreds with Merino and Rambouillet, born out of three mating seasons, viz., April–May, June–July and August–September (Gupta et al, 1974) revealed that the mating seasons influenced the birth to weaning weight trait of lambs significantly ($p < 0.01$) in all the genetic groups. The lamb crop produced from ewes bred during mating season I was heaviest at birth and during subsequent growth up to weaning (Fig. 9.5).

Major investigations into breeding season of sheep have been conducted in Australia on Merino and Border Leicester sheep. The results of phased mating of merino ewes over three different breeding periodicities presents an interesting picture (Table 9.1).

A gradual shift from non-breeding season and of different stages in the breeding season itself or occurrence of ovulation are reported in Merino ewes when these are moved from southern to northern hemisphere. Likewise when British sheep are carried from the northern to southern

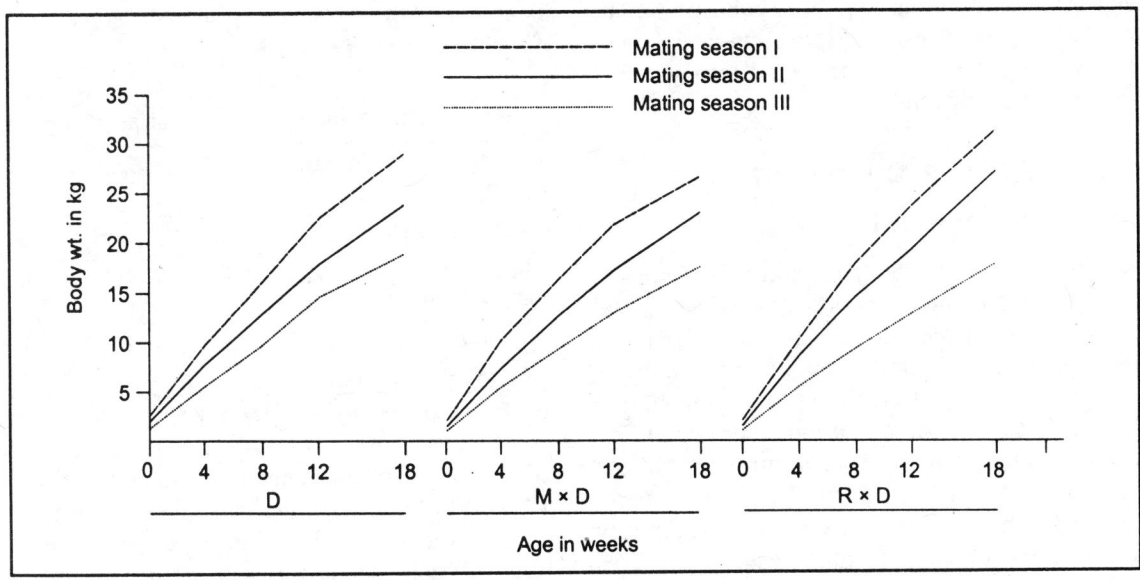

Fig. 9.5. Trends in body weight changes of Deccani, Merino x Deccani and Rambouillet x Deccani lambs born to ewes mated in different seasons.

Table 9.1: Fertility effect of mating periodicity in merino.

Fertility character influenced	Mating period		
	April-June	*August-October*	*December-February*
1. Mating	Mated readily	Mated readily	Mated readily after 3rd week of mating period.
2. Conception rate	Conceived readily after mating during one heat period	Did not conceive readily. Many ewes returned to service in later oestrus	Conceived readily after mating during first oestrus
3. Lambing	Most ewes lambed	Many ewes failed to conceive and lamb	Most ewes lambed
4. Multiple births	Highest propor-tion of ewes bore twins	No ewes bore twins	Moderate proportion of ewes bore twins

Source: Dhamale and Mooley (1963-64).

hemisphere the breeding season gets reversed. The periodicity of coming in heat shifts to March and July from October and February.

The Australian sheep and particularly the Merino have a longer breeding season and mainly breed from February-March onwards. The breeding season in Indian sheep conforms the one as of other north hemisphere breeds but there does not appear a uniformity in extent and seasonal occurrence. Female fertility in Marwari sheep is low during summer but quite high in autumn season. Some other strains of Bikaneri sheep like

Magra appear non-seasonal in sexual activity. The temperate zone and even eastern zone sheep reveal a tendency to breed predominantly from September to November.

PRE-BREEDING REQUIREMENT

Flushing management

It is the act of improving the condition of the ewes prior mating to achieve economical and biological gains. Increase in the number of ova shed, fertilised or implanted has often been claimed in ewes whose bodily condition is improving at mating time. It is also possible that the sound condition at joining stage helps in implantation of the fertilized egg and normal development of embryo in early period. Flushing at times aids in attaining puberty if protracted or delayed otherwise. It involves judicious feeding on a better plane of nutrition, avoiding over-conditioning. When the latter condition supervenes, loosing bodily condition for about 4 to 6 weeks before mating is essential, though advantage of flushing are not likely to reduce. However, fattening before joining may create problems of delayed conception or even temporary barrenness. Higher twinning rates as reported after flushing are missing in ewes in weak condition at mating. Favourable nutritional status before joining may provide opportunity for the ewe to express its twin bearing propensities.

Feeding for flushing

Main breeding season in the temperate region is autumn. The ewes returning then from alpine migrations are in the best of condition of flushing. Likewise the western zone flocks are in prime breeding state in both the spring and late rainy season. These are well flushed on a natural forage and availability of crop residues and stubbles. Addition of *Pala* leaves, small quantities of grains or better pasture may help to achieve flushing of weak flocks particularly when affected by drought.

Results of breeding performance of ewes fed different rations by Russian workers before mating season reveal that flushing reduces the number of

dry ewes and there is an increase in the percentage of multiple births (Table 9.2).

Table 9.2: Breeding of flushed Russian sheep.

Breeding performance	on pasture	Barley	Oats	Millets
% Barren ewes	19.5	12.7	15.7	15.9
% Ewes with multiple births	27.5	36.9	33.0	28.0
No. of lambs per 100 ewes bred	103.5	120.3	112.7	110.2

Source: Sheep breeding in Russia (1970).

It is usual to observe that a flushing period of 6 to 8 weeks leads to a gradual increase in body weight from 2 to 6 kg. The experiments have shown that by flushing the mating stock the percentage of ewes holding to service improves significantly. The lambing percentage and lamb marking percentages are also affected with flushing to the advantage of the sheep farmer.

Mudliar (1981) indicated that flushed ewes produced 12.19 percent more lambs than the unflushed ones. The duration of breeding days was shorter in flushed group. Prasad (1981) found out that in Marwari ewes ovulation after the onset of oestrus gradually improved from 22% at 12 hours to 90% and above between 36 to 48 hours. The number of follicles and the beginning of their pre-ovulatory development is determined by the combined action of FSH and LH on the ovaries of the ewe. Ovulation normally takes place about 24 hours after LH release. This generally coincides with the end of heat.

Synchronisation of oestrus

In world's one of the major sheep artificial insemination programmes in USSR. Professor Loparin used acetate of megestrol ($C_{24}H_{32}O_4$) for heat synchronisation in the ewes. Zanwar and Agarwal (1981) while synchronising oestrus in Polworth ewes used Estrumate, a synthetic Prostaglandin [Prostaglandin F_2 (PGF_2)] 2 ml solution i/m (final estrumate sol.). Ewes came in heat between 15th and 17th day. 79% of anoestrus and 92 percent of ewes of regular oestrus group came in heat. The use of serum gonadotrophin preparations Prolan-A (Bayer) and Folligon (Intervet) at the dose rate of 1200, IU in Polworth, Deccani and Chokla ewes lead to the recovery of 85%, 76% and 76.9% of ova respectively in the three breeds.

Towards synchronization of oestrus in ewes Umberger et al (1994) administered Melengestrol acetate (MGA) orally in seasonally anoestrus ewes at the rate of 0.3 mg over 10 days followed by Progesterone-600 at treatment withdrawal. Under tropical conditions Godfrey et al (1995) tried progesterone through injections as well as intravaginal sponges for oestrus synchronization in Awassi sheep and concluded that both the methods could be used without adversely effecting fertility.

Twinning and superovulation

Besides flushing, genetic and other environmental factors influence superovulation, twinning and lambing rates.

Breed differences

Certain sheep breeds like Romanov (Bulgaria), Welsh Mountain and Finnish Landrace (UK) are known prolific sheep, dropping 150 to 200% lambing. But for Patanwadi and Lohi which produce twins, there is hardly any sheep breed that drops more than 100 percent lambing in India. Even the imported Rambouillets that produce 25 to 30% twins in their homeland, are observed to drop just less than 10% twins under best managed farms in India. Selection experiments to evolve a twinner flock at sheep breeding and research farm Reasi (J&K) for five years yielded initial gains. Twin born ewes were mated to a twin born ram in an effort to construct a twinner ewes and high prolificacy flock, but the trend did not perpetuate further. The low estimates of repeatability ranging from 0.1 to 0.3 and heritability from 0.04 to 0.2 as reported from Australia for number of lambs born provides an indication of uncertain selection gains of the trait.

Seasonal and other factors

There is marked variation in the ratio of twins to single ovulation in Merino during the late autumn. During spring very few twin ovulations are observed. Other factors too influence the twinning rate under field conditions in breeding flock. Multiple ovulation as needed for twins is low at the beginning of breeding season, progresses with the advancement of season and declines towards the end of breeding season.

The age of the ewe and pregnancy sequence (1st, 2nd, 3rd and so on) also influence reproductive performance. Twining rates are higher in mature ewes than younger ones. In prolific breeds twin or multiple births are low at first lambing but sufficiently high for later lambings.

Beyond the existence of breed to breed differences in twining rates, even animal to animal differences have also been observed. A Rambouillet crossbred ewe of a sedentary flock in border belt of Jammu produced twins in all its five lambings from 1985 to 1990 while the rest in the flock were not regular twinners. Likewise in a migratory Bakerwal sheep flock of Ransoo-Pouni Block (J&K) 8 to 10 percent ewes dropped twins and triplets thrice in their life span. Twinning is a rare occurrence in these sheep otherwise. Such instances, however, warrant investigations in the prolificacy potential of indigenous and crossbred sheep in the country.

MATING SYSTEMS

Mating systems vary in field and farm conditions. Various farms too adopt different procedures depending upon the nature of project, stipulations of research scheme or the extent of availability of infrastructure and facilities.

Free mating

It is the simplest form of random mating where a group of selected rams remain running with the flock. Any ram has a chance to cover any ewe. Matching of breedable ewes with a particular sire, i.e. pairing of specific mates can not be ensured.

Generally followed in unorganised private flocks. The shepherd is unable to subdivide his flock for ram wise allotment on reasons of man power shortage.

Though the system is least labour consuming but the pedigree breeding can not be accomplished. Proper ram utilization is not possible. Improvement in productivity of progeny is difficult to predict. Possibility of spread of diseases looms large. Butting by rams is usual and such disturbances hamper normal breeding.

Controlled mating

It involves a scientifically sound system of effective utilization of pedigreed rams. Matching of animals and record maintenance is assured one, depending upon the type of method adopted.

1. Single sire mating: A single selected ram is used in a flock for breeding. Since the same ram is run day and night the pressure on the sire is more. Feeding is also hampered and rest to the animal cannot be ensured.

Even though paint on the brisket region or cradles with crayons are used on the ram for leaving an impression on the covered ewes, due to drying of paint or detaching of cradle in movement, the recording of mating may only be partial one. A few coverings are likely to go unnoticed. Uncertainties prevail about assured coverings. Running of ram after the ewes and pushing at times prove disadvantageous. Day's exhaustion of the ram makes it sit aloof at night.

2. Pen mating: In a given number of selected ewes a selected ram is put in a pen for service during night and withdrawn in the morning. Colour smeared on the brisket or a colour-cake, i.e. a crayon in cradle leaves an impression on the rump of the ewe covered. This practice is repeated daily in the evening when the animals return after grazing. Different breeding groups of ewes are sorted out in separate pens at the farm and the allotted sires are introduced in the respective pens. Rest and feeding of the rams is possible. Satisfactory mating record can be maintained. Pen mating is the most favoured practice at the sheep farms.

3. Hand service: An approned or vasectomised ram or a specially prepared teaser is essentially used in the flock to detect ewes in heat. Colour or paint may be smeared on the brisket of teaser for spotting ewes in the enclosures. Ewes in heat are carried to the closeby stationed breeding sire for covering. A perfect record of mating is possible. This system has a further advantage of utilizing proven sires to the maximum. It is a scientifically desirable mating system for the stud sheep farms. For artificial insemination too, the practice of heat detection with the use of a teaser is of great utility. This procedure is invariably adopted at sheep nucleus and research farms, but not at commercial farms.

Mating prerequisites

- Selection of fit and sound breeding stock in advance.
- The performance records scrutiny.
- Matching and flock constitution as per the breeding strategies.
- Ensuring proper availability of forage and suitable pasturage.
- Visualising the culling and replacement needs.
- Preparation of teasers and equipment like colour crayon and harnesses.
- Prior completion of deworming and vaccinations.
- Having determined the right and fixed time of the year when flushing and high fertility is possible, the pregnancy and lambing are correspondingly timed to season and marketing. The mating phase does not require any other special attention except that the rams and ewes are in fit condition and controlled service is ensured.
- It is advisable to mate maiden ewes to adult rams and older ewes to younger rams. The number of ewes allotted to younger rams is reduced to around 30 against the usual practice of 40 to 50 ewes per ram.
- In keeping with the breeding plan of farm the systematic mating of sheep through non-

random pattern may be classified into one of the following systems:

1. Mating of genetically related animals— inbreeding.
2. Mating of genetically unrelated animals— out breeding.
3. Mating of phenotypically alike animals— positive assortative mating.
4. Mating of phenotypically unlike animals— negative assortative mating.

Inbreeding and negative assortative matings are disfavoured in all earnest. Hardly any breeding manoeuvre at the sheep properties is aimed on these lines. Out breeding is the most preferred one for maintaining purity and constant improvement in the pure bred stock. On this very reason the nucleus flock of Rambouillet and other exotic breeds is required to be replaced by new stock after every three to four years either by interfarm exchange or through imports.

ARTIFICIAL INSEMINATION

Though not much popular among sheep farms, yet it is the most scientific technique of impregnating breedable sheep. At certain research centres neat semen, diluted semen or even frozen semen is being used. Unlike cattle however, it is the least practised method in vogue as far as private sheep flocks in India are concerned.

Erstwhile USSR. and some of other east European countries have produced astounding results through large scale artificial insemination. Australia, New Zealand, France and Germany too have exploited this technique for economic utilization of outstanding germ plasm. In fact main advantage is the proper use of superior rams, economy in the number of rams needed for breeding and disease control.

In India too, trials of artificial insemination in sheep were under taken at Reasi (J&K), Pune (Maharashtra) and at some other farms of the country under ICAR scheme in late fiftees of 20th century but ended abruptly, and without any supporting results. It was only in mid sixties that a couple of scientists and workers* after training in USSR practised AI on scientific lines in the sheep of north western region and elsewhere and made available results about semen attributes of rams of Indian and imported sheep breeds as well as the various diluents tried by them. Veterinarians from different states were imparted the specialised training of AI in sheep and thus a chain reaction to adopt this technology was set in motion. The years from 1966 onwards witnessed the development of country made AI equipment, standardization of techniques and upcoming of requisite infrastructure. The neat semen inseminations at Sheep Breeding and Research Farm Reasi J&K during 1974 to 1977 produced 58 to 63% lambing but with the use of EYC diluter it fell below 40%. The scientists in Rajasthan obtained almost 50% lambing. Though higher temperatures resulted into poor quality of semen, the autumn insemination of experimental flocks is reported to have produced even 70 to 80 percent lambing.

Beside egg yolk citrate (EYC), egg yolk glycerol (EYG), buffers combined with sugars + egg yolk; milk and a couple of other diluents are being tried. Undiluted semen should preferably be used within half an hour of its collection. Depending upon volume of ejaculate and its quality over 400 ewes can be bred with a single ram in a breeding season.

Feasibility

The low rate conceptions, transhumant system of sheep rearing and difficulties in observing sound hygiene and precision under field conditions have so far appeared deterrent factors. Thus the AI work in sheep could not take off with a bang as envisaged. Recent work at CSWRI and under various Veterinary faculties of the universities has again thrown an optimistic note. Synchronisation of oestrus is possible now. The excellent sheep germ plasm is available. The use of AI technique in sheep can be exploited for improving production

---

* Honmode, J.; Toshinwal, S.N.; Sahni, K.L; Luktuke, S.N.; Joshi, J.D., Ramamurthi, A, and others.

and economy of a flock. The whole process involves the technique of selection of performance tested or progeny tested sires, their preparation, teaser preparation, flushing of ewe flock, oestrus synchronisation, timely marking of ewes in heat, semen collection and its evaluation, proper equipment and its sterilization, selection of a suitable diluent, appropriate dilution, preservation, storage and transportation of semen, observing hygienic measures in handling and insemination and adopting proper posture of the ewe while inseminating.

Deep frozen (or nitrogen frozen) semen technique

This technique is widely practised in cattle in India. Little headway has however been made in deep frozen semen insemination as far as sheep and goat are concerned. There are no outstanding sires. The technique to preserve the semen of some good sires is needed to be standardised, further. The cost factor of top pure breed rams, their maintenance and acclimatization for successful breeding are quite prohibitive.

The frozen semen technique can play a major role in sheep reproduction. Firstly there is remarkable saving in the number of rams required and maintained. Secondly the quality semen remains available through out the year. If improvised handling cum transport facilities exist, the deep frozen semen has the added advantage of use under migratory flock conditions.

Embryo transfer technology (ETT) has also come to be talked about in pursuit of improving production but has not taken any practical footing in India in sheep as yet. Synchronisation of oestrus in sheep has however, been achieved with good success at certain experimental stations and at CSWRI.

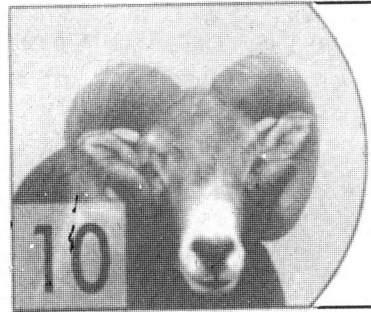

BREEDING STOCK MANAGEMENT

PREGNANCY

Pregnancy studies

Study and investigations into pregnancy in the ewes are aimed at understanding the:

1. Physiology of pregnancy and related factors that influence the commencement of oestrus, conception, development of foetus and termination of pregnancy.
2. Genetic factors likely to interfere with normal development.
3. Infections or metabolic diseases affecting the pregnant ewe and the foetus.
4. Economic aspects of obtaining a potential and viable lamb crop from the breeding flock. The importance of avoiding enormous wastage that occurs each year because of failure of ewes to conceive or to produce and rear a viable progeny.
5. Biological importance.

Gestation in sheep

The contribution of the ram to reproduction in a flock is comparatively over a short period. Reproduction in the ewes extends over several months. Oestrus, service, ovulation and fertilisation occur quickly. Implantation of fertilised ovum takes longer but with implantation starts the pregnancy. It terminates around 150 days later, with the birth of a normal lamb.

During gestation the fertilised and implanted ovum differentiates into numerous tissues as bone, blood, muscles, etc. and into organs such as heart, lungs, kidney, glands and skin. The embryo is contained in the foetal membranes which are attached to the uterine wall through cotyledons. The presence of blood vessels that pass from the membrane to embryo is through umbilicus. This is the guide to approach foetus proper. Twin embryos may be covered in one set of membranes. But multiple embryos may not always have separate membranes.

The rate of development of lamb foetus during pregnancy has an important bearing on its chances of survival, growth or its productivity as adult sheep.

These biological functions are comparatively easy to observe, but other more difficult to detect also occur or fail to occur during pregnancy. The foetal demands, the ewe's ability to meet them and the chemical changes that take place in the pregnant ewe's body may be reflected in reduced wool cuts, variations in the size and birth weight of lamb and milk yield of the ewe. Changes take place in the ductless glands of the ewe. The water requirements of pregnant ewes also change. These physiological changes associated with pregnancy return to normal ewe functions, i.e. nonpregnant level, within a few weeks after lambing. The successful, outcome of pregnancy depends mainly upon the ability of the ewes to provide a relatively stable environment for the lambs, they carry.

Unless drastic changes in environment overtake, the ewes meet the demands despite wide variation in air temperature, the amount of feed available or the distance traversed by the pregnant ewes for grazing. The management must, therefore, take cognizance of the biological demands of pregnancy and the factors that influence the same.

Foetal development

If gestation proceeds normally, the growth rate of the ovine foetus is often fairly uniform during the first three months of pregnancy though relatively less. Once the pregnancy enters the last 8 weeks of gestation and the placenta is extensive and firmly attached to the uterine wall, the foetus grows rapidly. In the last month weight may be doubled. It is from this period that individual lamb to lamb differences between birth weight develop. In Rambouillet and its crossbred lambs following pattern of foetal weight gain at various stages of pregnancy is observed:

Approximate age of foetus (days)	Weight of foetus (kg)
100	0.6
120	1.4
140	2.4
At birth (around 150 days)	3.2

Skin and wool follicle

The skin of the wool growing sheep is an important organ. The way the ewes are fed during the last two months of pregnancy, affect the life time wool production of the lambs they are carrying. The development of the follicle in the sheep skin can be divided into two main phases.

Primary phase: Commences on the most advanced regions of skin, i.e. over the face and poll as early as 35th to 40th day of gestation. By about the 60th day some primary follicles are established over whole of the body. During the next 20 days or so, further primary follicles develop in close association with those already present. The follicles are usually bunched in groups of three and referred to as trio-groups. The pair developing most recently being arranged on either side of the follicle that develop initially

between the 25th to 40th day. The primary phase is almost complete by the 90th day when the secondary phase commences.

Secondary phase: The main wool growing follicles develop during this phase. These are usually arranged around the existing trio-groups of primary follicles. The ratio between the primary and secondary follicles determines many of the characteristics of adult fleece. After commencing around 90th day, the secondary phase proceeds rapidly. By 120th day the secondary follicles attain their maximum density. Their final development and consequently the productivity of the lambs when they become adults, depends largely on the way the mother is fed while her lamb is developing its secondary follicles, i.e. during the last two months of gestation.

PREGNANCY DIAGNOSIS IN SHEEP

The sheep are generally run en-flock. Individual pregnancy detection is not carried out. Specialised technique to diagnose pregnancy in sheep have also not been put in practice. The general approach to detect conception and early pregnancy is based on the use of vasectomised rams to detect the ewes that return to oestrus between 15 to 19 days after service by an entire ram. A harness and marking crayon is applied to the vasectomised ram while allowing in flock for heat detection. This obviates the need to examine the ewes and the ram each day. The technique is beset with certain disadvantages like:

1. A pregnant ewe usually does not permit ram covering. The vasectomised rams may take advantage of the ewes when herded together or go through a gate. It may even jump at the pregnant ones and provide wrong indications.
2. The ewes that have conceived may return to service 17 days or so later. Pregnant ewes have been observed to return to service.
3. At times the unconceived and nonpregnant ewes may not return to service as has been seen to happen towards the end of breeding season. Non-return of oestrus may also happen in persistent or retained corpus luteum cases,

when even though pregnancy has not occurred, the next oestrus may not manifest.

4. Ewe may have conceived, but embryo fails to develop and is lost at about the 20th day making the ewe to return to oestrus by about 34 or even 51 days after service by a fertile ram.

Physical check up: Examination of udder development and abdominal or rectal palpation provide indications of pregnancy around 8 weeks stage to the expert hand.

Biological tests

The oestrogens circulating in blood at or near oestrus period stimulate the cervix to release salts that crystallise to form typical pattern arborisation. The mucous taken from cervix around ovulation time and allowed to dry on an unheated microscopic slide reveals a distinct fern like arborisation pattern. It does not happen at other times of the oestrus cycle due to inhibitory effect of progesterone or through lack of oestrogens. This condition does not appear between 3rd to 14th day of oestrus cycle when the corpus luteum is present and is secreting progesterone. However, if sufficient oestrogen is injected into the nonpregnant ewes on any day between 3rd and 14th day, the arborisation occurs.

During pregnancy the cervix loses its ability to secrete the salts that cause arborisation so that characteristic changes do not occur after the injection of oestrogen if the ewe is pregnant. The injection of Estradial benzoate on any date between the 12th to 25th day after service produces arborisation in the nonpregnant animals but fails to produce arborisation in pregnant ewes. The injection of oestrogen during early pregnancy can lead to loss of embryo. Besides, the anatomy of ewe's cervix makes it extremely difficult to obtain mucous that is not contaminated with cells from the lining of the vagina. The biological test therefore is not only cumbersome but unsatisfactory too.

Examination of vaginal mucosal cells: Nonpregnant ewes have more than ten layers of polygonal and squamous cells. But in the pregnant ewes the cells are usually cuboidal with fewer layers. Richardson (1972) reported an accuracy of about 90% in more than two month pregnancy by examining sections of vaginal wall mucosa taken from anterior to the urethral opening.

Hormone level testing: During pregnancy the progesterone blood level is always high, whereas it fluctuates with the stage of oestrus cycle in nonpregnant ewe. Progesterone level analysis of blood and even milk has been employed for this purpose.

Pregnancy detection based on Progesterone specific protein in blood around 4 weeks pregnancy has also been demonstrated by some workers. Diagnosis of pregnancy through urine hormonal assaying has least been reported.

Ultrasonic scanning: Ultra sonography technique in sheep is similar to the one adopted in doe by Mushtaq and Karl (1992). A small area of 5 cm × 12 cm is shaved from the right and left inguinal region adjacent to the udder. Transabdominal scans with the help of portable ultra sound system* are performed in the standing ewe by placing the probe in contact with the skin. Contact is accomplished by using a transmission gel (Echo ultrasound, Lewistown, PA, USA).

The 1st, 2nd and 3rd examinations are conducted at 40, 50 and 110 days gestation respectively. Besides determining the pregnancy of the ewe, examinations reveal number of foetuses present and their presentation. Foetal viability is ascertained from the individual foetal heart beats.

EFFECT OF ENVIRONMENT ON PREGNANT EWES

Climate

Atmospheric temperatures affect the pregnant ewes and the foetal growth directly as well as

---

* Like the Real-time Linear array US system with SMHZ transducer introduced by Technicare Denver Cap, USA.

indirectly. Direct effect of hot weather on the ewe and lamb is through endocrine system. The adaptability, growth, production and reproduction are all affected through an altered thyropituitary hormonal complex.

With the occurrence of hot weather there is decrease in lambing percentages, low birth weights and ewes' low rearing capacities. High temperatures may have an adverse effect on reproduction in the ewes. High temperatures and hot climates have also been found to impede the implantation of fertilised ovum in the tropical belt.

Nutrition

An unfavourable environment for sheep pregnancy would be a high temperature coupled with low plane of nutrition. The indirect effect on the grazing sheep is through the soil, i.e. the vegetation it supports and the nutrition that is available to pregnant sheep.

The outcome of poor nutrition is invariably low birth weight, smaller bones, an altered gestation period and low lamb viability. Experiments have shown that variation in the way the sheep are fed may influence the length of gestation period. Pasture effect may also be visible at times in more ewes needing assistance during lambing. Certain improved pastures predispose ewes to dystocia. Clover rich pasture produces a kind of infertility resulting into low conceptio ... ... due to oestrogenic contents.

LAMBING

Act of normal parturition

Parturition is the phenomenon of delivering a lamb by the pregnant ewe at the termination of pregnancy. Lambing is the common word in usage for this action and aims at delivering the foetus from the uterus and the body of ewe to the outside world without loss or damage, with expulsion of placenta in due course. Important factors involved in the process are the contractions or labour pains (a misnomer), the route and the foetal medium. In other words these are the *powers*, *passage* and the *passenger* as mentioned by some authors.

Uterine contractions (the powers): As parturition approaches, the uterus undergoes wave like contractions. These eventually become strong and painful. As a result the abdominal and thoracic muscles commence to contract. Intrauterine pressure gets built up under influence of oxytocin. The cervix, which has by now already relaxed due to secretion of relaxin hormone dilates a bit. Part of placenta is forced into it due to uterine contractions until the placental bag bursts and the fluid escapes. Once this occurs the normal birth of lamb soon follows. It, however, depends upon whether the powers continue to function. Some times the muscles become fatigued due to prolonged contractions and pressure.

The foetal passage: or route consists of two parts, the soft comprises of uterus, its floor, the dilated cervical canal and the vagina, where as hard one is formed of bony sacrum and pelvic opening. Normal lambing would further depend on whether the passages are adequate to carry the lamb and whether the foetal passenger is presented in a normal posture. There is a coordinated physiological action in the body at parturition, which proceeds in the following sequence:

- Foetus descends in the body of uterus.
- Approaches cervix.
- More stronger uterine contractions.
- Dilatation of cervix.
- Greater contraction of uterus.
- Pelvic floor muscles soften and urinary bladder draws down in the abdomen.
- Passage dilates and foetus slips through.
- Once the lamb head enters the pelvic passage the birth proceeds with reasonable quickness.

The hard parts of passage, the pelvis of female animals is usually broad and its opening funnel shaped. The exceptions of small pelvic opening in certain breeds and larger foetus with others, hamper normal parturition. Example in former case is South Down and in latter is heavy Rambouillet and Dorsets. When heavy exotic rams are used over small size sheep breeds, like Mandya and

Kashmir valley for crossbreeding, assistance is quite often required during parturition for safe delivery of the lamb.

From the time of bursting of foetal bag to the completion of normal lambing, 1 to 1½ hour time is spent. It is more in maiden ewes, less in subsequent pregnancies, but again more in old ewes where labour pains are feeble.

The lamb foetus: *Passenger* when in normal presentation, i.e. head first with lower jaw resting on its fore legs, the passage facilitates the slippage of rest of the foetal body. Larger shoulders and chest sometimes make parturition difficult. The head of the foetus protrudes or even hangs down, while the ewe exhausts or moves to another spot or even starts grazing. Head swells up. The cotyledonary attachments break. Umbilical cord becomes compressed between the foetus and the narrow hard passage. Such a dystocia results into death of the lamb. Similar type of abnormal presentations like bending of neck, turning back of one or both front legs, britch presentation, etc. do offer situation for veterinary assistance.

Lambing management

Lambing is the most important time bound operation of a sheep farm. Ill managed lambing can lead to high lamb losses. Postnatal mortality on ranches in advanced sheep rearing countries accounts for 10 to 15% in the very first week of birth and almost 20 to 25% of lamb crop up to weaning in the mismanaged farms. Any improvement in lamb survivability has therefore a direct bearing on the growth of a flock, availability of replacements and the economy of sheep rearing.

To achieve these objectives it is imperative to keep an attending shepherd and a paraveterinary hand for round the clock supervision during lambing. A veterinarian should also be available for guidance, to assist lambing at the abnormal presentations and other sheep gynaecological problems. A good light arrangement must be ensured to attend the ewes lambing at night.

Soon after birth the excessive chorionic fluid is drained off. Ewe is then allowed to lick the lamb to dry out the rest. Udder of the ewe be washed with luke warm pot. permanganate solution and towel dried. Milk out the first few strips of thick material from the teats. Watch for proper suckling and assist weak lambs so that the new born receives adequate colostrum, the immuno-protein rich first milk of the mother. This helps in clearing intestinal muconium. Weak lambs need extra feeding care and protection from cold.

Navel-cord is applied a week solution of iodine, preferably tincture of iodine or other antiseptics like Savlon, Povidin, etc. In case of disinterest of the ewe in the lamb or disowning rub lamb against the ewe or sprinkle a pinch of salt on the lamb to tempt licking by the mother. Once the lamb dries up, a temporary colour or paint mark is placed on the side of body for identification sake. Birth weight is taken as soon as it dries up and entries recorded. The ewe drops placental remanents within 3 to 4 hours of lambing. In case of delay, chances of septicaemia develop, hence steps and even veterinary assistance may be needed for timely expulsion before putrefaction sets in.

Open pasture lambing is common in private flocks in India and on commercial sheep properties abroad. This is beset with many hazards of inclement weather, mismothering, attack of predators, inefficient assistance, supervision lapses, etc. The lone advantage of open lambing is that no elaborate management and preparations may be needed. The nomads and migratory sheep rearing tribals follow such a system with the provision of ordinary low cost protection measures. The new born lambs after dissociating from the mothers are accommodated under a big bamboo basket, herded in a conical thatch (Kulla) or put in closure covered with a tarpaulin at 1 to 1½ metre height. Where constructed kacha or pucca shelter is available, ewe with lamb(s) is penned for first day. A couple of lamb-at-foot ewes* are then put together in a bigger pen for next two to three days.

---

* Recently lambed ewe with lamb.

Care is to be taken to avoid environmental stress. For various climatic regions in the country, the favourable ambient temperature during lambing is 5 to 20°C, low in the temperate and moderate in the western arid zone. Exposure of young lambs to high temperature leads to exhaustion, dehydration and stroke. Severe draft or humidity add to the problem of temperature stress. Under cold conditions exposure of tender lambs to wind is disastrous. Rainy season, high humidity, dingy-dirty housing environments affect the thriftiness of lambs.

Soon after gestation stress, lambing and lactation time is the most hard time for the ewe causing maximum strain on body system and reserves of the mother. For proper attention to rearing and saving lambs, the sheep farmer should also be in a position to spare enough time. Personal, keen and regular inspection of the farm management is vital for viable lambing and development of future rams.

Care and feeding till weaning

Sound lamb suckling is a precursor of good health and growth. This in turn is an indicator of better marking percentage and higher flock gains. The maiden ewes often show inadequate milk flow initially. Timely attention is needed towards the feeding of these ewes and their lambs. Fostering under other ewes does help a lot. Bottle-feedings is not as advantageous. Feeding the lean milkers on greens and maize results in improving lactation protential*. Elderly ewes of crossbred strains or even of pure-breeds maintained at private or public sheep farms have not been found to pose any problem of deficient milking on balanced feeding.

The young lambs attempt to nibble at when they are 8 to 10 days old. At two to three week age, lambs can be initiated to light type of starter. At four week age the addition of small quantities of crushed maize to the lamb feed proves useful. Additives like fish liver oils, liver tonics, vitamin and mineral preparations to the starter feeds at

Sheep Breeding and Research Farm Reasi produced higher weaning weights and higher survival rates of lambs during 1972 to 1978. Greens like berseem, lucerne or oats in small quantities when initiated at four weeks reduce the dependence of lamb on the ewe. Creep feeding is a scientific practice of developing healthy faster growing lamb crops, though not common in private sheep flocks in true sense. Shepherds allow the out movement of lambs with mothers at an early age. At organised farms the lambs accompany the ewes to pasture at 6 to 8 weeks age depending upon the terrain and manpower availability.

The ewe must also be watched for mastitis, teat injuries or other painful conditions. Unless treated in time, the ewes with mastitis do not make healthy and safe mothers. Contagious aphtha, sore eyes, joint ill, lamb dysentery, coccidiosis and diarrhoea are common ailments that afflict the lambs during early life and before weaning. When ewes have been vaccinated at right time, the hygienic measures, disinfection of premises, clean water and proper feed are helpful in preventing the occurrence of disease problems of parasitic and bacterial origin.

Other postnatal operations

Tail docking: Merino descendants, their crossbreds and a couple of other sheep breeds possess long tails. Soiling of long tails takes place during defecation, lambing, housing, etc. of sheep. The unhygienic condition attracts fly strike and even attack by maggots. In burr and thistle infested-pastures, burrs stick to long tails. These cause discomfort to the animal. During mating of ewes and artificial insemination long tails pose hindrance.

The tail wool is coarser and hairy. Wasting sheep energy on the growth of inferior coat is considered uneconomic. The sheepman therefore disfavours a long tail and often resorts to tail docking, i.e. the removal of extra length of the tail.

---

* The shepherds of north and south regions feed Methi and Kulthi (horse gram) fodder/grains respectively to low yielder ewes.

The tail docking operation is carried out in the first week of birth and preferably within 48 to 72 hours of lambing. At most of the sheep farms in India and in the flocks in Australia, New Zealand, USA, the surgical excision is practised. Either no antiseptic or only a light antiseptic is applied, not withstanding initial bleeding at times. On reasons of blood loss, pain and ethical considerations such a docking procedure is not liked. For a bloodless docking a rubber or elastic band is applied with an elastrator. An emasculator with crushing edges can also be used for sound docking.

In female lambs the docking site is between coccygeal vertebrae at the level of vulval tip. In males docking is conducted a bit higher so that the tail stump just reaches the anal region.

Lamb marking: Placing an identification mark on individual lamb is essential for its recognition and to trace its mother and pedigree besides maintaining various records (Fig. 41, PLATE 8). Initially a temporary paint marking is done on the body sides, differently for the two sexes. A number plate or a light plastic band/ring can also be put around the neck for identification.

Lamb marking is also accomplished by using ear tags as early as possible before paint marking fades away. For permanent and safer identification marking tattooing is inscribed at the bare chest region on the right side. This can be deferred till 6 to 8 weeks or even later. Number punching of ears and horn branding of horned stud rams is adopted at some of the sheep properties for life long identification.

While tattooing or other permanent marking number codes are used to express information with regard to:

- Farm/property
- Breed/genetic group
- Year of birth
- Serial register number
- Other vital particulars if any

The term 'Lamb marking percentage' implies the extent (%) of lambs surviving at weaning. This is considered a yardstick for flock growth and future replacements. The improvement in marking percentage can best be achieved through controlling postnatal death rate.

Castration: Unfit and off type male lambs are castrated while young. Method generally adopted is open surgery of scrotal sac. A crude way of severing the cord with teeth is stated in vogue at some properties. For bloodless operation, specially devised elastrator bands or emasculators serve the purpose. To avoid repeated handling sometimes docking and castration operations are performed simultaneously.

A scientific method of castration at a bit later stage or to prepare wethers is through the use of Burdizzo castrator. No injury or blood loss takes place. Pain and mild inflammation if any, too subside in a couple of days. Wet and fly season should be avoided especially in surgical castration. Winter season is preferred over summer to limit chances of infection.

Weaning is usually undertaken at 90 to 120 days age. Growth of lambs, lactation condition of ewes, forage availability, migrations and adequate dry period needed for restoration of condition of ewes before next mating are the main considerations while deciding suitable time and age of weaning. Recording of body weights at birth and subsequent weekly intervals is done as per stipulations of research project. In order to avoid repeated handling of lambs recording of birth and weaning weights only is advisable.

LAMB SURVIVABILITY

A number of infectious diseases are associated with sheep pregnancy that result into abortions and prenatal lamb losses. Congenital reasons for foetal deaths exist, though lack exhaustive study. A recessive lethal gene affecting the development of lamb has been recognised in merino sheep.

In the postnatal period lamb survivability rate of a flock is one major factor on which depends the progress and economy of a flock. Lower the lamb losses better the prospects of sheep rearing.

Consequences of lamb losses

- The lamb deaths defeat the very purpose for which the flock is intended, i.e. fat lamb, wool grower, breeding replacement or stud ram production.
- Pregnancy lowers fleece weight of ewes. The availability of lamb at *marking** is expected to compensate for the decrease of production of ewe. When the lamb is not reared, the loss of wool and lamb get added up.
- The feed, labour and money gone into producing lamb, is wasted.
- The ram fails to pay its full dividends. The biological importance of postnatal lamb deaths rests mainly in the loss of potential breeding stock, if genetically superior lamb is lost. This also reduces the chance of selection of superior animals.
- Natural selection is always operating. The lambs with coarse hairy birth coat may survive better than of desired characteristics. Thus the next generation flock may have uneven fleece coats and increased variability of fibre diameter.
- For a potential source of replacement and production, a lamb should not only be born but it must be capable of adjustment, escape predators, resist infection and grow optimally.
- The survival of lamb and its normal development depends on physiological development and normal functioning of ewe's motherhood capabilities like normal teats, sufficient milk production, mothering ability, etc.

Causes of lamb mortality

Mortality of lambs occurs due to a number of causes. In any flock the losses are usually highest at birth and during the first week of life and contribute almost to three-fourths of the total mortality. Range flocks in Australia, New Zealand, USA, and other countries are the ones where the early lamb mortality still continues to be a matter of anxiety

for the sheep man. Dystocia and lamb dysentery take a heavy toll. Predators, starvation due to mismothering and exhaustion rank as important causes of loss. Predators are invariably crows, vultures, hawk, foxes and other wild animals. Toxic vegetation and clovers also account for a sizeable lamb losses.

The general trend in private and public sector flocks in various regions of the country suggests that disease aspect is responsible for heavy mortality. The extent of losses due to diseases has to a great extent been controlled in the last two to three decades, yet it occupies a top killer position of lambs.

Investigations into mortality

The investigations into losses of sheep, importantly the young lambs are aimed at:

1. To find the trouble as soon as it occurs in the field and farm flocks to know the aetiology and epidemiology.
2. To examine system of husbandry and management that can be employed to check and reduce lamb losses.
3. To provide basic information that might be used for future, to define the cause of mortality as it occurs and to adopt immediate appropriate measures to control losses.

Losses of newborn lambs due to diseases

Diseases likely to cause losses of lambs in early postnatal age can be conveniently divided into:

1. Those infecting the ewes. The lambs pick up infection through blood circulation.
2. Those infecting the lambs directly after birth.

   Infection may be due to the following organisms:

   a. Anaerobic organisms like *Clostridium septicum, Cl. oedamatiens, Cl. chauvei, Cl. welchii* type D, etc.
   b. Salmonella, Pasteurella, Escherichia group of organisms.

---

* A higher % or number of surviving weaners (Lamb marking %) compensates the production loss (wool and body wt.) suffered by the lambing ewes due to pregnancy stress.

c. Viral origin-pneumonia, Enteritis and even other maladies of idiopathic or Mycoplasma origin.

d. Contagious ecthyma.

e. Coccidia and other protozoan organisms.

f. Pneumonia due to bacillary or other bacterial infections.

Unhygienic and damp environment is the most important predisposing factor for lamb deaths due to infections.

While investigating into lamb losses it is important to look for the probable cause of death. The appropriate specimens should essentially be collected and examined to confirm the diagnosis. Differentiation should be made between infectious and noninfectious causes.

The infective organisms responsible for lamb mortality may infect the lamb before birth or after birth. Those infecting lambs before birth usually infect the ewes. The lambs dropped, i.e. aborted in incompletely developed conditions reveal blood stained subcutaneous oedema, peritonitis, pericarditis, pleuritis, plaque formation on the sole or walls of hooves and necrotic lesions in the liver. Lambs from infected ewes may survive at birth but die soon after. Care has therefore to be exercised to examine placenta and if necessary, the ewes, that loose lambs after birth.

Postnatally infecting organisms gain an easy entry through the navel. Autopsy observations vary with the type of infection. Anaerobes usually result in gangrene of area surrounding navel. Oedema of the navel and belly wall may spread to the liver, kidney or urinary bladder. The oedamatous fluid may be clear, rosy, deeply blood stained or of gelly or gaseous nature. Salmonella group causes numerous small whitish abscesses in the liver of new births. Pasteurella results into severe peritonitis, blood tinged oedema, bronchopneumonia, fibrinous pleural adhesions with lungs, numerous small liver abscesses and enlargement of lymph glands. Escherichia group produce arthritis, purulent meningio-encephalitis, thick pus in the navel region and white scour.

Lethal factors in sheep

Lethal, and sublethal genes existing in the genetic pool of sheep germ plasm in various countries are an important source of loss of sheep. But for merino in Australia and some English breeds, little study in this regard has been made elsewhere. In India, there is hardly any reference to any investigations into the genetic abnormality or lethality having been made in sheep. Studies in Merino have revealed lethal genes for conditions like, Muscle contracture, Cleft palate, Paralysis, Rigid fetlock, Amputated limbs, Grey lethal. Dwarfism. Nervous incoordination, Congenital photosensitivity, and Blindness, etc.

In the first case the abnormal lambs are smaller than the normal ones. Their heads are narrower. The hind leg joints may also be flexed and distended. The back is arched and twisted. Although born alive, these lambs soon die. On postmortem, wasting of body muscles, enlarged liver, incompletely developed kidneys are the glaring features. Breeding experiments have revealed that this condition is due to a recessive gene.

Other factors contributing to lamb mortality

Exposure of ewes to high ambient temperature during pregnancy may lead to the production of under weight, undersized, abnormal lambs. Under field conditions climatic factors seldom act independently. High atmospheric temperature casts a direct effect on the pregnant ewe's physiology, but may exert indirect effect as well, through the amount and the quality of the feed, its digestibility, feed actually consumed and the distance walked during grazing.

Exposure of lambs to either heat or cold can be damaging and fatal depending upon the severity of change. At some of the sheep farms in subtropical part of India sudden deaths in healthy lambs take place in April, May in certain years as and when the mercury suddenly rises above 42°C. Heat stroke cases in young sheep especially of fine wool exotic and crossbreds is not an uncommon observation. In the first week of birth lambs may not withstand a two hour exposure to atmospheric temperature of 39°C under dry conditions and 33°C under wet conditions (humid conditions). Lambs deprived of shed or shade during bright sun days get exposed to solar radiation. Wider variations between day and night ambient temperatures (12°C or more) lead to adaptation stress on the new born lamb. Chances of exposure, respiratory problems and pneumonia increase.

Colour and length of the body coat and evaporation are the three factors that protect the lambs from tremendous heat. White coat of the lamb reflects a good deal of the radiant heat. Fortunately wool is a bad conductor of heat. Where the lambs have a long or compact wool coat at birth, lesser or little heat penetrates to the lamb skin. On the other hand if the lamb has a short curly coat, comparatively more heat may reach the skin and more chances of heat stress are there.

The movement of new born lambs with mothers for watering or grazing causes increased distress. This can lead to faulty mothering, disowning and increased losses from starvation or predators especially on the ranches.

Cold weather effect: The important factors that cause cold stress on a new born lambs are the low ambient temperatures, the wind or blizzard, the dryness of the air, rain and snow. The dryness and movement of air influences the rate at which the infant lamb dries up. The evaporation of fluid from the birth coat of a lamb requires a certain amount of heat. A part of it comes from the surrounding air. The remainder is provided by the lamb itself. For considering lamb losses due to exposure to cold, three aspects need attention.

1. The response of the lamb to increased heat loss on account of evaporation of amniotic fluid from the body coat of lamb.
2. Relative contribution of atmosphere and the lamb to the heat needed for evaporation of moisture from the coat of new born lamb.
3. The type of the birth coat and its effect on the relative contribution in evaporation by the atmospheric temperature and lamb itself.

A newborn lamb may have between 300 to 400 ml of amniotic fluid soaking its birth coat.

Some of it drains away. Some of it is licked off by the ewe. The rest evaporates. The coat dries quickly on a warm-windy day when atmospheric temperature range between 21-25°C and the relative humidity is 50%. The lamb is required to contribute 20-40% of the total amount of heat needed to affect evaporation.

At our farms and more so in open flock rearing in field conditions serious losses of new born lambs occur each year through exposure to cold and windy weather. Observations made in sheep advanced countries show that at birth the body temperature of the lamb is about 0.3°C above that of the mother. It falls quickly by about 2°C during first hour of life. Mostly it commences to rise again and returns to normal within about three hours of birth. But where the atmospheric temperature does not behave favourably, the lamb body temperature drops suddenly by about 4 to 5°C within half an hour post birth and the new born lamb may soon succumb due to failure of its thermoregulatory system.

Fall in temperature and cooling is more pronounced in light than in heavy lambs. Twin lambs which are usually lighter suffer greater fall in rectal temperature than single lambs. Thus the chances of mortality in twin born lambs may be more under unfavourable winter conditions.

Synergistic effect of exposure to cold weather and starvation

Lambs that have not suckled, if exposed to cold draught of air at about 5°C show the symptoms like coma, paddling leg movements, rolling of eyeballs and frothing.

Blood sugar level of new born lambs varies around 30 and 120 mg per 100 ml for fructose and glucose respectively. In starved lambs glucose level falls steadily and may be as low as 10 mg per 100 ml as death approaches. The rectal temperature too recedes below 35°C when death supervenes. Careful attention during lambing in the winter can reduce lamb losses. Early suckling of first milk, the colostrum, by the new born lamb is essential for survival.

CONTROL OVER LAMB MORTALITY

Multidirectional steps are needed to check lamb mortality. These include the following.

1. Proper feeding of ewes

It is important to maintain an ascending nutritional plain of pregnant ewes, during the last two months of gestation. Three salient aspects of ewe feeding are:

- Do not allow the pregnant ewes to lose too much condition during the first three months.
- Ensure that there is a steady gain in the condition of ewe during last two months.
- Avoid over feeding during the last two months of gestation lest the lambs may grow too heavy, exposing the mother and lamb to dystocia condition. As a consequence the lamb may be stillborn.

2. Maintain hygiene

Many disease problems of lambs during pregnancy and in early life are caused by the infections picked up by the mother from the sheds, barns and flock habitation grounds or polluted air and water. Cleanliness of pens and hygienic conditions of surroundings are prerequisite for healthy lamb crop. Sheep maintained on ranches and open dry areas are better placed with least chances of infection. Intensive housing breeds multiple disease organisms and parasites of animals. Disinfection of premises and shelters in advance is strongly recommended. Fresh and clean water to drink and air to inhale (free of smoke, dust, foul toxic gases, etc.) is essential.

3. Preventive vaccination of ewes in pregnancy

Some of the Clostridial diseases like lamb dysentery, enterotoxaemia, etc. overtake the lambs quite early in life. A better means of providing immunity to the lambs is through advance vaccination of mother ewes during gestation. The lambs so born to the vaccinated ewes carry antibodies at birth and are thus saved from immediate attack of the disease in postnatal state.

4. Help the lamb feed itself

Early disowning of lambs by mothers is a serious situation and results into loss of lambs. Careful handling of both the ewe and lamb is helpful. It is a accepted common practice in the shepherding communities to keep both together in a lambing pen or adjacent enclosure for a first few days after birth. The lamb may be assisted to suckle if it fails to do of its own. Shearing or crutching (of the udder) before lambing exposes the udder and makes the access of lamb more easy.

5. Protect lambs from exposure

The exposure of new born lambs to the extreme weather conditions, heat, cold and air draught or even unpredictable day to day variation in weather may cause lamb losses. At times the exposed lambs do not show instant adverse effect. A rise of temperature, indisposition or mild attack of pneumonia may go unnoticed. But subsequent unthriftiness, ill health and deaths reveal a protracted development of pulmonary adhesions, pleuritis, and severe lung involvement on postmortem. Providing sheds, shady sheltered paddocks and temporary cover arrangements can be considered. The proximity of the mother to the lamb is the best safe guard for the lamb against unusual cold weather. The general practice in the temperate region with the nomad shepherds and else where in some other parts is to fabricate large size bamboo baskets or cone shaped thatched shelters that can accommodate even twenty or more lambs together. Raising plantations for a wind break and erecting fences on the slopes is helpful.

6. Other essential provisions

Proper space and ventilation are essential. The floor should be dry as far as possible. A comfortable bedding of grass or bhussa free from dust and bristles is provided at times. Ample feed and water for ewe mother before lambing and after lambing in the pen has to be ensured. In fact this condition applies for the lambs also when they come up to starter feeding stage after a fortnight.

7. Watch for the unfit ewe mothers

Wool blindness as seen in merinos and introduced in other sheep through cross breeding hampers proper rearing of the lamb. To keep the ewe face open, *wigging* is resorted to.

Teats with cuts and mastitis condition need timely attention. Cuts or wounds should be dressed timely. Mastitis is amenable to early and immediate treatment. Any delay to attend may complicate the recovery process. Lambs attempting to suckle from mastitis suffering ewes either face starvation or pick up infection of gastro-intestinal tract and respiratory system.

8. Control predators

A large number of predators exist in the forest and bushy pastures in India. The birds of prey like crows, hawks, vultures, etc. on one hand and beasts like foxes, jackals, wolves, bears, panthers on the other, besides *pythons* too, are responsible for the killing of new born lambs. At times the predator losses may exceed disease losses. Since killing of wild life is forbidden, measures should be taken to make the lambs safe from the attack of such predators.

9. Watch for diseases

Possibilities of a disease overtaking the lambs in the early days of life should not be overlooked. Contagious ecthyma, coccidiosis, lamb dysentery do much harm at some of the sheep flocks. Investigations into mortality should always be expeditious and taken up carefully.

ABORTIONS IN SHEEP

Abortions due to pregnancy infections

At times abortions in a breeding ewe flock contribute to the prenatal lamb losses and thereby lower lambing rates and performance of the flock.

Feeding of fungus infested feed or grain, results into heavy abortions due to aflotoxins. Foot and Mouth Disease, Sheep Pox and Blue Tongue disease out breaks bring havoc in a pregnant ewes flock. Even the whole lambing is threatened at times.

Besides these maladies that are responsible for indirect abortions, a number of infectious organisms are known to induce foetal losses in ewes directly. The incidence varies. The main organisms associated with abortions are given in the following table.

Sl.no.	Name of infection	Organism responsible
1.	Brucellosis	Brucella ovis
2.	Listeriosis	Listeria monocytogenes
3.	Vibriosis	Vibrio foetus
4.	Leptospirosis	Leptospira sp.
5.	Toxoplasmosis	Toxoplasma sp.

The first time a flock is affected, serious lamb losses may occur. In subsequent year the same ewe may lamb successfully. There may appear little evidence of ewe having been infected earlier by an organism likely to cause abortion. The time of abortion may also vary. Sometimes ewes are affected early in gestation, i.e. between 1st and 2nd month, while others are affected later, i.e. during the last month. At times lambs develop to full term but die soon after, because of infections of one or the other organisms of abortions harboured by the ewe.

Brucellosis: Brucellosis has been reported in small ruminants in Europe, Mediterranean islands, New Zealand and Queensland (Australia). Isolated incidence of brucella infection in sheep in India has also been recorded over the years.

The most noticeable lesion is on the placenta which becomes oedamatous. Gelatinous swellings up to 5 cm thick are observed. Frequently one horn of the uterus is affected more than the other. Grossly diseased cotyledons are yellowish white in colour. As the condition advances the attachments between cotyledons and placenta may weaken so that the placenta becomes partially detached. Plaque like thickenings may occur in the placenta. Similarly lesions may also occur in the cells and walls of the hooves of the lambs, born to ewes suffering from Brucellosis. Attendants may also catch infection.

Listeriosis: The causal organism, the *Listeria monocytogenes* is also responsible for circling disease of sheep. Ewes experiencing abortions do not show early symptoms, but abort around 110 to 120 days' pregnancy.

Listeriosis is communicable to man and care is necessary in performing postmortem. Usually there is little to see after abortion. The walls of the uterus may be slightly thickened. There is often a yellowish fluid in uterus. Some ewes fail to expel their after-births. Circling disease of sheep caused by *Listeria monocytogenes* has been recorded in Australia.

Vibrionic abortions: Earlier reports reveal that in USA. 50 to 60 percent of the anticipated lamb crop used to be lost in some of the flocks. The disease would disappear only to reappear in a few years later in previously affected flocks.

Abortion due to vibriosis may occur early in gestation and continue for some time. The most characteristic changes are in the aborted lambs. The liver is invariably enlarged and shows necrotic pale areas. Body cavity contains a considerable amount of blood stained fluid. At times subcutaneous oedema may be observed.

Leptospirosis: A number of organisms belonging to Leptospira group infect domestic animals. In pigs the occurrence may pass off unnoticed as no symptoms appear. But in sheep and cattle disease appears with definite indications.

Abortions due to no other apparent cause lead to the suspicion of Leptospirosis.

In lambs the symptoms are mild with slight fever, off feed and haematuria like conditions. In cattle, fever, anaemia, red colour of urine and jaundice set in suddenly. Heavy mortality in calves may ensue. Abortions occur in pregnant cows which contract infection. A close association between cattle and sheep known to be suffering from Leptospirosis or presence of pigs and rats carrying infection provides an indication of leptospirosis.

The appearance of clinical symptoms among sheep, demonstration of organisms in the urine of affected sheep, sudden deaths without showing symptoms and typical changes of jaundice, watery blood, yellowish brown liver, brownish discolouration of kidney and blood stained urine in bladder are all suggestive of leptospirosis.

Toxoplasmosis: Toxoplasma is a protozoan parasite that multiplies in living cells. It has a small crescentic or spheroidal shape. Organism divides by binary fission. It has been isolated from rabbits, guinea pigs, mice, rats, squirrels, monkeys, a number of birds, dogs, cats and sheep.

The main symptoms in sheep are those of encephalitis and circling. The latter condition may resemble typically with *Listeriosis*. These symptoms appear due to the involvement of nervous system. Death of sheep due to acute illness and postmortem lesions of the placenta attached to the cotyledons in the uterus are an indication. Foetal cotyledons tend to be convex and bright red in colour. Numerous white flakes, soft white nodules, 1 to 3 mm in diameter amongst the soft tissue *pile* foetal cotyledons. History of abortions after about 15th week of gestation and continuing sporadically till lambing, is diagnostic of toxoplasmosis.

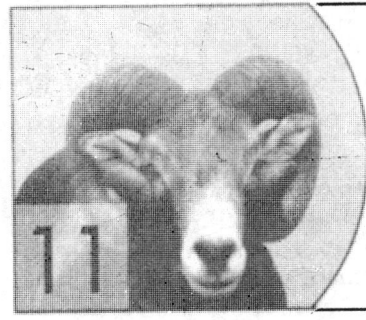

APPLICATION OF BREEDING PRINCIPLES

GENETIC ASPECT

A sound planning of any livestock improvement programme invites attention to the management aspects given in Chart 11.1.

Genetic make up determines the status and scope for improvement. In absence of genetic development the effect of improved feeding are not much pronounced in livestock production. Therefore a basic know how of type of germ plasm of population to be improved and its 'Genomics' is essential. Equally important is the aspect of breeding behaviour of the type of animals and their scientific breeding.

Species and breeds

A specie comprises of a population of similar genotype and individuals which interbreed and reproduce within. Different species have different chromosome number and gene pools. Breeding among species is mostly unsuccessful and where possible the progeny is invariably sterile, but for rarest of instances. A breed on the other hand is a group or population of genetically and phenotypically distinct individuals, that breed normally to produce fertile and reproducing progeny. Individuals of a breed share a common gene pool and their origin is traceable to common ancestors.

The diverse nature of breeds of livestock, particularly of sheep make it imperative to define the purpose and the direction in which improvement is desired. A wide range of genotypically and phenotypically different sheep types exist in the world. A distinction is generally made between woolly, muttonous, dual purpose or even milch and prolific types.

BREEDING SYSTEMS

Scientific breeding involves the study of following components.
- Breeding systems
- Breeding methods or mating systems

Chart 11.1: Livestock management

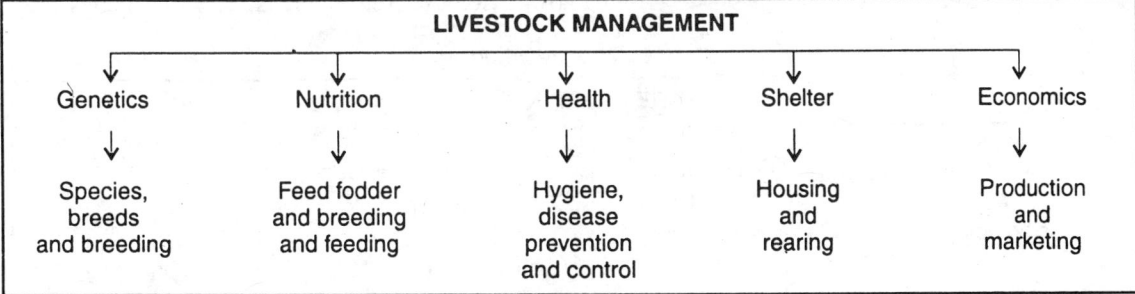

LIVESTOCK MANAGEMENT				
Genetics	Nutrition	Health	Shelter	Economics
Species, breeds and breeding	Feed fodder and breeding and feeding	Hygiene, disease prevention and control	Housing and rearing	Production and marketing

- Breeding behaviour
- Breeding advancements

The livestock breeding operations are conducted under one of the these breeding systems.

- Pure breeding
- Crossbreeding
- Species hybridization

Pure breeding: It is the mating of animals within the same breed. In other words it is the interbreeding of individuals belonging to a well defined breed. Breeding remains confined within the breed thereby the purity of the breed is maintained. Various forms of pure breeding are given in Chart 11.2.

Free breeding: Random breeding conditions prevail in village herds and among the flocks of the same breed, possessed by the breeders. The impact is difficult to assess unless relationship among breeding individuals and size of population are known. The large random mating population, when considered as base population, is a point at which there is least or no inbreeding. The chances of any deterioration in production, reproduction and vigour of animals in such large populations may be negligible over a period of time.

Many local sheep breeds have remained preserved and thriving in various tracts under free breeding environment in the past. The existence of true to breed/type sub-populations of indigenous livestock breeds and perpetuation of their age old purity is a consequence of random breeding.

Outbreeding: When the systematic mating of individuals through non-random pairing involves unrelated or less related animals on the average, it is out breeding. There should not be any common ancestor in their pedigree for five or six generations at least. The degree of outbreeding varies. Far off lines with no distinct or distant relationship when bred scientifically do not show any after effects of homozygous pairing.

Out breeding provides an effective system of genetic improvement of a population where genetic variability exists. Best selected animals of diverse groups/families of a breed on crossing, give excellent result at times. The merino stud production in Australia and the development of other specialised breeds elsewhere are such examples. When combined with scientific management and selection, out breeding is particularly useful for a gradual improvement in production traits.

Whereas this system takes care of inbreeding and overcomes its bad effects, the aspects of non-relationship and large population size can not be ignored. Within the same genetic framework the breeder is at times confronted with the situations of assortative mating, i.e. mating of phenotypically alikes or disassortative mating, i.e. mating of phenotypically unlike animals. On grounds of choice trait breeding, certain less advantageous effects can be corrected.

Inbreeding: is defined as the mating of more closely related individuals than are the individuals of the same population, selected randomly. In other words it is the mating of animals related through ancestry, i.e. having genetic homozygosity. The homozygous alleles may be either allozygous or autozygous.

Allozygous: These are the homozygous genotypes with alleles that have been derived from two different sources. The two genes may

Chart 11.2: Pure breeding

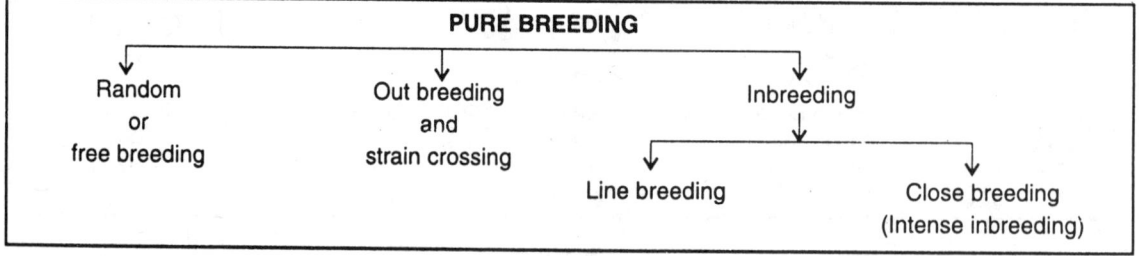

be alike and perform the same function, i.e. are alike-in-state. Means similar in effect and in nucleotide sequence.

Autozygous: These are the homozygous genotypes with alleles that are exact copies of the same gene derived from a common parent (ancestor), i.e. identical by descent, implying that the two alleles are replicate of the same allele. In the allozygous cases there may be no inbreeding even if there is homozygosity.

Degree of inbreeding: The impact of inbreeding and the consequences depend on the extent of inbreeding. While mating individuals of close strains the chances of inbreeding are remote though minimal levels cannot be ruled out in certain cases. The effects are, however, mainly discernible in respect of close breeding (Table 11.1).

An example of line breeding is given in Chart 11.3.

Likewise generation 4th rams may be born by mating rams Z_1, Z_2 and Z_3 to dams G_1, G_2 and G_3 which are not related.

When mated to unrelated dams the progeny of 4th generation rams would be distant related and not as close as x_{18}, x_{19} or x_{20}, thus giving rise to separate lines.

Consequences: In close breeding the level of homozygosity increases more than line breeding. The after effects of the former are therefore more marked than the latter type of breeding. Small size of flock with certain house holds and in confined pockets suffer deterioration in body size and other traits due to continued inbreeding unknowingly.

In general inbreeding leads to:

(a) Decrease in growth rate, (b) setbacks in reproduction, (c) reduced vigour and low survivability, (d) a decline in production might be visible, or (e) an increase in genetic disorders due to appearance of lethal and semi-lethal genes.

In view of these adverse effects a caution is observed in sheep flocks bred to limited number of one or two sires only. In commercial and below average producing flocks inbreeding should be avoided as far as possible. Breeding rams need to be changed after second breeding season. Of

Table 11.1: Close breeding and line breeding comparison.

	Close breeding	Line breeding
Mating example	Sire to daughter, son to dam full brother and sister.	Mating of other distant relations, or 4th–5th generation, individuals of various lines
Advantages	Undesirable recessive genes can be located and eliminated. Progeny becomes more uniform than out bred ones due to homozygosity	Increases uniformity. Dangers of close breeding are avoided to some extent
Disadvantages	Undesirable traits become more prominent, progeny becomes more prone to diseases. There is increase in reproduction set backs. Adverse effects of close inbreeding are difficult to overcome.	When the selection is pedigree based and individual merit is out of consideration, the advantage of selection in the next generation are missing.
Usage	May be recommended where both the parents are outstanding. However, the chances of undesirable recessive genes passing in the progeny in homozygous state, remain.	Is recommended where fixation of characteristics of outstanding sires are desired in the progeny

Chart 11.3: Line breeding example

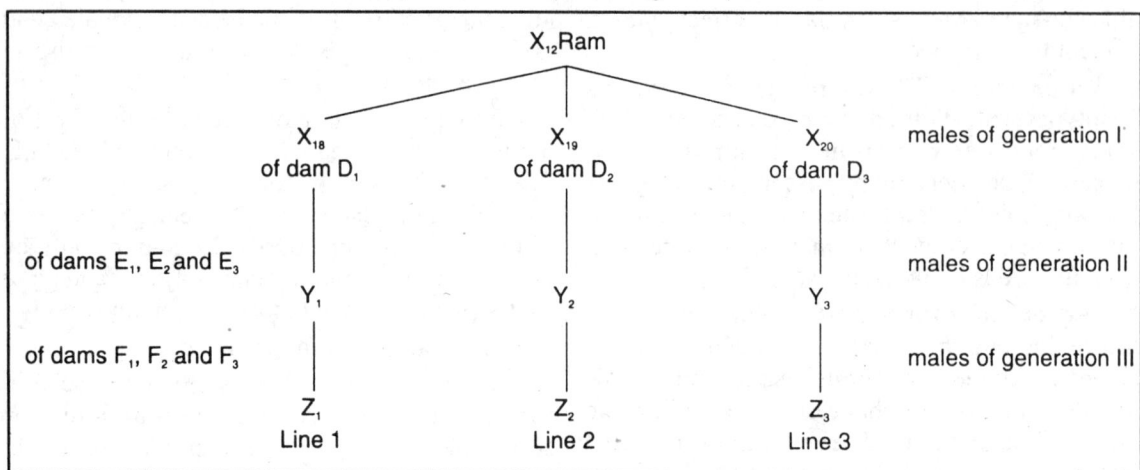

course, there are situations where the advantages of inbreeding can be exploited, viz.:

- To maintain purity of a breed, as maintaining pure lines of plants and animals meant for experimental purposes.
- When sires of outstanding merit are required to be used for transmitting the desirable characteristics in progeny
- Can also be practised in flocks having above average merit.
- And where a know how of inbreeding and checks to control inbreeding level are available with the breeder.

The tribal shepherd in India might have been conscious of the harmful effects of inbreeding. That is how within the parameters of pure breeding practised over the past centuries remarkable strains and sub-types of sheep breeds appear evolved in the country. Deccani breed in Maharashtra; Marwari in Rajasthan and Gujarat, Chokla in Rajasthan, Shahabadi in the fringes of MP, UP, and Bihar and Gaddi in Himachal Pradesh and Jammu and Kashmir offer best examples of sheep types without or with least inbreeding effects. Blood polymorphism and DNA studies shall further help to establish their entities in their respective breeding tracts.

Inbreeding depression

The over all effect of inbreeding leading to deterioration in size, body weight, reproduction, production, vigour and thrivability is due to inbreeding depression. This is dependent on the rate of inbreeding, which in turn is a function of population size (2N). Larger the population lesser the inbreeding.

The rate of inbreeding (ΔF) is therefore $= \dfrac{1}{2N}$

Genetic effects of inbreeding depression are:

1. Increase in homozygosity and loss of heterozygosity
2. Increase in homozygosity is accompanied by decrease in the mean performance of population.

   This decline in mean of population performance is further dependent on the degree of dominance. More the degree of dominance, more the decrease in mean performance of population after inbreeding. In small populations even if mating occurs in unrelated individuals, inbreeding cannot be ruled out.
3. Genetic variance in an inbred population may also be different from that in a non-inbred population. The effects of inbreeding on additive genetic variance (Falconer, 1981) are:

a. Genetic variance of the total population increases.

b. Genetic variance within lines decreases.

c. Genetic variance between lines increases.

Besides the general effects of inbreeding depression, Turner and young (1969) observed a fall in greasy fleece weight, clean wool (yield) percent, body weight at weaning and yearling stage in Merino and Rambouillet sheep. Inbreeding resulted into a decrease in staple length at yearling age, lambs born per ewe joined, lambs weaned per lamb born and survivability, aspects in sheep.

Inbreeding coefficient (F)

It is the probability that the two gametes which are uniting to produce offspring are identical by descent. In otherwords it is the probability of an individual to be autozygous for a given locus. As per Sewal Wright (1940) the correlation coefficient between uniting gametes is twice the inbreeding coefficient of the off spring.

Estimation of inbreeding

The degree of inbreeding over a period of time or generations is measured as coefficient of Inbreeding (F). Assuming the level of F, of random mating base population as zero, the maximum levels may be in selfing. These can be measured by:

1. Path method or Pedigree method, and
2. Co-ancestry method

Path method: A general formula for working out inbreeding coefficient is:

$$\Gamma_x = \Sigma \left(\tfrac{1}{2}\right)^{n_1 + n_2 + 1} (1 + F_A)$$

where F_x = Inbreeding coefficient x offspring

F_A = Inbreeding coefficient of common ancestor (CA)

n_1 = No: of segregation/generations from CA to one parent of x

n_2 = No: of segregation/generations from CA to the other parent of x

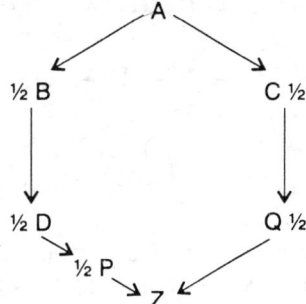

In the example given here, the Z individual has A as common ancestor. For calculating inbreeding coefficient Fz, the paths are:

$$Z \overset{1}{\leftarrow} P \overset{2}{\leftarrow} D \overset{3}{\leftarrow} B \leftarrow A \overset{1}{\longrightarrow} C \overset{2}{\longrightarrow} Q \longrightarrow Z$$

So, $n_1 = 3$

$n_2 = 2$

$$\therefore F_z = \left(\tfrac{1}{2}\right)^{3+2+1} (1 + F_A)$$

$$= \left(\tfrac{1}{2}\right)^6 (1 + F_A)$$

Where in such a system of irregular inbreeding the P and Q parents have x ancestors in common (in the above equation of total inbreeding, F_z of offspring Z) the cumulative inbreeding is determined by summing up the contribution of x common ancestors through all the paths connecting the two parents P and Q

$$F_z = \sum_{i=1}^{x} \left[\left(\tfrac{1}{2}\right)^{n_1 + n_2 + 1} (1 + F_{xi}) \right]$$

The below example illustrates various path sources of inbreeding:

Z offspring has P and Q parents. The common ancestor to both is A. The various paths are:

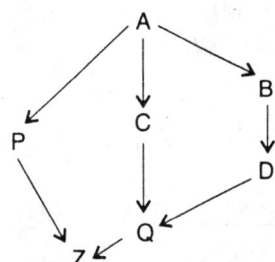

Path I $P \longleftarrow A \longrightarrow C \longrightarrow Q = (\frac{1}{2})^{1+2+1}(1 + F_A)$

Path II $P \longleftarrow A \longrightarrow B \longrightarrow D \longrightarrow Q$
$$= (\tfrac{1}{2})^{1+3+1}(1 + F_A)$$

$$\therefore F_z = \Sigma \left[(\tfrac{1}{2})^4 (1 + F_A) + (\tfrac{1}{2})^5 (1 + F_A) \right]$$

when the pedigree of common ancestor A is unknown or it is non-inbred the F_A is assumed to be o,

then the $F_z = \Sigma \left[(\tfrac{1}{2})^4 + (\tfrac{1}{2})^5 \right]$
$$= 0.0625 + 0.0312$$
$$= 0.0937$$

The other methods of coancestory proposed by Falconer (1981), Coefficient of parentage by Malecot (1948), Coefficient of Relationship by S. Wright (1921) are also employed for working out F values. As per Kempthorne (1957) in a regular inbreeding system where for the Z offspring its P, Q parents have the probability to possess genes *x*, *y* which are identical by descent, the coefficient of parentage (Fp) is equal to the inbreeding coefficient of offspring, i.e. $F_z = r_{xy}$.

Inbreeding due to small population size

In a small size population of N individuals (with 2N gametes) which is mating randomly, the gene and genotypic frequencies, variance and mean of population are effected. Let us consider the large and small populations where the gene frequencies p and q are in equilibrium, i.e.

$p = q = 0.5$

Large population	Small population
Size N = 5,000	n = 8
2N = 10,000	$2n$ = 16

When variance $\sigma_q^2 = \dfrac{pq}{2N}$

$$\sigma_q^2 = \frac{0.5 \times 0.5}{10,000} \qquad \sigma_q^2 = \frac{0.5 \times 0.5}{16}$$

$$\sigma_q = \sqrt{\frac{0.5 \times 0.5}{10,000}} \qquad \sigma_q = \sqrt{\frac{0.5 \times 0.5}{16}}$$

$$= \frac{0.5}{100} = 0.005 \qquad = \frac{0.5}{4} = 0.125$$

The distribution of the gene frequency in next generation is:

0.5 ± 0.005	0.5 ± 0.125
i.e. 0.495 to 0.505	0.375 to 0.625

The range is not much in large population but the spread or change in gene frequencies in small population is larger than in large population. The values may vary from 0 to 1 $(0 \rightarrow \leftarrow 1)$. When 0, the chances are for elimination of gene and as the value approaches 1, the gene get fixed. Any increase in homozygotes is at the cost of decrease in heterozygosity. The rate of change of inbreeding is dependent on N. The increment in inbreeding coefficient (ΔF) is given by $\dfrac{1}{2N}$.

In short, the small population or population broken down into sub-populations have the properties of:

- Sampling error results into elimination or fixation of genes, which is also a consequence of inbreeding.
- Sampling error results into reduction of heterozygotes and increment of homozygotes.
- The rate of change in gene frequency due to sampling is correlated with the rate of inbreeding. Both are in direct proportion to the size of population.

In livestock breeding programmes, a general approach is to avoid chances of inbreeding or maintain inbreeding levels at a lowest ebb. This makes imperative to plan the improvement programme with a large sample and population size. Limited numbers thwart random mating and are thus prone to inbreeding.

Degree of relationship or coefficient of relationship

Commonness of ancestors contributes to relationship among individuals. No common ancestor, no relationship. The progeny of a sire and dam is 50 percent related to each parent. The degree of relationship varies from 0 to 100 percent. Identical twins have all the genes alike and are 100 percent related.

Instead of being direct, the relationship may be collateral as for instance cousins are concerned.

Direct relationship	Collateral
A × B ↓ C 50% of A + 50% of of B relationship with each grand parent is 25%	A B ↑ ↑ ⌐——⌐ ⌐——⌐ C × D E × F ↑ ↑ M × H × N Here A and B are cousins by descent from common ancestor H

The relationship (R) between A and B can be worked out by following the steps to common ancestor (s)

$$R_{AB} = \Sigma \left(\tfrac{1}{2}\right)^{n_1 + n_2} (1 + F_a)$$

Where Σ is summation of contribution of all common ancestors through all paths.

$\tfrac{1}{2}$ = the factor of halving inheritance per generation.

n_1 = No. of generation between A and common ancestor.

n_2 = No. of generation between B and common ancestor.

F_a = Inbreeding cofficient of common ancestor, H, in the present case.

Method:
1. First find the number of common ancestors.
2. Calculate contribution through each of them
3. Then sum all the contributions.

Values of R, i.e. coefficient of relationship, among relatives is:
- First cousins 12.5 percent related;
- Half first cousins 6.25 percent related;
- Double first cousins are 25 percent related.

The illustrations of the three cases are given in Chart 11.4.

Chart 11.4: Illustrations of three cases

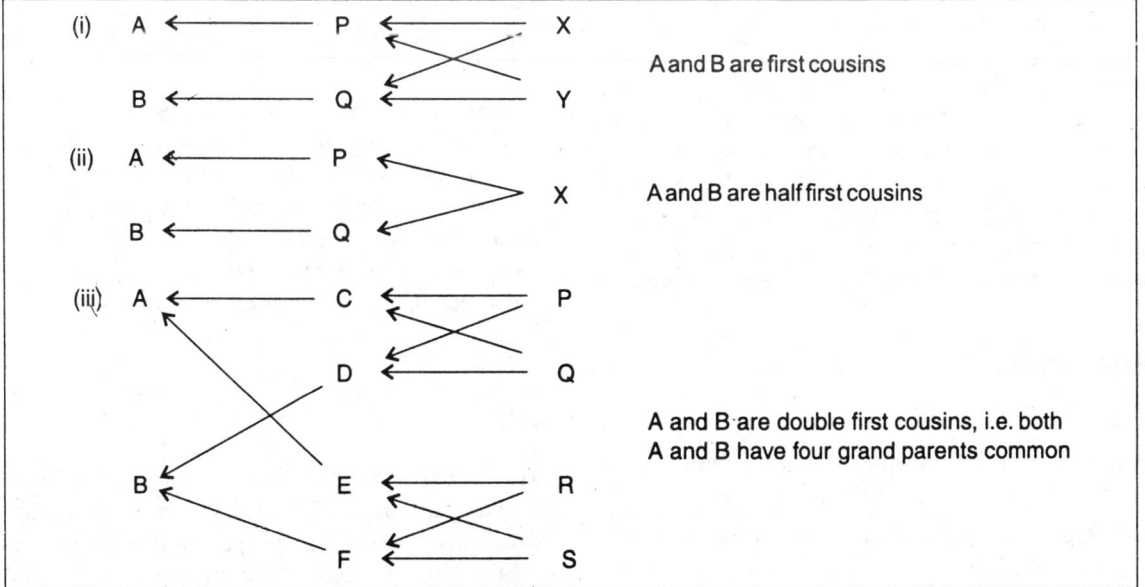

This coefficient of relationship provides another method for determining Coefficient of inbreeding.

Crossbreeding

Is the mating of animals of two different breeds of the same specie. The result of mating of individuals of two or more varying breeds leads to the formation of new gene combinations at various loci. A stable pure breed is normally considered homozygous in respect of certain alleles and characteristics controlled by them. With crossbreeding the homozygosity existing in the breed individuals gives place to heterozygosity in the progeny. Besides gain in heterozygosity the mean and variance are also affected in the crossbred progeny. The extent of change in the genetic parameters depends on:

- gene frequencies of alleles controlling a trait of economic importance.
- degree of dominance.
- epistatic effects among genes controlling that particular trait.

In the aegis of plant breeding and livestock development the tool of crossbreeding has been employed most commonly. In the last century especially, this served as a means to improve inferior breeds faster enough than the traditional manoeuvres available with the breeder. Choice traits were introduced in certain Indian sheep breeds through crossbreeding. Breeds like Merino, Rambouillet, Stavropols, Corriedales, etc. have helped to raise the status of many indigenous sheep breeds in respect of wool quality and quantity.

Advantages

Crossbreeding is used for:

- Transforming the low producing breeds into more productive crossbreds.
- Upgrading of existing breeds is the main advantage.

- With new gene combinations, evolution of new breeds is possible by imposing and combining other genetic measures like selection, interbreeding, etc. Kashmir merino, Bharat merino are some examples.
- In many cases improvement in disease resistance, adaptability, vigour and reproduction is possible.
- Like enhancement in broiler production in poultry, the faster marketable lamb production can be achieved by exploiting heterotic effect for quick gains.

Disadvantages

- A prerequisite of crossbreeding is the maintenance of animals of two pure breeds and additionally the crossbreds.
- A knowledge of the genetic make up of two breeds, their adaptation, genetic compatibility and behaviour is necessary.
- The crossbreds have a heterozygous, rather a disturbed genotypic array. Due to disruption of gene combinations all the offspring may not be up to expectations. Wide variability in the cross breds often calls for rigid selection. Only a small percentage may be fit for retention.
- Due to many enviro-physiological interactions in the crossbreeding, the sure success in onground achievements is often thwarted. For local sheep cross-breeding in Jammu and Kashmir nine exotic breeds were initially suggested. After trials with five a workable and beneficial success came with one breed only.

Utility

Crossbreeding affords a convenient tool for improving quality and quantity of wool in sheep breeds. It is generally employed in grading up the existing scrub breeds and evolving new breeds through selection. Visible heterotic effects are often exploited for improving vigour and other economic traits. It further helps in the study of trait transmission and other hereditary aspects.

Forms of crossbreeding

Like inbreeding there are varying forms of crossbreeding. From breeding among two or more widely different or dissimilar breeds, i.e. non-assortative out crossing like, Merino x Indian coarse woolly breeds to milder type like mating Nali x Lohi which have more resemblance to each other than the former ones. Even the genetic levels may vary in a flock/herd like quarter breeds, half breeds, three quarter breeds and so on.

Thus besides direct crossbreeding other different forms, used in livestock development and breed improvement are:

1. Crisscrossing

When in a usual crossbreeding programme, the two involved breed sires are used alternately. It is also called alternate crossing. This way a varying genetic level or contribution of either breed is maintained. Breeder takes advantage of maternal heterosis from both the breeds used in the crisscrossing. Examples are shown in Chart 11.5.

2. Triple or multiple crossing

Certain animal breeding plans envisage the incorporation of characteristics of more than two breeds. Such breeding operations involve the use of three or more breeds at regular or irregular sequence. In USSR it is named *mutative* crossing. When breeds are used at regular rotation it is also called *rotational* crossing.

3. In-crossing (incross breeding)

It is one time crossing for introduction of a desired trait of other breed in an otherwise normal population of a breed. Incrossing is resorted to when it is essential to impart a choice characteristic in a flock/breed to enhance utility, while preserving the inherent traits of that breed. The sires of the breed possessing wanted trait are withdrawn and their female off springs are further bred with the mates of their original breed.

Such an infusion of germ plasm is also called *instantaneous* or *introductive* crossing. Sal breed of sheep in Russia is one such example of Incrossbreeding. It is believed that the progenitors of highly prolific Booroola merino flock in Australia might have got an infusion/dose of some prolific sheep germplasm. For improvement of staple length of crossbred wools to make them more

Chart 11.5: Examples

Crisscrossing	*Triple/Rotational crossing*
Two breeds	(Three breeds A, B, and M)
A × B	A × B
↓	↓
A × C 50% A + 50% B	C × M — 3rd breed
↓	↓
B × D 75% A + 25% B	D × A — Ist breed
↓	↓
	E × B — 2nd breed
↓	↓
E 37½ A + 62½% B and so on	F × M — 3rd breed and so on

lucrative, a trial introduction of Lincoln blood on this vary anology has often been advocated by the experts in Jammu and Kashmir state as illustrated here in the breeding plan (Chart 11.6):

First generation male lambs to be used for breeding of original (base) population flocks. Vitally needed gene for lustre in wool and heavy weight trait of Lincoln is intended to be introduced simultaneously in the incrossed progeny in addition to fibre length.

4. Grading up (upgrading)

A common way to improve a scrub, non-descript or low productivity breed is to cross the females with males of a superior breed and then back cross the progeny to the sires of superior breed successively to 3/4th, 7/8th or any such desirable level to approach the superior breed in performance as illustrated in Chart 11.7.

The level of superior breed inheritance increases at every step. It is however observed that the graded up progeny do not exhibit corresponding increments in production due to adaptability problems. There is rather reduced resistance beyond 3/4th bred level, resulting into lowered survivability.

HETEROSIS

When on crossing of individuals of two unrelated strains, breeds, varieties or even certain species, the resultant progeny is superior to the mid parent value the phenomenon is called heterosis. It is associated with heterozygous state of the crossbred-progeny. A cross between Desi sheep and Rambouillet breed exhibits heterosis in respect of body weight and greasy fleece weight. Mean value of the traits in offspring is above the mean of the parents in some crosses.

In rare instances the cross bred may even be superior in certain economic traits to the parent with the higher value. Such a heterozygous state is termed 'true heterosis' and is synonymous to *hybrid vigour*. The crossbreds of Merino and Border Leicester sheep exceeded the mean of pure breds by 0.47 for number of lambs weaned per ewe joined and also exceeded the pure breds by 10 percent in clean wool weight (Turner, 1969). In extreme heterosis cases of mule production the progeny is hardier and more vigorous than the two involved equine species.

Estimation: The extent of heterosis in respect of any economic trait can be reasonably worked out by considering the difference between the mean of F_1 progeny and the mean of parents belonging to pure bred strains, breeds or species.

Chart 11.6: Breeding plan

Fine wool crossbred ewe A × B Less coarse Lincoln ram
↓

C.B. Generation (1)　　Lincoln C.B.　　　　　　C　usually males culled except selected ones.

	Option I	Ewe		**Option II**
	Ram of breed/genetic group	A × C ↓ D_1	C × C ↓ D_2	Lincoln crossbred ram used for interbreeding
Generation (2)				The interbred D_2 is 50% longwool (Lincoln)
	Incross backcrossed progeny D_1 is 25% longwool (Lincoln) bred.			

Chart 11.7

Desi or scrub breed A ♀ × B ♂	Superior breed
↓	
½ bred ♀ C × B₁ ♂	–do–
↓	
3/4 bred ♀ D × B₂ ♂	–do–
↓	
7/8 bred E × B₃ ♂	and so on

$$\text{Heterosis \%} = \frac{\text{Mean of } F_1 \text{ offspring} - \text{Mean of parents}}{\text{Mean of parents}} \times 100$$

Basis of heterosis

Dominance deviations and epistasis are known to cause heterotic effect. The additive gene action results into coinciding of mean of F_1 progeny with the mean of parents, if environmental variations are excluded. Gene action of this nature does not give rise to heterosis. Various explanation offered from time to time for heterosis are:

- *Physiological basis:* Sufficient metabolic system variations as observed in top cross pigs and some excellent crosses of poultry, sheep, etc. may be due to lower maintenance requirements or less energy loss during growth and fattening phases.
- *Genetic basis:* Heterosis is caused by heterozygosity involving genes with nonadditive effects. Such gene action includes:
  1. *Dominance:* Crossing offsets the effect of pairing of inbred homozygous alleles in the crossbreds, i.e. intergenic complementation.
  2. *Over dominance:* Interaction of allelic gene pairs, i.e. inter-allelic complementation.
  3. *Epistasis:* Due to interaction between pairs of genes that are not alleles (nonallelic).
- *Biochemical basis:* Heterosis appears as an expression of the activity of favourable concentrations and combinations of chemical growth factors produced as a result of complimentary gene action in hybrids.
- *Enzymatic action:* The oxidase enzyme action on the crushed growing tips of corn varieties and their hybrids is found to have an altered oxygen consumption and utilization.

Utility

Remarkable revolution in crop production, viz. maize, tomato, cotton, etc. has been possible through exploitation of heterosis in various outbred-inbred lines. It is of importance in improving the production status of certain mediocre animal breeds and employed to produce commercial high producing animals. Heterotic effects are also exploited to evolve new strains and breeds of poultry and livestock for better performance.

Exploitation of heterosis however demands continued crossing of the strains, breeds, etc. This in turn necessitates the maintenance of pure bred lines. Sizeable/large population of respective germ plasm becomes imperative. This usually seems costlier than improving through selection within one group or breed. Therefore a prior or timely study of comparative gains of hybrid vigour *vis-a-vis* expected estimates from other breeding plans is desirable while launching any such programme.

SPECIES HYBRIDISATION

It is a phenomenon restricted to certain special species of animals, where two species with different chromosome numbers (2N) but having some alikeness do reproduce when mated. The breeding outcome, a true hybrid, is potentially hardier and vigorous.

The progeny of such interbreeding species is invariably sterile though physically superior to parents and better suited for tough job like draft, ploughing and pack purposes. True animal hybrid examples are:

Mare × Male ass (Jack) ⟶ Mule

Female ass (Jannet) × Horse stallion ⟶ Hinny

Local cow (Demo in Ladakh) × Yak ⟶ Zo, Zomo

Male (Zo) is sterile where as female (Zomo) is fertile when back crossed. Same is true of progeny of a cross of American Bison and European cattle.

Hare (Lepus 2N = 48) and rabbit (Oryctolagus 2N = 44) species are also reported producing viable hybrids in a crossbreeding instance (Gupta, 1994). A couple of hybrids of wild life animals reported by Osamu Ishikawa (2003) are:

Donkey mare × Zebra stallion ⟶ Zenkey (sterile)

Zebra mare × Donkey stallion ⟶ Zebroid

Lion (male) × Jaguar (female) ⟶ Liguar

Any viable hybrid between sheep and goat is a rare phenomenon.

SELECTION

It is the process of choosing the breedable males and females to be parents of next generation. For improvement of production levels in live stock, selection is an effective tool. Basic principle applied is to retain the superior and discard the inferior animals. In sheep, selection for economic traits, viz. body weight, growth rate, fleece weight, wool characteristics, dressing percentage, etc. is generally practised at various regional and central sheep research farms of the country and in private flocks.

Method of selection in combination with mating system constitutes a breeding plan. Selection and mating system are the two tools in the hands of an animal breeder for genetic improvement of live stock. Variability in turn enhances the scope of

selection for raising production potential. To produce better genetic/breeding value animals various methods of selection are:

Showring selection: Where individual animal's phenotype is observed by the expert selector in the race, showring, exhibition or competition yard. Opinion is framed depending upon general appearance, ideal conformation, trueness, qualities of productive animals and existences of correlated traits to production abilities.

Performance selection: Individual's own performance is the guiding factor. Instant record of measurement, and preferably repeated recording of the trait on the same animal provide the data inputs for correct decision. Performance test is an accurate measure of the genetic value of the animal. Its effectiveness depends on the heritability value of the trait under selection, Higher the heritability better the results of performance selection.

It is also termed as mass selection in plants and lower organisms as the selected individual are put together enmasse for mating. Technique may involve individual's one measurable characteristic or summation of a number of economic traits which go to form the phenotype of the individuals.

Family selection: It is applied in two ways:

1. *Pedigree based:* Genes of parents are transmitted to offspring, resulting into resemblance between the two. Thus goes the saying, 'like father like son'. The expressed performance of the progeny much depends on the genetic make-up of the parents.

   Selection based on the information of sire and dam or grand parents helps better in determining the breeding value of the animal under selection. This method is of particular importance in sex limited characters and in estimating carcass qualities which involve slaughter. Pedigree selection is virtually performance selection based on the records of ancestors. It enables selection at an earlier and younger age.

2. *Progeny test:* It is the selection of animals 'the parents' on the basis of performance of

progeny. The underlying principle is 'select thy parents'. That is selecting the seed/plant on the basis of fruits it bears. The merit of the offspring provides an estimate of breeding value of parenting individuals. However, a generation gap elapses before the performance results of the progeny are available. In animal breeding the duration between two generations is long. This limits and reduces the future utility of the parents under test. The advent of artificial insemination and the deep frozen semen technique in sheep have overcome this problem to some extent.

In pedigree selection records of parents are preferred over grand parents, whereas in progeny selection records of offspring are preferable over cousins and other collaterals.

Aids to selection

Important criteria that serve as useful guide before selection are economic and genetic aspects of traits under improvement.

1. Economic factors

A well defined target: Fleece weight (greasy as well as clean), staple length, fibre diameter, body weight, growth rate, dressing percent, etc. are some choice traits for which selection is aimed at in sheep production.

Cost involvement: A prior consideration of financial inputs of conducting a selection programme is essential.

Anticipated returns. Economical value of improvement of each trait and anticipated returns need assessment and comparison. Traits of low economic value can be ignored easily.

2. Genetic parameters

The outcome of selection in an animal breeding programme depends on genetic parameters, i.e. heritability, repeatability and genetic correlation among traits to be selected. As aids to selection, information on these is too relevant.

Measurement of trait values: This includes mean and range of variation in the trait in the population. Higher mean value of the trait in selected population augurs better results. Variability provides for fair amount of selection. For wool production the mean and variability are low in desi sheep. Raising production through selective breeding in local breeds is thus a slow and longdrawn process. Crossbreeding with exotic breeds alters both the mean and variance of wool production and other traits in the crossbred progeny.

Heritability: The transmissible fraction of the phenotypic variance (σ_p^2) which is due to genetic differences among individuals in a population is expressed as heritability. The total observed phenotypic variance for a metric trait in a population may be split-up into the components shown in Chart 11.8.

Lush (1940, 1948) defined heritability as degree of genetic determination (H^2) in the broader

Chart 11.8

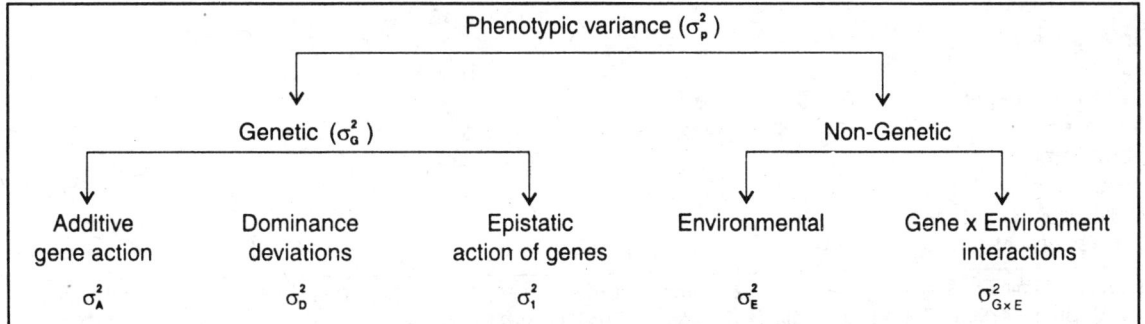

sense, i.e. $\dfrac{\sigma_G^2}{\sigma_P^2}$ and genetic transmissibility (h^2) in the narrow sense, i.e. $\dfrac{\sigma_A^2}{\sigma_P^2}$

In the first case it is the total genetic variance as a fraction of the observed phenotypic variance, whereas, in the latter it is only additive genetic portion of the variance to the total phenotypic variance assuming that dominance and epistatic effects of useful gene combinations may not persist in further offspring due to segregation and recombination.

Since h^2 value takes into account the transmissible part of genetic variance, this parameter provides indication of superiority of parents and is helpful in prediction of gain in the progeny.

A quantitative trait when influenced strongly by environmental effects has low heritability. But in another population with a rigid physical control (where σ_E^2 is low), higher estimates of heritability

for the desired character are obtained. Therefore the h^2 values of the same trait for two populations or for the same population at varying periods shall differ. The values of h^2 range between 0 and 1. Table 11.2 shows heritability values for important production traits in sheep.

Heritability values below 0.1 are considered low, 0.1 to lower than 0.3 as moderate and above these as high. Traits with low heritability values, viz. fertility or twining rate (where h^2 is generally < 0.1) do not show as good response to selection. If the value is moderate to high as in traits like post weaning and yearling body weight, greasy fleece weight, fibre fineness, etc. selection provides a direct basis and yields faster and desirable results.

Estimation of h^2: Direct observations on the values of quantitative traits on the individuals of a population provide estimates of total phenotypic variance (σ_A^2). The estimates of additive genetic variance (σ_P^2) are worked out from correlations

Table 11.2: Heritability values for important production traits in sheep (exotic and Indian).

Trait	Merino and other exotic breeds		Indian sheep breeds Arid region	Evolved cross-bred types	
				1/2 bred	3/4 bred
Body weight at:					
*Birth	0.1–0.3		0.15–0.64	0.17	0.02
			0.10–0.27		
*Weaning	0.2–0.3	0–0.4	0.50		
			0.10–0.7		
*Six month	–	–	0.36	0.24	0.19
			0.37–0.74		0.30
Yearling to					
18 month	0.3–0.5	0.1–0.7	0.25–0.72	0.28	0.54
			0.15–0.48	–	–
Greasy fleece	0.3–0.5	0.2–0.7	0.2–0.6	–	–
weight			0.5	–	–
Clean wool weight	0.3–0.4	0.1–0.6	0.8	–	–
Staple length	0.4–0.5	0.2–0.9	0.6–0.75	–	–
Fibre diameter	0.3–0.5	0.1–0.7	0.33–0.95	–	–
Medullation	0.5–0.6	–	0.65	–	–
Prolificacy	0.1–0.3	–	–	–	–
Carcass weight	0.4–0.5	–	–	–	–

Source: Columns 1- Botkin et al (1988); Col. 2 - Turner and Young (1969); Col. 3 - Basu Thakur and Acharya (1972), Acharya (1972), Chopra (1968); Col. 4 and 5 Malik (1972), Khan (1972), Gupta (1972).

between parents and offspring or between relatives as suggested by Falconer (1981) and Turner and Young (1969).

The realised heritability (h_r) can however be estimated if we know the genetic gain (ΔG) and the selection differential (SD), where

$$h_r^2 = \frac{\Delta G}{SD}$$

The difference of trait value of parents (unselected and selected) gives the selection differential and the difference in progeny gives genetic gain. Since the estimate of realised heritability is based on actual genetic gain, it differs from the expected estimated value. Realised heritability is generally lower than the estimated (expected) heritability.

In sex limited quantitative traits like prolificacy, milk production or egg production in poultry, for which selection is practised in one sex only the realised heritability is given by:

$$h_r^2 = \frac{2\Delta G}{Sel.\ differential}$$

Repeatability

Certain traits viz. milk yield, wool yield, etc. can be recorded many times on an individual during its life time. The total phenotypic variance can be partitioned into between animal variance (σ_B^2) and variance within animal (σ_W^2) The ratio of between animal component of variance and total phenotypic variance provides another estimate known as repeatability. Repeatability can be defined as intra class correlation of repeated records of individuals. High repeatability values suggest that the trait is least influenced by environmental effects. Early record of an individual's performance expresses its real producing ability which helps in early selection of an individual.

Characteristics like greasy fleece weight in sheep besides having high heritability, show high repeatability as well. This parameter therefore is equally helpful in early selection for such traits of economic importance. In 10 to 18 month age group sheep, Turner and young (1969) reported following repeatabiilty values for the important traits, viz.

Greasy fleece weight	0.5 to 0.8
Clean wool weight	0.5 to 0.7
Fibre diameter	0.5 to 0.6
Staple length	0.6 to 0.8
Body weight	0.5 to 0.7

Correlations

Genetic correlations among various characteristics viz., correlated characters provide an indirect basis of selection. Depending upon the nature of correlation, positive or negative, selection for one trait results in gain or loss in the other correlated trait.

High positive correlations exist between certain traits in sheep, viz; body weight and wool production, post-weaning weight and further growth, fibre density and greasy fleece weight, etc. Selection for one trait leads to simultaneous improvement in the correlated trait. The effect may however be slow and transitory in certain cases. In negatively correlated characteristics the values range from -1 to 0, whereas in positive correlations range varies from 0 to 1. Estimates of genetic correlations between important economic traits in sheep are presented in Table 11.3.

Mode of Selection

Direct: Where phenotype of the animal, i.e. the measurement/records on particular characters of economic value are available. Observations on traits like body weight, body size, milk and wool production, wool yield and fibre quality can be made directly on the animal. Selection response is better in traits having high heritability values. Sire scores for body conformation, trueness to breed; soundness of genitalia, semen quality, etc. are additional useful parameters for direct selection.

Indirect: Is considered when certain information is not available from the animal and the observer has to depend on other sources,

Table 11.3: Estimates of genetic correlations* between important economic traits in sheep.

Characteristics	Exotic sheep (Merino)	Indian Sheep		Rambouillet Cross-bred sheep	
				½ R	3/4 R
	1	2	3	4	5
Birth weight and six month weight	–	0.38	0.79	0.66	–
6 month weight and yearling wt.	–	0.74	0.87	–	–
Body wt. and Gr. fl. wt.	0.3	0.98	0.53	0.35	0.44
Gr. fl. weight and clean fleece weight	0.65 to 0.82	–	0.77	0.42	0.96
Greasy fleece weight and staple length	–0.02 to +0.70	0.87	0.47	–	–
Greasy fleece weight and Av. fibre diameter	0.13 to 0.19	0.50	0.40	–	–
Greasy fleece weight and density	–	–	–	0.42	0.59
Av. fibre diameter and staple length	0.11 to 0.44	0.23	–	–	–

particularly information from collaterals and relatives as in respect of:

- Sex limited traits, like milk production, fertility, prolificacy, twinning, etc.
- Traits involving slaughter. For once life time data availability, viz. dressing percent, meat quality, bone-meat ratio, fat or pluck component of carcass, one has to base observation on collaterals or individuals closely related to the animal under selection.
- Correlations between traits as discussed earlier. In case of traits having high correlations, pedigree record of ancestors and information/ measurements of relatives enables to take decision especially where the trait under selection is difficult to measure. Information on other trait is made use of if easily measurable.

Relative selection efficiency

The relative efficiency of indirect selection compared with direct selection can be estimated by the method suggested by Turner and Young (1969)*. Genetic gain calculation for this purpose is prerequisite which further depends on the heritabilities of the two traits and the genetic correlation.

$$\text{Thus R.S.E.} = \frac{\text{Genetic gain in 2nd trait under selection for 1st}}{\text{Genetic gain in 2nd trait under selection for 2nd}}$$

$$= r_G \sqrt{\frac{h_1^2}{h_2^2}}$$

---

* Turner and Young (1969), Acharya (1972), Basuthakur and Acharya (1981), Gupta (1972).

Where r_G = genetic correlation between 1st and 2nd trait and h_1^2, h_2^2 are heritabilities of trait 1st and 2nd

Selection for more than one characteristic

In livestock improvement programmes invariably it in imperative to take up selection for a couple of traits. In woolly sheep for instance, greasy fleece weight, body weight and fibre quality traits are considered together. While increasing milk production, the fat content is also attached importance. To achieve such objectives three methods of selection are in vogue:

- Tandem selection
- Independent culling levels and
- Selection Index

1. Tandem selection: As suggested by Hazel and Lush (1942), one trait is to be considered for improvement at a time for couple of generations. Then the second trait is taken up for one or more generations, followed by the third trait of importance and so on. The relative economic benefits of the trait and the personal preferences of the breeder determine the priority.

Only one particular trait is measured over a period of time so minimum record maintenance is needed. Individual identification of animals and their ranking in the descending order is imperative. Repeated handling of animals is not required. A know-how about genetic parameters of the trait and basic selection is beneficial. The expected genetic gain (ΔG) in the particular trait per generation depends on the heritability (h^2) of the trait.

While taking up important correlated traits, the change in one might lead to economic loss in the other in the long run. Turner and young (1969) pointed out that, "wool weight and crimp number are negatively correlated and h^2 values of the two traits are almost same in Merinos. The economic weightage of the former was however four times the weight of the latter trait. Continued selection for wool weight in Australia lead to a decline in wool count". That is likely to deteriorate wool quality and thus a fall in wool prices.

2. Independent culling levels: Generally normal or desirable production/performance levels for various traits are defined first. Culling for a particular trait is taken up when any individual falls in its measurement for a particular trait below certain fixed standard. Some animals may be culled on one trait at first, some others for the next trait at the second occasion of measurement and so on for the 3rd trait. This enables selection for higher production level animals. At one of the research farms in Jammu and Kashmir (Reports, 1974 to 1978) such a selection of Ramoubillet maiden ewes above a fixed norm of 33 kg body weight in the first instance and then for annual greasy fleece weight of above 2.2 kg tended to produce a 1½ year age ewes flock of 35.3 kg average body weight and 2.6 kg fleece weight. In all 27% of animals (19% for 1st trait and 8% on 2nd trait) got excluded from elite breeding flock on two accounts.

Two different situations are likely to arise in respect of uncorrelated characteristics and correlated characteristics. Instances, are that of body weight and wool quality. While affecting simultaneous selection, the genetic gain in such cases in economic units is the sum of gains from selection in individual trait. The intensity of selection for any trait is related to its contribution to the total gain. Higher the contribution, greater the selection pressure.

3. Selection Index or Total Score method: This method involves simultaneous consideration of a couple of traits of high utility and economic importance together. Each trait is given due weightage for selection. Such weighted values when summed, provide a total score of each animal in the form of an individual merit or index, called selection index.

Let the traits under selection be $x_1, x_2, x_3 \dots x_n$ with their respective weightage factors as $y_1, y_2, y_3, \dots y_n$. The selection index so framed is,

$$SI = x_1 y_1 + x_2 y_2 + x_3 y_3 + \dots x_n y_n$$

The assigned weightages are dependent on the relative economic importance or utility of the individual trait and heritabilities and genetic correlations among traits. In otherwords it represents the genetic value of the respective characteristic. The selection index so framed is an expression of the total breeding value of the animal. The selection index values may show a fairly normal distribution pattern. Best score animals are selected.

The pattern adopted for prime importance traits in sheep breeding in Australia has played a significant role in improving the production levels. Similar but a simple index adopted in the selection of breeding rams and ewes at sheep farms in Jammu and Kashmir takes into account only two important traits recorded at 1½ years age.

S1 for ewes = Body weight (kg) + 10 × Annual greasy fleece weight (kg)

S1 for rams = Body weight (kg) + 10 × Clean fleece weight (kg)

Total score of each animal is arranged in descending order and higher ranked animals are selected.

Another comprehensive index for selection of performance tested and progeny tested breeding animals is being employed at Texas (USA) Research Centre (1991-92). So named Registry of Merit (ROM) Index, takes into consideration the important relevant traits with weightage to evaluate the merit of breeding animals.

The undesirable characteristics like face cover and skin folds lower the over all merit of fine wool sheep. Both positive and negative correlated characteristics receive due weightage as may be perused in a typical scoring like the one cited here under:

I *(ROM) = 60 × Daily body weight gain + (plus)
4 × Staple length + (plus)
4 × Annual clean fleece weight – (minus)
3 × (face cover score) – (minus)
4 × (skin fold score)

Coarse britch and higher fibre diameter variability of fleece contribute to unsoundness of fleeces. Thus bring down the merit. A suitable weighage for the defects is incorporated for final scoring.

To make the ROM performance test more feasible and ensure animal to animal comparison a value known as Index ratio is worked out.

$$\text{Index ratio} = \frac{\text{Actual index value}}{\text{Average index value}} \times 100$$

The index ratio permits ranking of animals around a mean with above average animals having values greater than 100 and vice-versa. Such index values are utilised for selection of a definite percentage of animals for the certified Ram classification and Stud Ram Registry.

Ercanbrack and Knight (1996) suggested a new selection technique based on selection for reproductive efficiency in sheep and showed it as highly effective under highly extensive grazing conditions.

Comparative merit of selection techniques: The culling level method is better than tandem selection. The superiority of it depends on size of population and selection intensity. Higher the number and the selection intensity better the efficiency of this method. The selection index surpasses in efficiency over tandem selection and independent culling level methods.

Sire Index

A sire or for that matter a breeding ram specifically, is half of the flock. As a sire leaves a large number of progenies in comparison to a female, selection of a sire is more important than females. Emphasis as such is laid on proper sire selection. Due attention is given to each trait of economic importance. The selection index so framed as to represent various prime importance characteristics with due weightage to each considered trait is known as sire index. In fact

---

* I-stands for Index (Selection Index).

this function represents the genetic value of the breeding male.

At the stud ram production centres the sire selection entails an exhaustive exercise. Regular data maintenance is necessary right from birth. Body weights, body measurements or growth rate recording at vital stages, wool production, wool yield and wool quality attributes are major production traits. In mutton sheep dressing percentage is an important trait. Being once life time record the observation made on the parents or the collaterals are made use of. Other relevant characteristics for consideration are the size and weight of pelt of slaughtered animal and the weight of abdominal viscera. Because of comparatively higher weights of these two items in the Rambouillet crossbreed sheep and lesser utility of pelt than the desi sheep, the economic advantage of heavier weight crossbred sheep are partly out weighed.

Scoring of ram with regard to body con-formation, trueness to breed, genitalia, semen quality and libido is essential and score value is incorporated accordingly. In sex limited traits like reproductive rates, fertility, twinning or prolificacy, dam performance and pedigree records of ancestors and relatives provide the necessary information. Progeny testing though more accurate, may not be of much utility when selection at early stage is desired.

Turner and young (1969) suggested a practically workable sire index computation as

$$I = b_1(x_1 - \bar{x}_1) + b_2(x_2 - \bar{x}_2) + ... + b_n(x_n - \bar{x}_n)$$

Where $b_1, b_2 .... b_n$ are the weightages attached to various measurements of characteristics included, viz. $x_1 x_2, ... x_n$ The weightage depends on the heritability values of the traits and whether the trait recorded on the same animal or the record of relatives/collaterals are considered.

$\bar{x}$ is the average (mean) value of the respective trait in the population or the flock.

Taking the individual phenotype and performance data into account, scoring of sires on a set index pattern enables selection of best among the available lot of breeding males.

Selection differential

It is an important measure for evaluating the selection results in animal breeding. Precisely, the difference between the average production of selected population and the average of the unselected base population for that trait is the selection differential. The following example shall explain the SD computation with reference to lamb weaning weight trait.

1. Mean weaning weight (of ewes)   = 22.5 kg
   in the random population (P_0)
2. Mean weaning weight of
   selected (ewes) group of
   animals at weaning stage (P)   = 24.5 kg

   SD = 24.5—22.5   = 2.0 kg

The deviation when recorded in measurable terms gives standardised selection differential and expressed as selection intensity.

Response to selection or genetic gain

The effect of selection made for the parents in a particular population is reflected in the progeny. The prediction of response in a selection trial is measured as genetic gain (or ΔG). In other words this is a measure of genetic improvement caused by selection in the next generation.

In the earlier cited example for selection differential, the mean weaning weight of progeny (P_1) of the selected ewes (of mean P) was 25.4 kg ($\bar{P}_1$)

Thus the response to selection, ΔG, expressed as percent is given by $\dfrac{\bar{P}_1 - \bar{P}_0}{\bar{P}_0} \times 100$

$$\therefore \Delta G = \frac{25.4 - 22.5}{22.5} \times 100$$

$$= 12.8\%$$

In direct selection, genetic gain expresses the improvement in the characteristic in the progeny over the parents. Traits of economic importance usually considered are body weight, wool pro-duction, mutton production, dressing percentage and fibre characteristics. Response to selection in such cases depends on heritability. Higher the heritability of trait better the genetic gain. In low heritability traits like twinning rate or prolificacy there is poor response to selection.

Response is measurable per generation or per unit of time (per year).

Per generation gain may be estimated as;

$$\Delta G = \bar{P_1} - \bar{P_0}$$ where $\bar{P_0}$ is population average value of the trait.

$\bar{P_1}$ is average value in the progeny at the same age.

$$= P_0 + h^2 i\sigma$$ where, h^2 is the heritability in narrow sense, i.e. $\dfrac{\sigma_A^2}{\sigma_P^2}$

and $h^2 i\sigma$, is the realised heritability (Lush, 1945).

i, is the standardised selection differential or selection intensity.

σ, is the standard deviation of the trait.

Per year gain

The generation gap is the interval between the average age of parents and the identical age of offspring. Total genetic gain divided by the number of years of generation gap gives the annual genetic gain. In sheep the same trait measurements in parents and progeny are usually available at almost two to four year gap.

The expected and realised response to selection is the effect of a package of various aids to selection, their values and selection intensity. It is desirable to confine selection intensity on a few highly correlated and economically important traits. Higher the number of traits included, lesser the selection response to individual trait. Relative contribution of ram is more in a breeding flock. Selection of ram therefore leads to higher genetic gains as compared to selection of ewes.

Genetic gain due to single trait selection is the sum of direct gain in the trait under selection plus correlated changes in others, if those are genetically correlated with it. Main emphasis should be on one or two economically important traits of high heritability which respond to selection. Unimportant traits are not included and better considered for exclusion.

Open nucleus breeding system

The concept is not new to livestock development in India. It has now been re-oriented to ensure for better and larger germ plasm availability than one dependant on government farms. In various regions or livestock breeding zones there do exist superior stud producing farms. Open nucleus breeding (ONB) implies the establishment or formation of large scale associated flocks/herds in the breeding zone in private sector. In fact it is the creation of a network of superior sire producing sub-farms or centres that are owned and maintained by the breeders under proper scientific and technical supervision (Chart 11.9).

Screening of the progeny is accomplished at the associated flocks at post weaning stage. Best animals are selected and reared at a central nucleus breeding station or feeding centre. Their growth and fitness is monitored under uniform maintenance conditions. Sound breeding animals are ranked on merit basis. The top ones are then redistributed among the existing and new associated flocks/herds. This avoids within line or herd selection. The random distribution further minimizes chances of inbreeding.

The second best-sires are utilised for upgradation of other common or commercial flocks/herds. The over all below average or inferior males are culled. The stud sires of the institutional or breeding project/farms are provided replacement at some intervals to avoid inbreeding. Likewise a change of rams is also considered at better managed and selected associated flocks.

Culling levels

An initial visual observation is employed in culling. In the quantitative traits, the measurement aspect is essential. Either Independent culling level method or application of selection index system is generally used. Percentage of culling may vary.

Chart 11.9: Open nucleus breeding system

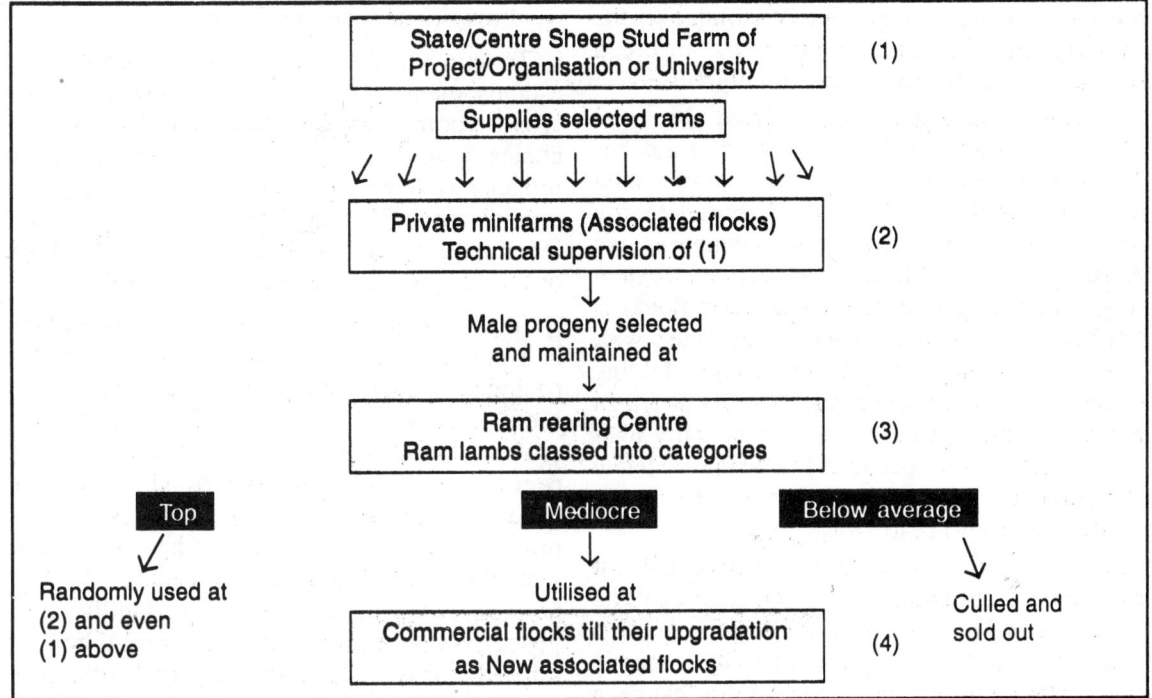

While considering a single characteristic an independent culling level of 4 to 5% is appropriate. The precondition is that the measurement of the trait is below a certain standard regardless of its merit in others. Genetically superior animal may get culled because of lower phenotypic value of characteristic under selection. In the latter method the culling rate may go up to even 20% depending upon the level of various parameters.

Culling rates however depend on lambing rates, weaning numbers, survivability till joining and availability of replacements. Regular culling of low performance animals in each generation helps raise the productivity level of a flock. Besides, it reduces pressure on grazing pasture, feed and manpower resources. A sound practice is to affect disposal of culled and surplus stock before the onset of winters. This enables better care of the left over pregnant and lambing ewes.

In the migratory flocks the usual routine is to carry out culling twice a year, preferably before undertaking down and up migrations. These coincide with breeding season in autumn and post lambing period in spring. Thus sheep below farm standard, and unfit for breeding or unable to undertake long migrations safely get excluded. As an aid to selection the culling practice serves as good tool for raising average body weight and average wool production of the flock and performance improvement in future generations.

EVOLVING NEW BREEDS

Improved varieties of livestock and new breeds of choice traits and better production have been evolved the world over in the last few centuries. In India too a couple of new sheep and other livestock breeds have come into being in the 20th century. This has been possible through a combination of various breeding principles/methods and concerted scientific approach. Various breeding systems put in practice are as follows.

Inbreeding: Mainly utilized to improve a pure breed or evolve a more productive strain over the existing one. The method adopted is to breed selected top breds that are less closely related.

Outbreeding: Mating of unrelated pure bred animals or strains of the same breed is a better tool to achieve a defined goal. Such outbreeding measures appear to have contributed to the development of merino in various countries like Australia, USA, South Africa, etc. To some extent raising of productivity of Chokla sheep flocks is attributed to this method when combined with selective breeding. Introduction of high yielding bucks of Changthangi pashmina goats at Upshi breeding station resulted into substantially high producing Changra goat herd. Practising moderate selection further raised the average pashmina production from 118 to 180 g.

Crossbreeding: Is the most effective and fast tool for transformation of less productive local and scrub breeds. This is accomplished by introduction of breed of superior and high productivity economic traits in the inferior breed. Crossbreeding has been widely used in India in the last century in cattle as well as sheep breeding. A significant improvement in production, and evolution of new breeds has come about through breeding manoeuvres like the following.

1. *Backcrossing* to raise the inheritance level of the superior breed.
2. *Grading up* towards the superior breed is generally restricted at 3/4th bred level or even earlier. The attainment of desired trait and productivity status is the main criterion besides adaptability and survivability of the progeny.
3. *Interbreeding* is a measure of stabilization of inheritance (at the desirable level of superior breed) is brought about by interbreednig of the individuals of same inheritance avoiding inbreeding as far as possible.
4. *Incrossing* is one such aspect of crossbreeding that has helped to produce strains/breeds with

a difference in the major productivity trait through one time infusion only.

To sum up, the usual technique adopted for establishment of new breeds is through initial crossbreeding among selected individuals of choice breeds. Back crossing or grading up the progeny is undertaken to produce the targeted type of animals. Importantly, levels of superior inheritance, productivity, survivability, suitability of the progeny, etc. are the main considerations.

Imposing selection at every step or generation is a prerequisite. Stabilization and fixing up of desirable characteristics to evolve a uniform type/breed is achieved by interbreeding the selected crossbred/graded progeny. While interbreeding, regular selection for five to six interbred generations and pedigree scrutiny are essential to minimise chances of inbreeding. New gene recombinations through crossbreeding introduce heterozygosity and increased variability. The progeny in certain instances might behave unpredictably in growth, survivability, productivity and reproduction aspects.

The extent of improvement in the crossbreds depends on the combining ability, which may be general or breed and trait specific. Merino has shown general combining ability for fine wool. In India its use to produce fine wool crossbreds with the native breeds has been appreciated in the last century. Hissar dale, Kashmir merino and Bharat merino are such breeds evolved through crossbreeding of indigenous breeds with merino. Chart 11.10 clearly illustrates this.

Merino inheritance maintained at 3/4th level by inter-se breeding of selected G_1 (75% merino graded) animals for a couple of successive generations with the objective of stabilising desired characteristics in the progeny. Selection in each generation has to be rigid and is invariably higher in case of 7/8 or higher inheritance graded animals to bring in uniformity.

Chart 11.10: Crossbreeding of Desi sheep with merino

Desi sheep		Merino	
A	×	B	
	↓		
F_1	C ×	B	Back crossing of C to merino
		↓	
3/4th merino graded		G_1 × G_1	Interbreeding at 3/4th merino level
		↓	
2nd generation		G_1 × G_1	
3/4th merino interbred		↓	
3rd generation		G_1 × G_1	
3/4th merino interbred		↓	and so on

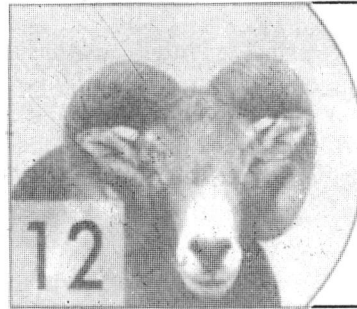

SHEEP CLASSING, CULLING, AGEING AND BIOMETRY

SHEEP CLASSING

It is the operation of classing or grouping of the breedable ewes and selecting sires on similar quality attributes. This involves individual assessment of qualities of the animals based on visual and phenotypic examination. Bonitation, as it is named in some of the east European countries is considered an essential part of development of a flock. Main objectives are:

1. Weeding out the animals showing marked deviation from the desirable types or least profitable sheep.
2. Grading and grouping of the breeding flock on consideration of both constitution and fleece covering.
3. Affecting improvement and uniformity in the breeding quality of the flock through a certain level of culling.
4. Enabling the flock to be more easily managed through elimination of defective ones or those causing difficulty in movement and handling.

For the classing of the individual fine wool sheep and assigning it a particular group, observations are made about breed, type, general constitution and conformation, staple length, fineness of wool, amount of suint and conditioning, evenness and uniformity of wool and body wool cover. An appraisal of apparent reproductive capacity is also essential. Generally speaking the experts assign +, ++, +++ and ++++ gradations to important individual traits while classing. But the whole exercise is more of

experience and evaluation expertise of the sheepman or the classer. A mark is usually kept on the ear or forehead of the class assigned while releasing the animal after assessment or appraisal. Keener the expert eye, better the results.

The sheepman ought to know the requirement of his country and industry, the breeding policy, type of suitable sheep, pasture and seasonal conditions, etc. before deciding upon grades and standards of classing. Maiden ewes are preferably classed at 12 to 15 months age in local breeds and at 15 to 18 months in cross breds. By this time most of the basic data of the animal is available. Once thorough grading has been accomplished at right age, it is customary to perform subsequent classing in the progeny at an earlier age. Final classing at lamb wool or earlier age is however, not advised otherwise. The position of maiden ewes classing takes into account the:

- Culling levels and culling age
- Suitable age at first mating
- Mortality among the ewes
- Lambing percentage
- Replacements
- Feed and Pasture availability.

Having decided on conformation and production standards, the grade assigning is taken up in respect of individual sheep. Best suited time for the operation is full fleece condition or when the sheep have 9 to 12 months wool in fine wool breeds and 5 to 6 months wool growth in crossbreds or local woolly sheep. To gain some

151

idea, it is advisable to make thorough examination of a portion of the flock. Culling of young ewes in maiden stage should be fairly good to avoid entry of inferior animals in the breeding group.

The top best and the worst can easily be marked out. Taking the rest as mediocre or doubtful, the classing is directed towards identifying the:

1. Serious conditions, including hereditary constitutional faults.
2. Ewes away from general standards and inclining towards inferior standard.
3. Flock type ewes that can be retained.

At most of the sheep farms the nature of birth coat, birth weight and subsequent growth data are also considered for final grouping after visual classing of ewes. The final selection of rams, involves laborious scrutiny of pedigree, performance, index score, laboratory investigations into semen quality, fleece analysis, etc. over and above the classing by a conversant observer. The criteria and yard sticks of standards of classing vary from breed to breed and the purpose for which the sheep breed is maintained.

Class criteria

Quite often purebred or crossbred sheep of fine wool lines are presented for classing. Through classing the sheepman attempts to produce a flock of sheep of uniform fine fleece of compactness, good staple, shinning nature with minimum conditioning. The latter aspect tends to produce higher clean wool weight fleeces and thus better returns. Where to draw the border line for various classes is a matter entirely on the classer's own judgement. He should decide actual standards of conformation and various characteristics that are under consideration.

The classer is also expected to take note of the seasonal and management conditions to make necessary allowance in grading so that some of the otherwise suitable or choice animals do not get rejected or downgraded. The constitutional defects and wool faults of genetic origin tend to perpetuate and should not escape the notice of

classer. The initial classing at birth on the basis of birth coat nature does serve a useful purpose.

Having taken into consideration all the points, an overall visual grade is allotted to the individual sheep. A common pattern for classing of fine wool cross bred sheep can be developed on the following lines:

Class I: Animals of excellent constitution, growth and type; fleece with desired fineness of over 60's, staple length 6 to 7 cm on annual clip basis; no hair, least conditioning of wool, fleece coat compact and uniform; wool cover extending over legs and belly. Midside wool clean white and glistening.

Class II: Good constitution and development; wool quality approaching 60's and the quantity as well as quality is not inferior to class I. Neck and britch region may have sparse sprinkling of coarse fibres; legs and abdomen area have shaggy fleece coat; over all coat appearance lacks good compactness, a moderate degree of yolk persists. The wool length is 5 to 7 cm.

Class III: Animal is of moderate constitution and fair breed appearance. Partly open fleece coat; staple length is around 7 cm and wool is of 56's quality; heterotype fibres scattered over neck, back and other body parts and in certain cases medullated fibres predominate. Yolk content is less, in a few animals, but in majority the conditioning is as good as in the former two grades.

Class IV: Animal may or may not have good constitution or breed type. Appearance of body coat is coarser and ruffled; compactness is lacking. Heterogenous fibres present all over the body; belly and legs have lesser or no wool cover, staple contains long medullated fibres of over 8 cm and shorter fine fibres of 5 to 7 cm length; conditioning at par with class II and III but with expected better yield.

Lamb classing

Various patterns are followed for grouping lambs. After a lamb dries up after birth, its body coat is observed in fine wool breeds and following procedure of grading adopted:

Wool cover (coat)

A type   Where the whole body coat of lamb is fine.

B type   A few coarse fibres are present over head, neck and down britch region.

C type   Coarse fibres intermingled with fine fibres cover the whole body.

D type   Wool cover is predominantly or wholly coarse.

The newly born lambs of evolved fine wool breeds like Kashmir merino, Bharat merino and Hissardale are also classed on the same standards.

Colour pattern

White: The whole body coat is white.

Coloured: Black, brown, fawn, tan or grey body.

Spotted or pigmented: Either the face, head, ears, nostrils, lips, fetlocks, etc. may be partly coloured or colour spots (black or brown) or patches exist over the body.

Body weight

Heavy weight, medium or average weight and low weight lambs.

Nature of birth

As singles, twins or triplets.

Genetic grouping

Pure breds, crossbreds and graded as 1/4th, 1/2, 3/4th interbreds, etc. specifically indicating the breeds involved and the level of inheritance.

Selecting breeding flock ewes

Should take cognizance of the type of flock to be maintained, whether stud, nucleus, or commercial. Following points are of prime importance in selecting breeding ewes.

- One of the first consideration in selecting the ewes for particular type breeding flock is uniformity.

- Ewes selected should be well grown and thrifty, free from hereditary and constitutional defects.
- Breeding ewes should also bear evidence of strong constitution, active in movements, alert to strange sights and sounds. They should carry their heads well up.
- Chest should be wide and brisket full. Legs should be wide apart. The general appearance of style, compactness, capacity and utility must emanate at first sight.
- Ewes desired for the farm flock should have dense compact fleece and not ruffled coat as, far as fine wool sheep and their crossbreds are concerned. In case of local breeds the typical nature of fleece coat of that breed is the working criterion.
- Quiet disposition for flock mothers is rewarding.
- Udder and teat should be sound.
- Teeth should be in intact condition and not worn out, irregular, or short.
- Ewes selected for raising lambs for the market should be in prime condition and possess sound mutton form at the time of purchase or selection.
- Above all the selecting sheepman must know his needs well.

After the intended type of flock has been established the further approach is to:

1. Increase the size of flock and
2. Replace poor individual by rejecting.
   a. Ewes not bearing lambs regularly,
   b. Ewes habitually bearing late lambs, and
   c. Ewes failing in general condition.

CULLING OF SHEEP

Culling or weeding out is the process of discarding of unproductive, substandard off-type or defective animals from a flock to improve the production status and uniformity of flock in a desired direction. Culling is complimentary to selection. A sound sheep improvement programme has a fair provision of culling of inferior animals.

A regular system of discarding of animals in a developing flock is undertaken at various ages and stages, viz. lamb, weaning, hogget or maiden ewe age. Sometimes the culling is necessitated at premigration, prebreeding, deteriorating pasturage stage, shepherding (man power) problems or under apprehensions of a approaching disease. Distress culling and sales are resorted to under abnormal conditions. The breeder may then retain only a couple of excellent performers. In routine culling, the following reasons are considered:

1. Off type: Off colour, pigmented 'baldy or badger' lambs and those not true to type or breed. Kashmir merino or crosses of it or of Merino, Rambouillet, etc. lacking pink nose, and pink skin (which is characteristic of these fine wool breeds) are regarded off type.

2. Defective conformation: Body conformation defects are quite common in sheep, congenital or otherwise. Face cover, chalky face and body wrinkles in fine wool sheep are negative aspects.

3. Defective wool: Sheep possessing heteroptype coat, containing highly medullated fibres and kemp, mercury wool, etc. are to be rejected in apparel wool sheep flocks.

4. Sub-standard: Sheep showing slow growth or underweight, low production and performance that fall below certain prescribed norms or standard. Selection index application or truncation type selection yield satisfactory results.

5. Uneconomical sheep: High feed consumers but low yielders or those showing low feed conversion efficiency are not a fit lot for retention.

6. Cast for age and gummy mouth sheep: After 6 to 7 year age a decline in production and reproduction comes in local sheep and the crossbreds. The teeth show wearing in certain sheep even at an earlier age, thus incapacitating proper feed utilization by the adult animal.

7. Irreparable growths and incurable diseases: Rams with cancerous horns, fibrosed prepucial sheath, orchitis, cryptorchism Actinomycosis, sternal fistula and other irreparable condition of genitalia or those causing breeding problems are discarded. Ewes having blocked or cut teats and bad udders are unfit. Abnormal physical formations like exostosis, overgrown digits, flat pasterns, blindness, pendulous abdomen, etc. are a couple of disqualifications for breeding stock.

8. Infertility: Poor semen quality, reduced libido, difficult covering in rams, habitual aborters, prolapse of genitalia, regular repeaters and barrenness of ewes are serious draw backs.

9. Vices: Rams in certain cases have the bad habits of butting co-rams or even the shepherd and children. Masturbation and licking of urine or eating abnormal objects like soil, bones, are noticed at times.

Rare instances of allergic skin scratching or addiction as of consuming Ipomea leaves renders the animal finally crippled. Detection of it at earlier period may be amenable to medication but subsequently the culling of such patients is the only way out.

10. Surplus stock: Any number over and above the requirements of the scheme, more than the stipulated replacements, above the carrying capacity of a property, farm or pasture is surplus and hence culled on lowest performance or below average basis.

11. Potbelly condition: Is a common feature in ill fed and parasitic infested animals. It should not be mistaken for healthy sheep or construed as a voracious eater.

12. Some other aspects: The occurrence of parrot mouth condition, i.e. under short jaw, is almost 3 to 4 per 100 sheep particularly in Rambouillet crossbreds. The defect becomes visible right from a few weeks age to hogget stage. A thorough examination takes into account the other anatomical and physical faults like cow hocks, pigeon toes, narrow chest, devil's dip, camel neck, weak hind quarters or Roman nose, etc. paraplegia and 'swayback' conditions usually call for disposal.

Detection of wool faults requires experience as many abnormal wool conditions exist. Knowledge of the same and regular handling of sheep of woolly breeds obviates any chances of wrong selections. Rambouillet sheep appear less subjected to as rigorous wool standards now as the merino in Australia. This has resulted into arrival of certain sheep with heterotype coats, mercury wool or doggy wool, etc.

AGE DETERMINATION

For estimation of age of sheep as of other animals, it is essential, to understand the dentition phenomenon right from birth. Like all other ruminants, in sheep too, two sets of teeth appear in its lifetime.

1. Milk teeth or temporary, deciduous ones appear when the lamb is a month old.
2. Permanent teeth. The temporary incisors get replaced at almost a definite sequence and interval by the permanent ones. The identification of this type of teeth lies in these being broader and longer than the temporary teeth.

The incisors in both the cases appear on the lower jaw. The upper jaw has no incisors but only a dental pad. For the approximate age determination the four pairs of incisor teeth provide the major information though not always reliable one. The arrangement of incisors is given in Fig. 12.1.

At times the incisors do not appear in regular order or at proper age when due. Breed to breed differences markedly alter the eruption and thereby the age estimation. All the temporary incisor teeth are evident at about 4 to 5 weeks age. The central pair is the most conspicuous. The first two pairs, viz. centrals and intermediates are often seen protruded at birth of the lamb.

Besides the incisors, the lamb possesses three temporary molar teeth on either side of upper and lower jaws. From one month to about 18 months age the various changes comprise of:

1. Eruption of 4th molar around 3 months age as a permanent tooth.
2. The third temporary molar wears out.
3. As the jaw grows and elongates in the next six months, the 5th molar (permanent) is cut around 9 months.
4. By this time the temporary central incisors loosen and make way for the pair of central permanent incisors to emerge between 12 to 18 months age.
5. 6th permanent molar (the last one) is cut around 18 months age approximately.
6. Around two years age the 2nd permanent pair of incisor is cut.
7. At 2 years the 6th molar is freely protruding.
8. The 1st and 2nd temporary molars show wearing and are replaced by the permanent molars.
   The condition of molars and shedding of premolars provides additional information in determination of age between 1 to 2½ year age.
9. The lateral or 3rd pair of permanent incisors erupts at about 2½ to 3 year or may be delayed to 3½ year in the cross bred sheep.
10. The final permanent 4th pair or corner incisors pushes out the temporary counter parts at 3½ to 4 year age.

A sheep at this age carrying the full set of teeth is called '*full mouth*'. Table 12.1 gives the complete sequences of eruption.

Formula of dentition for sheep

A full mouth sheep has 8 incisors on lower jaw and 3 premolars and 3 molars each on both sides of the upper and lower jaws. Canine (c) teeth are

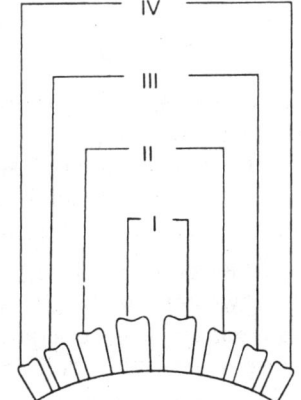

I. Central pair
II. Intermediate or medials
III. Laterals
IV. Corners

Fig. 12.1. Incisor teeth on lower jaw of sheep

Table 12.1: Eruption of teeth in sheep.

Incisors	Cutting age	Molars	Cutting age
Temporary Central and Intermediate	At or soon after birth	**Temporary-premolars** 1st, 2nd and 3rd pair	At birth or within 1 to 1½ month age.
Permanent Centrals Medials Laterals Corners	1 to 1½ yr. 2 to 2½ yr. 2½ to 3 yr. 3½ to 4 yr.	**Permanent molars** 4th 5th 6th Replacement of temporary 1st, 2nd and 3rd premolars by permanent premolars	3 to 6 months 9 to 12 months 18 to 24 months Takes place around 1½ to 2 year age

absent in sheep like other true ruminants. These can be represented by:

Temporary (T) or milk teeth

$$2\left[T_i\frac{0}{4} + Tc\frac{0}{0} + Tp\frac{3}{3} + Tm\frac{0}{0}\right] = 20 \text{ teeth}$$

Permanent (P) teeth

$$2\left[P_i\frac{0}{4} + Pc\frac{0}{0} + Pp\frac{3}{3} + Pm\frac{3}{3}\right] = 32 \text{ teeth}$$

In practice the age determination through dentition reveals marked variation in the period of replacement or cutting of teeth in individual sheep or different breeds. Type of pasture and feed too have a considerable role to play. At some of the institutions where hard pelleted feed or whole maize is fed the wearing and even shedding is observed earlier. The teeth decay is quite earlier in certain sheep rearing areas where pasture and water have higher fluorine content as observed in certain pockets of Ladakh.

Occasionally the shedding of permanent teeth starts at around six year age in our sheep and this masks the job of age approximation beyond this age. Certain animals have been found to have intact dentition even at 8 to 9 year age. Such a vast variation often results into erratic age estimation. The broken or worn out teeth conditions appear at any time after 4 to 5 year age under ill-fed or unbalanced feeding conditions. Gummy mouth condition of course, speaks of the old age and senility.

SHEEP BIOMETRY

Growth

Is a phenomenon of change in size, weight, shape, composition and structure of body. In general there are two aspects of growth, accretion of body substance and alteration of form and function which proceed largely independent of changes in the size and weight of body as a whole. These two aspects are often distinguished as growth and development (*Fuller, 1969*). *Acharya et al (1982)* observed that growth has mostly been studied in terms of body weights at birth, weaning, six months, nine months and twelve months of age.

Information about body measurements of sheep are vital from various angles, viz.

1. For knowledge of growth of the animal, which is reflected in the increase in body weight and size.

2. For physical definition of a sheep breed. Body size and weight are characteristic of each breed.

3. To gain an idea about the production and reproduction potentials of the animal, and

4. For selection and further scientific breeding.

The exhaustive studies involve assessment of body weight, length, girth, and height of the animals of a particular genetic group and sex at different age periods. While defining a particular breed the additional measurement of body frame, limbs and appendages like tail, ears, horns, etc. are also mentioned. For similar and true to type animals measurements are recorded and mean values reflected for individual parameters. Recording of measurements is regarded as an important aspect of biometric and population genetics studies.

For proper description of local sheep breeds, some of the states as well as ICAR initiated surveys and body measurement estimations in pre-independence era and seriously followed after 1948. This provided distinctive phenotypic identification of various sheep breeds of the country like Deccani, Marwari, Nali, Chokla, Magra, Patanwadi, Gaddie, Mandya, Nellore and other western and peninsular India sheep breeds.

Body measurements—mode and method

Body weights

1. Birth weight: The lamb after birth is allowed to be licked by the ewe and made to dry up. It takes 4 to 6 hours. The weighment is then taken by using a standard 5 to 10 kilogram spring balance or a pan balance. Weight is recorded to the nearest hundredth of a kilogram or even in grams with the help of a sensitive balance. In no case the period between birth and weighment should exceed 12 hours. A thin, light but strong tape or rope net or a sling is employed to secure the lamb and hold it on the hook or pan.

2. Pre-weaning and weaning body weight: To avoid daily handling the usual procedure is to weigh the lambs at weekly intervals at the farms, till weaning. Research stipulations at times specify daily weighment for some initial period or duration of experiment. A pan balance or spring balance shall suffice during first few weeks. For recording weaning weight a 25 to 50 kg spring balance is generally used. As the lambs grow a weigh bridge or any other platform type scale becomes essential. Such a scale is normally fixed in a shed or by the side of sheep race in such a way that the lambs or sheep enter into it directly from the shed or sheep closure. Before weighment it is desirable to maintain the animals without food or water for at least 6 to 8 hours. At commercial farms or private sheep properties frequent weighment of lambs is neither practicable nor advisable. Weight at weaning is however, an essential feature.

3. Hogget weight: Post weaning weights are usually recorded at monthly intervals till the yearling stage. Usual routine at the farms is to weigh with a bigger 100 kg spring balance. A strong but light sling made out of jute or nylon serves the purpose of securing and tortioning at the hook.

4. Adult sheep weighment: Quarterly or half yearly weighing invariably at shearing time or pre-breeding occasion is resorted to at research farms till 2½ year age. Weight recording is not advocated at later age till shearing, culling, sale, etc.

Slaughter age body weight do provide a tentative assessment of mutton value. The butchers or buyers on their behalf affect purchase from the shepherds just through assessment of weight by hand lifting of the animal.

At certain established properties or big farms a bigger platform weigh bridge is installed in a room or walled surroundings to collectively weigh 20 to 30 or even more sheep at one time to have average assessment of weight of desired category of sheep.

Manpower requirement for weighing

For the platform weighment, in all, three persons and in spring balance weighing five persons are needed.

1. Two persons are required to catch and bring the sheep from closure to the cage of the platform balance and calling out the tag/tattoo number.
2. Another man observes the reading on the scale and records entry in the weighment sheet or register.
3. Two assisting hands are additionally required while conducting spring balance weighment, i.e. to raise the bar or the animal in the sling on to the hook of the balance. The operation is laborious and only 50 to 60 sheep, can be weighed per hour.

Body size: Size of the body frame provides indication of growth and extent of area or body barrel that grows wool and is also of interest to producers. Any change in body condition has a marked bearing on the width at ribs. Various body dimensions are therefore incorporated to ascertain body size, a salient characteristic of each breed. These measurements of body serve the purpose of animal size and breed description.

For body size of the sheep the measurements are recorded in terms of

- Length of body from point of shoulder to pin bone.
- Girth of body at withers, i.e. just behind point of elbow.
- Height of body at withers, i.e. highest point of withers vertically down to ground level.

Measurements for breed description

Besides the primary dimension of size, other characteristic measurements of body are also important in respect of individual breeds.

1. Length from withers to pin bone, i.e. point of withers, the anterior most spinous process of thoracic vertebra to either ischiatic tuber.
2. Length from elbow to coronet: From the top of olecranon process to the mid lateral point of coronet.
3. Depth of chest: The vertical distance from the highest point of withers to the ventral surface of sternum. It is depth of body barrel just behind shoulders. One of the purpose of recording wither height is to find the ratio of chest depth to the length of the leg, viz, elbow to coronet. Its measurement error is lesser than that of wither height.
4. Width at shoulders, i.e. from the lateral tuberosity of one humerus to the corresponding tuberosity of the otherside.
5. Width at ribs. Maximum width is at the level of last but one rib. The tips of callipers should rest on the rib and not sink in between ribs.

6. Width at hip from one point of ilium to the corresponding point on the opposite side, away from tuber coxae.
7. Depth of body at the last rib.
8. Depth of body at flank, i.e. at the site of last vertebra of loins.
9. Length of body from point of breast to pin bone.
10. Girth of body at flanks—the paunch girth.
11. Height of head from ground, while in normal standing posture.
12. Length of face from point of poll to the point of mouth.
13. Distance between the inner canthus of eyes.
14. Distance between the horn buttons.
15. Size of horns with a mention of formation, curves, twists, etc.
16. Length of ears—from base to tip.
17. Breadth of the ear at the mid region.
18. Length of tail from base to tip.

Table 12.2 gives biometrics of adult sheep of some Indian breeds.

For recording measurements it is essential that

- Sheep be held in natural position and posture.
- Sheep be held on level ground or on a platform.
- Practice of measurement recording be preferably adjusted in post shearing time.
- Equipment like measuring stick, callipers, graduated tapes, etc. are available at hand.
- Measuring equipment marked in metric system be quite legible.
- At least three operators are available. One to catch the sheep and hold in right posture. The other one to take measurements and call out the same to the third assisting hand who records the data in a register against the animal number called.

Change of operators can lead to errors in the standard practice. Measurement differences may arise to the extent of 2 to 4 percent in general measurements. With regard to width at shoulders, width at ribs, and depth at hip the error due to operator's change might escalate to 6 to 7 percent.

Table 12.2: Biometrics of adult sheep of some Indian breeds (recorded at Govt.. farms in the country).

Sl. no.	Item of measurement	Breed						
		Gaddie	Deccani			Mandya	Nellore	Marwari
1.	Sex	Ewe	Ewe	Ewe	Ram	Ram	Ram	Ram
2.	Age:	FM	2T	4T	FM	FM	FM	FM
3.	Body wt. (kg.)	27	23.8	25.0	43.0	52.0	40.0	57.5
4.	Distance between two eyes (cm)	10.2	10.1	10.5	12.0	13.0	12.0	15.0
5.	Distance between horn buttons (cm)	Polled	Polled	Polled	10.0	9.0	4.0	9.0
6.	Ear-length (cm)	15.5	16.2	15.7	14.5	15.0	16.0	14.5
7.	Ear breadth (cm)	8.0	8.1	8.1	9.0	8.0	8.0	5.5
8.	Length from poll to point of mouth (cm)	21.5	21.9	23.5	29.3	28.0	34.0	30.0
9.	Height of body at withers (cm)	56.6	58.6	59.6	63.2	59.0	72.0	76.5
10.	Depth of body just behind shoulders (cm)	24.4	25.2	25.1	30.0	32.1	30.0	32.2
11.	Depth of body at last rib (cm)	–	16.5	28.6	29.7	29.4	27.5	32.5
12.	Depth of body at flank (cm)	–	26.1	24.4	27.8	25.5	26.0	31.6
13.	Width of body at shoulders (cm)	–	17.1	16.7	21.4	25.0	17.4	21.7
14.	Width at last rib (cm)	–	22.4	23.2	25.2	28.3	21.5	26.0
15.	Width at points of hip (cm)	–	18.2	19.1	21.5	25.4	20.5	22.3
16.	Length of body from breast to pin bone (cm)	–	65.0	65.3	78.0	88.0	74.0	82.0
17.	Length of body from withers to pin bone (cm)	55.5	57.4	57.1	64.0	62.0	70.0	67.0
18.	Length of body from shoulder point to pin bone (cm)	–	62.5	62.7	76.0	78.0	71.0	71.0
19.	Length of body from pt. of elbow to coronet (cm)	–	37.1	37.1	39.5	35.0	44.0	43.0
20.	Girth at withers (cm)	74.4	74.7	77.5	90.2	95.0	86.0	100.5
21.	Height of head from ground (cm)	–	72.2	72.1	74.8	83.5	90.0	91.5
22.	Tail length (cm)	11.0	13.1	12.6	15.3	12.0	12.0	26.0

FM: Full Mouth
T: Teeth

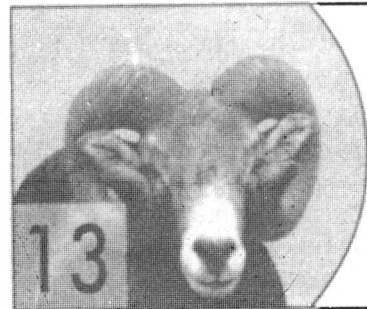

PRODUCTION IMPROVEMENT PERSPECTIVES

SHEEPMAN'S WEALTH

To the farmer the improvement of his livestock implies cost effective production and better returns. The salient yardstick is the corresponding reflection in production per unit of investment. The criterion is however foregone in stud or nucleus stock breeding which demand liberal inputs. The maintenance of exotic and superior pedigree animals definitely costs much more on better care management and feeding. Yet in all earnest, economy in rearing and production of commercial flock is the main guiding consideration with the sheep owner.

Wool, mutton and skins are the major items of sheep production that fetch income to the sheepman. Milk production of sheep, though a source of shepherd's family sustenance in the tribal belt, has not gained much commercial importance in India as is in some countries of eastern Europe. Sheep manure is an invaluable material for soil enrichment but its proper utility and applicability is hardly ensured. Lamb and mutton production is the main revenue earning source for the shepherd in the western states of India but being monopolised affair the share of the sheep farmer is just nominal. Sheep skins and other byproducts of sheep and wool production offer potential industrial base. Besides generating employment avenues these can benefit the producer if tapped properly. Whereas the Australian sheepman calls his flock as 'property' a tribal shepherd in India names his sheep as *Dhann*.

Future prospects

After synthetic fibre introduction, its competition with wool fibre and gradual averseness of public to red meat the future of sheep and wool is being debated at times. Comparatively low increments in pricing of sheep products, fast squeezing forage resources and harsh life conditions of a shepherd are proving deterring to sheep rearing. Current global recession in wool market and cheaper bulk imports of desired quality wool in the country are cited other reasons for the emerging gloomy situation.

Notwithstanding the depression being projected, the ground position speaks otherwise. A significant increase in sheep population has been recorded in the country in the past twenty five years resulting in increased wool and mutton production. Demand for wool, mutton, sheep skins and other sheep byproducts has risen substantially. Cold and temperate area population of the country can hardly go without wool and meat. Indian carpet wool and carpets still hold sway in the international market. As an apparel and blending material, qualities of wool fibre are unsurpassed. In fact true substitute to wool fibre is yet to arrive.

The oft stated slogan for sheep, i.e. 'millions fed, millions clothed and millions employed' holds out more relevant in India now than ever before. Millions of tribals, small and marginal farmers and landless labourers are directly dependant on sheep for earning their livelihood. Millions more are engaged in wool and woollen industries, meat and meat processing and leather and leather products.

The sheep sustains in various regions under adverse and unfavourable conditions and sheep rearing provides an excellent means for the upliftment of rural poor. As a stubble and crop residue utilizer or as close grazier no other ruminant can compete sheep.

ECONOMICS OF SHEEP REARING

Profits from sheep have often been dwelt upon. Sheep rearing has been a sole vocation with nomads and tribals in India for generations providing them livelihood, though the returns are only at a lower ebb. The hard labour put in by the sheepman is hardly retrieved in commensurate terms. Thus the sheep rearing vocation has failed to compete with other alluring and remunerative professions. Reasons generally assigned for this hapless situation by the production experts are:

1. Low productivity of indigenous sheep in terms of wool and mutton. The average wool production of our sheep is lowest among the main sheep rearing countries.
2. The comparative appreciation in the price of wool in India has been dismally poor.
3. Sheep and wool development and marketing have received a late start and that too on low priority.
4. Wool, woollens and the sheep serve as a major earner of foreign exchange but the incentives offered to this industry and the shepherd are no

match at all in comparison to other industries, crop production or horticulture.

But for isolated attempts no elaborate exercise appears to have been made to determine economic viability of sheep with the Indian farmer. At the government farms the cost of production of rams is worked out quite high. The reason attributed for that is the quality management requirements to produce and maintain pedigreed and genetically superior rams. The higher investments at the farms are compensated by curtailing importations of exotic germ plasm leading to enormous savings in foreign exchange.

While working out the pros and cons of a small sheep unit (20 females + 1 male) for introduction among small/marginal farmers or landless families, Kumar (1992) reported the cost-benefit position for six years as given in Table 13.1.

In addition to these profits the complete loan amount will be liquidated in the six years. The sheep farmer shall own almost three times the initial strength and a regular source of income for family subsistence.

The success stories of at least ten sheep unit-holders of plain belt of Jammu reveal that after starting with a unit of 10 sheep (under centrally sponsored programme) the owner repaid the loan with interest in five to six years out of annual savings and further accrued a profit of Rs 800/- to 10,000/- from 4th year onwards on an increasing trend. The breeding ram and health cover were provided by the Sheep Husbandry Department free of charges. By the beginning of 6th year the

Table 13.1: Cost-benefit position of 20 sheep unit rearing.

Item	1st year	2nd year	3rd year	4th year	5th year	6th year
Total Receipts (Rs)	960	1150	1350	2450	2800	3050
Total Expenditure						
Small farmers	800	718	770	760	744	672
Marginal farmers	700	635	695	690	680	585
Net Income						
Small farmers	160	432	580	1690	2056	2378
Marginal farmers	260	515	655	1760	2120	2465

farmers possessed a flock of 40 to 50 sheep even after a sound culling percentage.

An exercise, about economy of migratory and stationary sheep rearing was made in Pune in 1962-63 which showed that migratory system paid better annual dividends per sheep (Table 13.2a).

For the sheep maintained on grazing alone, Acharya and Saksena (1972) reported the average annual income of Rs 3881/- and Rs 5640/- of a flock of 100 Chokla and Nali breeding ewes respectively. This estimation is based on the assumptions of fixed size and composition of flock; fixed birth and death rates; 1:1 sex rates; fixed reproductive period; continuous replacement of old by newborn at a fixed rate; no purchase of breeding ram and thrice shearing a year.

Yet in another study Choudhary (1985) worked out the following returns from large and small flocks in the two regions (Table 13.2b shows the economy of a flock of 200 sheep).

Flock of 25 sheep: Against 100 or 50 sheep a small flock of 25 can be managed with ease. This is normally a situation in the case of stationary rearing, where there is no land holding and the sheep are run on village grazing lands free of cost. The profits are stated around Rs. 34.40 per sheep per year in the South-Eastern region. Though no wool is obtained from the southern sheep, the higher receipt from them may be due to cheaper labour and lesser feeding costs.

Economy in sheep rearing like other livestock farming is subservient to genetic cum production potential and judicious management so as to reduce feeding cost without lowering nutritional level. Prolificacy, lambing percentage, survivability or in otherwords lambs born per ewe joined and lambs weaned per ewe lambed are basic components to determine progress of the flock Rate of growth of lamb, related to body weight, size and muscle gain is an important factor. The quality and quantity of wool produced and proper marketing contribute to the profits from sheep.

CONSTRAINTS IN SHEEP PRODUCTION IN INDIA

The fast changing scenario of country's development has affected the sheep and wool production as well. Hardly there is any state in India where significant deviations from the traditional pattern have not been observed. Broadly, the following factors are considered responsible for slow growth of sheep population and production.

Table 13.2: (a) Comparative economy of migratory and stationary sheep rearing.

Type of flock	Gross income/ sheep/year (Rs)	Gross expenditure/ sheep/year (Rs)	Net income/ sheep/year (Rs)
Nomadic/migratory flock	8.97	2.70	6.27
Stationary flock	8.39	6.40	1.99

Table 13.2: (b) Migratory and semi migratory nature—large flock.

Region	Gross income/ sheep/year (Rs.)	Gross expd/ sheep/year (Rs.)	Net income/ sheep/year (Rs.)
South eastern	178.00	137.00	41.00
North western	82.50	54.80	27.70

Declining pasturage

Vast and open grazing areas once existing around the villages in India as common grazing grounds, Kahcharai or Shamlat Deh, now stand either encroached upon or utilised for cultivation, forestation and habitation. Pasture land in the peripheral areas to townships have been brought under industrialisation or developed into colonies. Extension of irrigation facilities has further lead to reduction in grazing area.

Unmanaged pastures

Wherever and whatever grazing area is available, it is in a neglected and mismanaged state. Conservation, rest and rotation, reseeding, fertilization or deweeding efforts are hardly taken up. Because of complete apathy of silviculturists and foresters towards pasture resources and ignorance and non-involvement of livestock men, most of the pastures now, have a mixed cover of toxic and obnoxious weeds and un-nutritious vegetation.

Creation of closures and reserves

Large pasture and forest grazing grounds have been converted into wild life sanctuaries, national parks and forest enclosures. The livestock has, therefore, been deprived of free movement and grazing in such big chunks of pastures.

Sheep a close grazier

All the soil conservation, forestation and eco-restoration programmes lay emphasis on plantations, with little stress to improve surface grass cover. The sheep is a close grazier. For want of a good surface vegetation, the sheep suffer irreparably year in and year out.

Sheep flock migrations

Many problems of migratory sheep rearing are inherent in the transhumant system itself. Open, insecure life conditions, weather vagaries, rain and snowfall, predators and poachers, sheep thefts, distress disposal of sheep and wool, prolonged absence of shepherds from families, their inattention towards health of families and education of children are a few glaring ones to mention. Transit problems of carriage of young and weak animals, lack of grazing and watering facilities enroute, long stopovers and road side accidents often add to the anxieties of shepherd.

Uncertain grazing destinations

In Jammu and Kashmir, Himachal Pradesh, parts of Uttaranchal and other hilly states, flocks migrate to alpines with the onset of summer and move down to foot hills in winter. The Haryana, Rajasthan, Gujarat, Maharashtra and Karnataka sheep population in part undertake even interstate migrations. They do not have permanent grazing rights or fixed grazing areas. The district to district and area to area movement without a sure destination compounds the problems of a sheep-man. His animals have at times to go without a mouthful grazing under such precarious situations.

Unforeseen calamities

Natural calamities like droughts, lean period, floods, lightening and epidemics cause heavy loss of sheep and lamb crop. Under disturbed and scarce conditions, poor families and tribals restrict the sheep number or even abdicate their flocks and sheep rearing vocation.

Professional toughness vis-a-vis alluring vocations

Shepherding is a tough job. Because of unsettled life conditions of the sheep breeder, the profession is looked down upon in the society despite an angelic back ground. New takers are few. Even the traditional flock holders and their children are in look out for other alluring and economically viable jobs.

Lack of skilled labour

Sound shepherding is a highly skilled job. Traditional vocationalists are getting rare. The art of tending sheep, lamb rearing, shearing and flock maintenance is gradually waning. For fear of social stigma attached to sheep rearing (*Bheden paalna Khanabadoshon ka kaam hai*) in India the educated and elite sects of society do not come forward to establish sheep farms.

Heavy taxation

The high levy on grazing of sheep imposed by some states on migratory flocks has proved detrimental to migrations and sheep rearing.

Wool importation

Free wool importations from abroad and disguised importations (like the fine wool for shoddies) have hampered the growth of wool production at home. The organised woollen sector in India has its own preferences. In view of liberal availability of wool from other countries there is no eagerness to utilize Indian wool. Thus the indigenous produce is not well priced.

Low returns

The hike in prices of wool and mutton over the last decades have not been commensurate with agricultural produce and other commodities. The returns to the farmer from sheep and wool sale have not registered a favourable trend. A skin or fur of a sheep ordinarily fetches just Rs 40/- to 60/- in the local market. But the same piece after preliminary treatment values over Rs 100/-. Cheap forage and labour for sheep tending is only a nightmare now.

Desired wool types—production

May it be carpet wool or fine wool development, the proper thrust towards the production of an ideal type of wool in India is still not visible. The quality of the wool for industrial consumption too has not improved in the existing sheep. But for Bikaneri wool the indigenous carpet wool falls short of competitive international standards. Likewise the fine wool produced in North-temperate region suffers from defects like short staple, uniformity, pigmentation and lower yield. After an initial

initiative to evolve better producing sheep for different environments in the country, a stalemate period has set in. No where any better adapted and better producing sheep has made appearance in any state over the last two decades.

Marketing

Various states like Rajasthan, Gujarat, J&K, Maharashtra, Karnataka, HP, UP, etc. have set up their sheep and wool marketing boards or federations. But a long term rational system of price protection and watching the interests of sheep and wool producers has yet to be adopted.

Disease problem and control measures

Obscure diseases are taking a heavy toll of sheep and lambs thus hindering growth in sheep population and level of optimum production. Production of biologicals for effective prophylaxis against Ecthyma, Viral Pneumonia, Sheep Pox and emerging diseases like Blue Tongue, PPR, Mycoplasma, etc. are lacking. Worm infestation of sheep is quite common. The imported anthelmintics are too costly for the sheep owner to use. Worm resistance to these drugs as observed lately is a matter of serious concern. Safer treatment or prevention of mange is possible through highly expensive imported parasiticides only. Pollution and carcinogenic aspects of free use of these chemicals are forbidding factors.

Industrial raw material

Sheep is providing raw material like wool, skins and mutton, etc. for the industrial utility, but fails to enjoy the incentives as being provided to other industrial sector in the country. The subsidies, attractive credit facilities and compensations and relief during drought and other natural calamities are not readily forthcoming.

GENERAL CORRECTIVE MEASURES

At various fora in the past two decades, solutions to the problems faced and suggestions to improve sheep production have been advanced. Excerpts of recommendations and observations made there in* are presented here:

- Sheep and goat need to be given due priority under Central as well as State Plans so as to raise per animal production.

- Sheep are not responsible for the degradation of ecology and should not be labelled among animals responsible for eco-destruction. They are in fact economical and eco-friendly.

- Emphasis should be on quality improvement of the animal rather than numerical numbers. Sheep of improved genetic make up and production potential may be introduced among small and marginal farmers, landless labourers, some social tribes, etc. as income generating units after purchase from large flock owners and within the same district or area.

- Sheep and wool development in the country is intimately connected to livestock husbandry, forestry, agriculture, rural industry and environment. Their sectorial approach and work in isolation has bred interdisciplinary apathy with restricted benefit to the society. Hence in pursuance of the recommendations of the National Commission on Agriculture, committees should be constituted in various states of the connected departmental heads as members and minister for agriculture/animal husbandry as chairman to oversee feed-fodder resource development and allied problems.

- In the states where small animal (sheep, goat and rabbit) rearing is of any consequence, separate departments should be created or carved out to provide proper and exclusive attention to sheep breeding, management and health.

- Since interstate sheep migrations are becoming problematical and grazing levy unbearable by the shepherd, the matter should be brought in the purview of interstate councils or Central Advisory Committee for small animal development. The pattern of reduced rather nominal Kahcharai (grazing) tax adopted in certain states for the improved sheep can be a sound way out for other states, considering the low economic profile of a shepherd.

- The tendency to make a scape goat of a sheep and the shepherd for the ill designs of contractors, forest exploiters, ignorant public and neo-ecologists needs to be checked. In fact the cooperation and education of the sheepman can help check vegetation destruction and eco-restoration. Awareness of the shepherd is of foremost importance.

- The tribals and nomads are the main sheep rearers in India. Most of them follow the traditional migratory system. To improve their lot, the pasture development, grazing area allocation, health cover and marketing of produce require priority attention. Facilities like establishment of fodder banks, shelter sheds, development of migration tracks, reservation of grazing strips along the route, provision of halting stations, watering facilities, veterinary aid camps, low cost durable tentage, proper security for the flocks and tending persons are essential. Spain, the pioneer of Merino sheep development had enacted a 'Transhumant Law' a couple of centuries back to facilitate and regulate flock migrations.

- Controlling long and interstate sheep migrations is being advocated at times. This demands garnering of local and state's own fodder and grazing resources, silvipastoral measures, restructuring of flock size and composition. A lesser number of improved sheep can generate better income than a large flock of old, uneconomical and scrub animals.

- The grasslands can be improved tremendously by reseeding, fertilization and proper management. Generating a three tier surface cover is admittedly a scientific and healthier recourse for the livestock and improving ecology. The Task Force set up to study the impact of small animal introduction in ecologically fragile zones further recommends the plantation composition as 80% fodder and fuel trees,

---

* Bandey (1981); Task Force Report (1987); Golden Jubilee Seminar Proceedings (1992); Gupta, (2001).

20% timber trees. It is a pity that unacquainted environmentalists while emphasising the plantation drive ignore the grasses and edible shrubs. The tree plantations only cannot be a potential check against soil erosion and for moisture conservation. In the afforestation programmes the growth of underneath vegetative cover of indigenous grasses, creepers and bushes should find precedence.

🐑 There is no denying of facts that overgrazing and undue pressure of unproductive large animals is a cause for irreparable damage to regeneration of natural flora of pasture lands. Any guidelines or control from a remote, apex system may not be workable. Therefore, coordination committees at local village or panchayat level and then at district and regional level need to be set up to study, monitor and take steps to regulate grazing and improve the utility of available village pasture lands.

🐑 Mis-utilization of common village grazing grounds, (the Shamlat Deh), forest area pastures or culturable waste lands by way of *Noutods* or reclamations on slopes for agronomical operations is a source of enormous loss of forage material and to the ecosystem. Such unauthorised actions can only be prevented through enforcement of law. A proper land use policy for hills and fragile topography is of paramount importance all the more, to protect the environment and pasture lands from degradation.

🐑 Sheep dung pellet is indispensable manure to improve soil and its productivity. The old system of night penning of sheep in the cultivable fields is unique to impart lasting fertility to the poorest of soils.

🐑 The introduction of small animals under the poverty alleviation programmes in various regions of the country suggests beyond any apprehensions, the viability of it as an income generating unit and employer for rural youth and have-nots.

🐑 A dependable marketing system is a boon for any industry or production unit to flourish. The establishment of Sheep and Wool Production and Marketing Corporations or Boards by various states has assured a better deal to the wool producers to some extent. These institutions require further strengthening. Besides, a chain of Sheep and Wool producers cooperative societies in different areas must be considered to assist proper marketing.

🐑 Due to odds and harsh life conditions in transhumant system, the sheep farmers are feeling disenchanted with migratory rearing. A trend towards semi-migratory and sedentary pattern of rearing is imminent. Larger flocks are giving place to smaller ones in many areas. Under such husbandry practices a semi-intensive rearing, i.e. pasturage + stall feeding is a plausible solution. Thus sheep rearing if encouraged on mixed farming system would bring many takers of sheep. The population and production would thus not be affected substantially with a shift as anticipated above.

🐑 A step towards supplementation of feed-fodder resources would be proper utilization of crop residues, silage preparation, reprocessing of industrial waste like sugar cane tops, bagasse, apple pomade and mango seed kernels, etc.

🐑 For the production of adequate quality fodder, seeds, seedlings and cuttings of grasses, shrubs and fodder trees, large scale farms should be established.

🐑 The vast pasture lands which hitherto before served as grazing grounds for the livestock have been usurped by unscrupulous growth of weeds, and obnoxious and poisonous plants. The programme of their eradication needs to be initiated on a long term basis on regional or even national level. The areas so reclaimed shall provide additional grazing or fodder resource.

🐑 Under the Integrated Water Shed Development programme the cut and carry system of grass is permitted to the beneficiary farmers from the conserved enclosures. These areas providing surplus fodder can further be utilized for Fodder Bank reserves. Once the plantation are out of reach of livestock the surface grazing by sheep would benefit both, i.e.

1. Enrichment of pasture without detriment to it or the ecology.
2. Augment fodder resources.

The procedure may also be applied mutatis-mutandis to forest enclosures, village gochars/ Kah-charai areas or any other enclosed reserves.

🐑 The organised slaughter houses for small animals in the main rearing pockets and centralised ones nearer the towns and cities shall not only be beneficial to the producers but also provide wholesome meat. Pollution shall also come down. These will open up avenues for judicious industrial exploitation of slaughter house products. Losses incurred during long transportation of live sheep shall be avoided.

🐑 In the sedentary and semi-migratory flocks, the use of artificial insemination has been advocated for better utilization of valuable exotic sheep germ plasm. This would obviate the importation and maintenance of large number of studs. Now, even the introduction of biotechnology advances like super ovulation and embryo transfer is being suggested by the scientists.

🐑 There is an increasing demand for genetically superior rams in the sheep rearing states. Besides the improved rams production at the government farms, some progressive private sheep flocks have also come up as potential ram producing units. The selected rams are purchased at young age from them by extension agencies of the government departments, corporations or social organisations. Such an open nucleus breeding system should be encouraged in all the sheep rearing areas.

Research and development

There is a need for the field oriented research rather than the academic one. The thrust on breed development and disease control that was witnessed in the early decades of independence appears subdued now. In fact the large scale importation of sheep, allocations and development infrastructure in the last twenty years could have helped to transform the sheep and wool industry of the entire rearing zone. The epic performance of IVRI in animal disease investigation and control is well known. The other prestigious institutions and multitude of Agricultural universities can put in a coordinated effort to give new directions by developing better technologies.

Health cover

1. Preventive and curative health cover measures should be made available at the door steps of the sheep farmers. Mobile Veterinary units as set up by some states like Jammu and Kashmir, Rajasthan, etc. for the migratory sheep and goat flocks are proving quite effective.
2. To meet the requirement of vaccines for all the prevalent and emerging sheep and goat diseases, there is a dire need to strengthen the existing biological production units in the country and even to establish newer ones on latest technology.
3. Effective anthelmintics are generally imported. Availability as such is scarce and cost very high. Indigenous resources and technology can be of better use. The use of neem and other local dewormers would be worth investigation for common worm infestations.
4. Epidemiological surveys may be taken up seriously and on perpetual footing.

Training and supervision

1. Sheep and wool production is a coming up scientific field and a means for rural poverty alleviation in India. Training centres for the work force of various categories on modern and practical lines are of priority. The facilities existing with the states, CSWRI and other institutions to produce well trained sheepmen, supervisory cadres and veterinarians require strengthening and proper utilization.
2. Regular exposure of the in-service hands to latest techniques and advanced knowledge is a prerequisite. The need for training within the country or abroad coupled with their inter-

actions through attending of seminars, conferences, workshops and refresher courses has been impressed at various occasions.

3. But for Rajasthan and J&K, hardly any independent or exclusive administrative and technical set up is available in any other state to oversee small animal development aspect. Separate infrastructure for the overall development of these species is desirable in the states having sizeable population of sheep and goats.

Sheep breeding policies

Sheep and wool development is a state subject. In addition to the broad national level guidelines, it is desirable to set up state level committees of experts to advise on the sheep breeding strategies and to take time to time appraisal. The policy should be dynamic one conforming to the changing scenario of demand and supply.

Incentives

1. Majority of Indian wools are carpet type. Defects and deficiencies in the wool quality of different zones require study and corrective measures. Selective breeding has been recommended for north western arid zone carpet wool sheep and cross breeding of hairy breeds with woolly breeds for improving the wool quality in addition to growth and body weight. In certain areas where wool is finer but shorter, cross breeding with Lincoln or Leicester is suggested to impart length, lustre and appropriate thickness or diameter.
2. Liberal imports of carpet wool should be discouraged.
3. The drawbacks of fine wool produced in northern temperate region need immediate review and steps to improve the quality in the desired direction. To make it remunerative it is essential to regulate the direct and disguised imports of fine wool in the country.
4. Proper testing of wool consignments at the landing seaports and airports need rigid enforcement.

BREEDING AND DEVELOPMENT STRATEGIES

Approach and general recommendations

Since the time the idea of improvement of production of indigenous sheep struck to the breeders and scientists in India, two schools of thought have mostly reigned.

1. Improvement for existing traits of carpet wool in most of the Indian sheep through selective breeding particularly in Rajasthan, Gujarat, Maharashtra and north arid zone sheep.
2. Others felt that cross breeding for improving quality and quantity of wool with the superior exotic germ plasm could be a better solution. The chief breed to be imported was the Merino and the area, the northern states. In view of embargo on Australian merino, the German merino, Spanish merino and Russian merinos came under consideration. Small consignments of such sheep were procured by different states up to middle of 20th century for limited trials.

Ad hoc committee on Sheep and Wool (1970) and subsequently the National Commission on Agriculture (1976) elaborated specific recommendations for genetic improvement of sheep in various regions, viz.

🐑 Crossbreeding of northern temperate region sheep for production of fine wool.

🐑 Selection amongst ideal carpet wool breeds of northeastern region and crossing of very coarse and hairy local sheep breeds with better wool sheep with the following objectives.
   1. Transforming the local coarse hairy sheep into woolly sheep, and
   2. Improving their body weight and mutton producing potential.

🐑 For the southern peninsular region the approach was again two-fold:
   1. to practise selection among better indigenous breeds like Mandya, Hassan, Nellore, etc. and
   2. to upgrade the rest of the inferior breeds with the above indigenous breeds.

The Commission laid further emphasis on the provision of improved health cover, disease prophylaxis, development of feed-fodder resources, improvement of management, introduction of better production technology and strengthening of marketing and extension network in the country.

A study of overall outcome reveals that selection process has not received a serious consideration and sustained effort any where. What ever little work was done did not yield tangible results. It is the cross breeding aspect that has been favoured by and large in all the zones. Thrivability, reproduction and production of some exotic sheep breeds in certain areas posed problems. Much remains to be assessed with regard to other aspects like suitability of particular germ plasm for a specific environment, its combining ability and feeding and management requirements. As a result the fruits of cross breeding have not been harvested in right earnest in totality.

For carpet wool

The northwestern arid zone is known for carpet wool. The plainer belt sheep including that of Deccan plateau can be developed for mutton and carpet wool. A number of schemes have been launched in this direction by the concerned states, the I.C.A.R. and the Central Government.

Contrary to the general feeling of superiority of fine wool over carpet quality, the actual trend reveals a better market for the carpet wools in India than apparel wool. For finer and valuable carpets the Australian and New-Zealand wools of 27 and 28 micron are presently finding way in the Indian market. Out of a total production of 22 million kilograms of good quality carpet wool in India about 10 million kilograms is consumed by the indigenous carpet industry. Therefore, any further import of carpet wool can lead to slump and jeopardise the interests of the wool growers. Replacement of imported medium and fine carpet wools is being sought for. Many a scientists are advocating the introduction of long wool blood in the heterotype cross bred woolly sheep. The idea in mind appears to exploit

the qualities of both types of germ plasm to synthesize local substitutes for imported carpet wool raw material by:

- Sacrificing fineness of cross bred wool from 24-28 microns to 30 to 34 microns.
- Improve staple length. Due to short length, variability and heterogeneity the cross bred wools in the country are not suitable for carpets.
- To impart lustre to this wool.
- Keep medullation within prescribed norms.
- A simultaneous attention to parameters like;
  1. Increase in body weight of progeny.
  2. Faster growth rate.
  3. An increase in clip weight, and
  4. Improvement in yield percentage, i.e. clean fleece weight.

Limited cross-breeding with Lincoln in fine cross bred sheep might hold a promise towards improving attributes like fibre diameter lustre and staple length. It is contemplated thereby to produce a suitable raw material for fine carpet manu-facturing as well as woollen system.

For apparel wool production

As per recommendations of NCA the temperate region is the only potential fine wool producing area. Though a good headway has been made to develop fine wool sheep in some states, yet the quality of the wool produced and availability of wool for the organised sector is not up to the mark. The worsted industry continues to face shortage of indigenous fine wool. As a result huge quantities of fine wool are imported. Out of total wool production of the states of temperate region, the apparel quality wool accounts for just 50%. The main characteristics of such wools for con-sideration are the fibre diameter and crimps; mean fibre/staple length; medulation, uniformity and density of fibres per unit skin area.

Elimination of heterotype and medullated fibres and pigmentation occupy prominent approach in the strategy to develop an apparel wool producing sheep. The results achieved so far in fine wool production suggest that with the available germ plasm in the temperate zone the production of apparel wool can be doubled in the next decade without corresponding increase in sheep numbers.

Breeding sheep for mutton

Growth pattern

The growth rate of some Indian sheep breeds is shown in Table 13.3.

Improvement efforts

Prior to 1960, limited and isolated attempts to improve muttonous status of indigenous sheep through selective breeding were made in certain parts of India. Carpet wool sheep breeds like Deccani, Lohi Nali, Malpura and hairy breeds like Sonadi, Nellore and Mandya were subjected to selection in the respective states of Maharashtra, Punjab, Rajasthan, Tamil Nadu, Andhra Pradesh and Karnataka to achieve weight gains in the progeny. Over all results of improvement of mutton production did not prove fruitful. The body weight gains and early physiological maturity of the progeny was partly attributed to improved feeding and management. Cross breeding among

the local sheep breeds too showed no faster gains or better growth of progeny.

Introduction of exotic mutton sheep for crossbreeding of local sheep started after sixties of 20th century. Main imports consisted of Romney Marsh, South Down, Polled Dorsets, Suffolk, Corriedale, etc. For the production of mutton and dual purpose sheep following attempts had been made. Malpura, Sonadi, Muzzafarnagri, Mandya and Nellore crossed with Dorsets and Suffolks; Coimbatore, Bellary, Nellore and Muzzafarnagri bred to Corriedale rams as well. These breeds have produced heavier crossbred animal than the locals in general. Higher carcass weight and overall increase in meat production is observed in the half-breds of Sonadi, Mandya and Nellore with Suffolks and Dorset rams. Polled Dorset and Corriedale cross breds of local sheep of Jammu and Kashmir reveal better weight gain and carcass formation. Corriedale crosses with Bellary and Nellore are significantly superior over their contemporary natives. Romney Marsh also produced identical results. Avimaans sheep synthesized by C.S.W.R.I. possesses the desired growth, body weight and characteristics of a mutton sheep.

Table 13.3: Average body weights/growth rate of some Indian sheep breeds (kg).

Breed	Birth weight	Weaning weight	6 mth weight	9 mth weight	12 mth weight
Gaddi	2.52	7.44	10.81	12.26	14.29
Lohi	2.81	10.88	14.34	16.47	19.57
Nali	2.88	10.19	13.30	14.54	17.74
Magra	2.98	11.70	20.14	21.82	27.99
Deccani	2.80	10.56	11.88	13.10	—
Muzaffarnagari	3.01	10.80	16.54	18.39	25.01
Nellore	2.74	11.98	16.60	17.08	22.72
Madras Red	2.61	13.50	15.72	21.70	21.89
Bellary	2.60	11.09	16.28	—	18.68
Ramnad	1.68	7.31	8.45	14.50	16.30
Mandya	1.94	8.05	17.76	15.08	21.02
Cross Breds					
Gaddi Synthetics	3.5	20.23	22.74	23.6	24.92
Malpura/Sonadi X Dorset/Suffolk	2.89	12.05	22.03	23.78	24.48

The thrust towards wool production in the temperate region revealed that the crossbreds of indigenous sheep and exotic fine wool breeds were heavier and faster growing compared to their local counterparts/contemporaries. Besides wool improvement, a usual increase of 15 to 25 percent in mature weight was observable in the exotic cross breds and graded sheep at various stations/farms. At different levels of exotic inheritance of various genetic groups, the actual mutton gain ranges from 10 to 20 percent only.

Essential features of mutton production

For production of mature mutton and lamb, improvement in following parameters is considered:

- Higher weaning weights
- Faster subsequent body weight gains at 6, 9 and 12 months.
- Optimal growth and production cost exercise vis-a-vis earlier slaughter age, viz., lamb, hogget or yearling stage.
- Feed conversion efficiency.
- Maintaining intact or improving other production traits like wool production status, mature weights, meat yield and other attributes of meat quality, etc.

To achieve these, attention to following basic aspects is quite imperative:

- Selection of suitable breed (s).
- Designing of appropriate breeding plan.
- Providing improved feeding, management and health care.
- Adopting a proper rearing system.
- A record of meat production is essential.

'Crossbreeding for fine wool' programme in the northern states has opened vistas for higher meat production. The practice of feed-lot system produced encouraging results. The Rambouillet crossbred male yearlings attained 50 to 55 kg weight. At 18 months the feed lot wethers and even males retained for breeding gained weight around 70 kg at farmers' house hold. Nutritious fodders and grasses, top feeding, crop residues and protein rich cheaper compounded feeds are

a prerequisite to fat lamb production in absence of improved ranches. Rearing of mutton sheep on migratory pattern is not a profitable proposition. Loss of energy under prolonged journeys and transportation is not recouped or compensated economically.

Mutton system approach

Research work at CSWRI. specifies following possible production systems:

- Early maturing lamb—marketed below the age of 6 months.
- Late maturing lamb—marketed between 6 months and 12 months of age.
- Yearling mutton production-between 12 to 24 months of age.
- Mature mutton production—when marketed after 24 months of age.

Good mature mutton production is reported possible from Nali, Marwari, Magra, Jaisalmeri, Pugal and Jalauni breeds which are also good carpet wool producers. Selection for higher weaning weight and lower slaughter age is advisible.

In semi-arid zone, for yearling mutton, Magra, Malpura, Patanwadi, Deccani and Muzzafarnagri having faster growth potential have been suggested. In semi-arid to humid regions the development of Shahbadi, Belangir, Ganjam, Bellary, Mechari, Kilakarsal, Coimbatore, Ramnadwhite and Kenguri for yearling mutton production and the Nellore, Vembur, Madras red and Bonpalla for late maturing lamb are advocated. For early maturing, the suitability of Mandya, Hassan, Chotanagpuri and Tiruchy Black is considered in their home tracts.

Yearling mutton from wethers of migratory flocks is possible. In the temperate high lands of north, production of mature mutton from existing wool producing genotypes like Gaddi, Bakerwali, Rampur Bushair, Poonchi, Karnah, Gurez, and Changthangi and in southern hills from Nilgiri breed is in vogue. In the Gaddi and Bakerwali flocks the surplus wethers are maintained for their wool crop and disposed when they are invariably over two years of age.

The successful production system demands priority to management, healthcare programme and marketing besides the attention to breeding and feeding. The crux of a specialised mutton production programme lies in the introduction of mutton breeds for crossbreeding and consolidation of body weight gains of the programme of 'crossbreeding' for wool. The superior native sheep germ plasm needs preservation. The 'selective breeding' of it may be of some utility. Selection index in this case must take due care of higher body weight and faster growth rate.

In both the above cases*, the aspects of feed conversion efficiency, carcass quality, yield, weight of abdominal viscera and skin weight deserve proper attention. The prolificacy and survival rates are other important parameters. The two such major components are;

1   Lambs born per ewe joined, and
2. Lambs weaned per lamb born.

These indicators reflect on the availability of lamb for the market. A favourable index value indicates augmented mutton supply. Age, sex, season, feed quality and quantity affect the carcass quality and the dressing percentage. In view of limited information available on the subject, further study and investigations are called for into various facets of mutton production system including optimum slaughter age in the local and crossbred sheep of Indian origin.

SECTORAL SCHEMES

Multidirectional schemes aimed at achieving a breakthrough in sheep and wool production stand launched at the state and central level. Major thrust is provided in the Annual and Five Year Plans of those states which have potential and sizeable sheep population.

State sector

- Breeding—In accordance with NCA recommendations and the States' priority, selective breeding, crossbreeding and upgradation of local flocks is implemented.
- Importation of superior sheep germ plasm and its multiplication.
- Stud ram production at the nucleus farms of the states.
- Production of cross bred rams at the farmers flocks.
- Extension organisation and establishment of service centres like sheep extension centres, ram centres, sheep sub-units, etc.
- Intensive sheep development projects for migratory sheep flocks including mobile centres, transit camps, etc.
- Disease investigation and research.
- Health cover—disease prevention and control.
- Wool testing laboratories.
- Wool shearing and grading.
- Artificial Insemination and ETT in sheep.
- Training of sheep supervisors, basic sheep workers and farmers.
- Feed and fodder resource development.
- Sheep and wool marketing, establishment of wool boards/corporations and federations, etc.

Central sector schemes

Under five year plans a number of sheep and wool development schemes are in operation, such as:

- Establishment of Central Sheep Farm at Hisar (Haryana). To cater to the additional requirement of exotic and cross bred rams of different states.
- Grants in aid to large scale sheep breeding farms for ram production on 50:50 share basis. Various states that have availed the scheme benefit are AP, Bihar, Karnataka, MP, Rajasthan, UP, Gujarat, Maharashtra, Haryana, J&K and HP.
- Establishment of Central Wool Board under Ministry of Textiles and strengthening of Wool Boards/Corporations or Federations of the states.

---

* Indian sheep breeds and their crossbreds with exotic breeds.

The Central Wool Board has taken up a number of programmes for sheep and wool development, wool utilization, training and marketing. Besides, it has helped in strengthening of wool boards/corporations/federations, etc. of AP, HP, UP, J&K, Rajasthan, Gujarat, Karnataka and Maharashtra since 7th Plan. The scheme aimed at providing central assistance on 50:50 pattern has also been operational.

➡ The Market Intervention Operation (MIO) scheme is the one to check the fall in wool prices and resultant loss to the producers. The MIO scheme can be operated in any state which is willing to share cost and losses on 50:50 basis.

➡ Integrated Rural Development Programme and other Rural Poverty Alleviation Schemes.

The facilities under these programmes are available to the poor sheep rearing families, sheep unit holders of the states on usual terms envisaged under various schemes. The small and marginal farmers, landless labour, border area farmers, poor S/C, S/T families and destitute women have been benefited in various states by opting for small sheep units.

ICAR schemes

The involvement of ICAR is mainly in Research and Development of the sheep and wool. The IVRI carried out the major task of research and investigation into sheep diseases. Study on animal fibre like Pashmina and wool too were undertaken. After mid sixties the CSWRI and agriculture universities over the country shared the work of research and development with regard to disease, nutrition, genetic and production aspects. Sponsoring of schemes under the All India Coordinated Research Projects have provided new direction to research in various states. The guidelines and breeding strategies have been planned and suggested for various regions. Efforts have also been put in over the last forty years to synthesize woolly, muttonous or dual purpose sheep genotypes. As a result a good number of cross bred sheep like Bharat merino, Avivastra, Avikalin, Avimaans, etc. have come into existence by eightees of the 20th century.

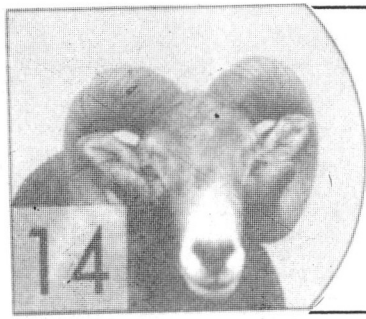

SHEEP MEAT, MILK AND MANURE

14

MEAT

Mutton and lamb are the terms normally in usage for the respective end product of slaughter of adult and young sheep.

Main product

Native sheep and goat in India are maintained by the shepherds and farmers primarily for meat. The major income to the owners of these small ruminants particularly the sheep, come from sale for slaughter. Invariably the sale proceeds of live animals account for almost 80 to 85 percent of the total receipts from a sheep flock which include other byproducts like wool, milk, manure, etc. Though the profit share of the sheepman is only marginal, these animals always offer a flourishing business for the middleman on obvious reasons of illiteracy of the producer and absence of any organised effort in meat trading in the country. Sheepman is just complacent that with his 'sheep possession' he can tide over his financial problems in all eventualities. Any surplus sheep (wether or cast for age) is his 'traveller's cheque' for encashment as and when necessity arises. Customers visit his door steps, the pastures and even transit routes for a deal. With this satisfaction he is not much concerned about loosing substantially in the hands of middlemen, butchers or others in the trade.

Consumption trends

Mutton is not in much demand in USA. and parts of Europe, viz. Italy, Belgium, Holland, etc.

Russia, China, Middle East and even South East Asian countries offer a lucrative mutton market. The growing dislike of health conscious consumer for red meat is giving place to fish, poultry, turkey and a marked yearning for the lamb. The production of lean, young and fat free lamb for slaughter augurs brighter prospects for sheep. Lamb rearing industry in Australia, New Zealand, Argentina and in certain other countries occupies a special place.

In India mutton or lamb production has not received as much exclusive attention as wool production. Overall awareness of common consumer about quality and type is lacking, with certain exceptions. Sheep rearing for mutton purposes still occupies a back seat. Live sheep and meat transportation and trade on modern lines or even a change over of slaughter technology is taking off at a slow pace.

Per capita meat consumption in India is just 1.57 kg per annum as per recent estimates by Arora and Garg (1998) and 1.3 kg mutton reported earlier by Carles (1983) which is far less than most of the developed and even some developing countries of the world. New Zealand, Greece, Bulgaria and Ireland are the countries which stand on top of per capita mutton and lamb consumption in the world (Table 14.1).

With a sizeable population of the country being non-meat eaters, low meat consumption is at times attributed to socio-religious and climatic conditions. Because of climatic reasons and food habits the demand for animal proteins is more in

Table 14.1

Country	Per capita mutton consumption (in kg)
New Zealand	32
Greece	16
Bulgaria	11
Ireland	10

northern states like Jammu and Kashmir where per capita consumption of meat is substantially higher than the national average. Annual per capita consumption of mutton and chevon together is around 3.5 kg. The small ruminant population of the state can not meet the required quantum. So animals are imported from outside the state for slaughter. During the last decade of the 20th century 1 to 1.2 million live sheep alone arrived annually in the state for slaughter besides 10 to 15 percent goats. Almost identical number of animals are available for slaughter out of the sheep and goat population of the state (Gupta, 1993).

In Central and Western India, population is mostly vegetarian and meat consumption is far less than the north and north eastern states. In the latter states piggery, poultry and fish form the main animal protein source. The coastal belt meat requirements in the country are by and large met by poultry, fish and partly goat.

Choice: The people in the warmer regions of India have a general liking for 'chevon', the goat meat. In cooler regions like Kashmir mature mutton is preferred over goat meat due to fat content. The taste and preference for Kashmiri Wazwan meat preparations or Punjabi mutton cuisines is known since ages. Various delicacies and varieties require the meat of specific parts of

a carcass. An old Punjabi saying interprets this tendency glaringly, viz.

Leyameen Puth, netaan aamein uth,

Leyameen seena, panwain lage meheena.

'Bring back-meat or else come back; bring brisket meat even if it takes a month'

The quality of mutton depends on type of sheep breed, condition, conformation, health and age, i.e. young, fat lamb, mature, old, lean, etc. Well developed muscles with short fibres, interspersed fat and limited connective tissue add to the juiciness. Slaughter of mature or adult sheep produces a carcass of poor taste and undesirable characteristics. Proper slaughter age (under local conditions for desi sheep) to provide a tender, juicy well developed muscles is considered around hogget to yearling stage. Many consumers prefer even smaller weight lambs and this mutton is called '

Hulvan. It is delicate and relished much. Early slaughter is, however, discouraged at times on ethical and economical considerations.

Composition of mutton

The factors that influence the quality have also a bearing on the composition of mutton, though fluctuations are less marked. A mature mutton has a composition as shown in Table 14.2 (A); its values are given in Table 14.2 (B).

EFFECT OF MOVEMENT/TRANSPORTATION ON SHEEP

Routine grazing of sheep involves a daily movement or journey of a few kilometres distance in our conditions. The transhumant sheep are in

Table 14.2(A): Chemical composition of mutton (%)

Item	Moisture	Protein	Fat/Ether extract	Mineral matter	Carbohydrate	CA	P	Iron
Sheep liver	70.4	19.3	7.5	1.5	1.4	0.01	0.38	6.3
Mutton muscle	71.5	18.5	13.4	1.3	–	0.15	0.15	2.5

Table 14.2 (B): Values/100 g

Item	Calorific value	Vit. A (I.U)	Vit. B (mg)	Vit. C (mg)
Sheep Liver	150	22,300	120	20
Mutton Muscle	194	31	60	–

Source: Report on the marketing of meat in India.

the habit of regular walking over long distances. Trekking to far off pastures in pursuit of grazing is not unusual to sheep in the arid regions of Rajasthan and Gujarat or in cold desert of Ladakh. The unimaginable effect these walks have on the body weight of sheep has hardly been assessed.

It is usual in certain cases especially migration, sale, purchase or despatch to slaughter houses to resort to vehicular transportation of sheep. In the long sojourn the condition of animals deteriorates. The appreciable loss in body weight at times renders the deal uneconomical.

While transporting the Rambouillet sheep (Reports 1976-77 of Reasi farm flocks in J&K) from winter to summer stations, stretched almost 200 km away, a marked change in general condition came to light after 8 hours on board the double decker trucks. This necessitated a trial recording and observation. Results are presented in Table 14.3.

Further observations revealed that the fall in body weight ranged higher in younger and older lots. Proportional loss of weight in lambs per unit body weight was considerably higher. The jolting and exhaustion in transportation affect the young animals more than the adult sheep. These transportation losses of weight were regained in a month's period of grazing in the summer pastures.

The loss is more pronounced in unsound vehicles and recoupement is quicker in the sheep that have an easy access to adequate watering and good grazing after unloading. Over packing and congestion in carriers and rough roads contribute more towards loss in condition and weight due to wear and tear of tissues, dehydration, stress, exhaustion, sweating, etc.

Rail transport of 140 Mandya sheep from Bangalore to Jammu and Kashmir in January 1978 resulted in an average body weight loss of 0.8 to 1.5 kg in various age groups and sexes (Gupta 1978). Comparatively lesser fall in weight than trucks is ascribed to good condition of wagons, least jolting, beside adequate feed, fodder and water facilities enroute. Almost similar observations have been made in a 30 hours air transport of over 1500 sheep in a chartered Jumbo flight from Houston (Texas) to Delhi in 1988.

Transportation to slaughter houses

At least ten truck loads of sheep and goats arrive at various locations in Jammu and Kashmir state daily. The origin of the despatch is roundabouts of Delhi or even beyond that. Each truck carries 150 animals or more. The distance of over 800 km is covered in almost 30 hours. The body weight loss in transit has never been investigated even though it appears of very high order. A couple of

Table 14.3: Results of vehicular transportation

Type of animals	No. loaded on one deck	Age group	Body wt. (kg) (range)	Av. B.wt. at des-patch (kg)	Av. B. wt. after unloading and movement to Base camp (kg)	Av. wt. loss* (kg)	loss %
Rambouillet rams	21	Adult	58 to 76	65.5	58.8	6.7	10.2
Rambouillet ewes	28	Adult	39 to 55	44.2	38.6	5.6	12.6

*Including excreta voided in transit on board.

sheep and goat die during transit and many others are found too debilitated to stand up on disembarking.

Elsewhere in the country too the road transport of sheep to slaughter houses is a common feature. At occasions the sheep purchased and collected from interior villages are made to traverse sufficiently long distances on foot to road heads often deprived of proper food, water or even rest. The animals are pushed or dragged, causing bruises to the tissues and muscles. The middlemen and traders have little or no knowledge about the adverse effects on the meat content and carcass quality.

Live sheep and mutton marketing

The purchase of sheep and goat in the production pockets is made by the agents of the wholesale merchants, kothedars and contractors on arbitrarily negotiated rates. The middle man, therefore, rules the roost, by exploiting the shepherd about market rates. The producer's share of the end sales at butcher's shop are hardly 45 to 55%. Rest of the profit is shared by the chain of the intermediaries.

The live-sheep marketing is highly monopolised. Strangely an animal produced in a Rajasthan village moves over to Kashmir and another one coming from Madhya Pradesh or Haryana reaches its destination in Maharashtra metropolis. The situation of exploitation of the producers is expected to improve with the institution of sheep and wool boards and corporations.

Rajasthan did make a headway in procuring contract for export of live-animals and meat to Gulf countries. Some multinational concerns have also ventured into meat trading and processing recently. But mutton and chevon export industry in India needs sound planning and scientific management for acquiring a place in international arena. For meeting export requirements as per their specifications and to provide hygienic meat within the country it is essential that:

1. System of sheep and goat transportation be improved.

2. Slaughtering technology be updated.
3. Modernisation of slaughter houses be taken up.
4. Meat inspection system be strengthened. Ante and postmortem examination should be compulsorily adhered to.
5. In rural areas, especially in the small ruminants rearing zones chain of abattoirs is required, preferably nearer to major townships.
6. Along with modernisation of abattoirs, facilities for production and processing of better hides, skins, meat and meat products, animal casings, recovery of slipe wool, etc. are required to be developed. Salvaging of these byproducts shall open up varied fields of industry.
7. The development of satisfactory storage and refrigeration facilities for meat should find priority.
8. Awareness about meat hygiene through veterinary public health is highly important for internal and outside market.
9. Standard specifications as existing for other commodities should also be laid in meat trade. Age, weight at slaughter, dressing percentage, fat content, bone meat ratio and freedom from disease are some such parameters. In other words strict quality control measures for exports should be introduced.
10. Transportation of live animals over long distances should be avoided. To overcome marketing problems and exploitation of farmers it is advisable to have sheep breeders cooperatives/or mutton producers cooperative societies.
11. Above all, the acts of cruelty on animals during transport, handling and slaughter should be banned.

SLAUGHTERING AND DRESSING OF CARCASS

For study at research stations it is necessary to adopt a well defined procedure for recording meat and growth. A few lambs or kids are generally slaughtered first for carcass evaluation before the marketable crop of lambs or kids is sold.

1. Slaughter procedure

As a matter of fact proper handling during transport and in the yard attached to the slaughter house is essential. Slaughter should not be resorted to soon after arrival at the abattoir.

- The animals should be slaughtered in the morning to avoid moisture loss. A day prior to this, the sheep and and goat should be weighed and fasted. They should have access only to water. Prior to slaughter, details of condition, age, breed, etc. should be recorded.
- The humane slaughter requires that animals must be stunned prior to slaying.
- The throat of the animal should be cut at the level of occipito-atlantal joint and the blood collected in a pre-weighed basin and weighed. The head is then severed and weighed.

2. Dressing technique

- The skinning of the carcass is done according to the generally accepted practice. The skin is weighed immediately.
- The offals (stomach and intestines) are removed, weighed full and then cleaned and weighed again. Caul fat (fat on the stomach and intestines) may also be separated and weighed.
- Liver, spleen, diaphragm, kidney alongwith kidney fat, fore and hind cannons, four hooves below the cannon bones, i.e. metacarpals and metatarsals are weighed separately. So should the chest cavity contents, viz. lungs and heart (pluck) removed and weighed. Skin is also weighed in fresh condition.

3. Linear measurement records

The external measurements as specified below are taken on the intact carcass as skeletal growth records are necessary.

After de-skinning the carcass is suspended from a standard gambrel, i.e. hooks placed at a specified distance which are not to be changed through out the operation. The distance between the two hooks on the wooden plank of the gambrel is generally 15 to 16 cm. The standard width between the two hooks is necessary to avoid error in measurements. The following measurements help in the study of skeletal development.

- BODY LENGTH (DORSAL) is taken with a tape from the base of the tail to the base of the neck, i.e. at the junction of first thoracic and last cervical.
- LENGTH OF THE NECK (DORSAL) is taken with a tape from the junction of 1st thoracic and last cervical vertebra to the atlas joint.
- BODY LENGTH-LATERAL, from the anterior edge of the symphysis pubis to the mid point of first rib.
- DEPTH OF THORAX is the measurement taken with sliding callipers dorsoventrally perpendicular to the long axis of the carcass and the maximum depth of chest.
- HIND-LEG LENGTH is measured from the anterior edge of symphysis pubis to the anterior edge of the distal end of the metatarsal. Use sliding callipers for this measurement, so that the value is unaffected by the contour of the body.
- FORELEG LENGTH is taken with a tape in straight line from the crutch of the flesh between the two legs to the anterior edge of the distal carpal.
- THIGH WIDTH is measured by using sliding callipers across both the thighs at a point where the body is widest laterally, i.e. take the width of gigots.
- THIGH DEPTH is the measurement whch relates to the depth of gigots and is taken by sliding callipers behind the tail, based to the line perpendicular to the long axis of the carcass and from the dorsoventral side.
- FULLNESS OF THE THIGH is thelength taken from a point just below the patella on one side and the tape to be passed under the tail to the corresponding point on either side.
- TIBIA LENGTH is taken by steel dividers from tubercle on the proximal end of tibia to the anterior edge of the distal end of tarsal plus the length of tibia.
- LENGTH OF HUMERUS is measured by steel dividers.
- LENGTH OF FORE AND HIND CANNONS is measured as above.

🐑 EYE MUSCLE AND OTHER MEASUREMENTS: If the growth of the eye muscle (back muscle-*Longissimus dorsi* at the 12th rib) is to be studied, then take a transverse cut at 11th, 12th and 13th rib and measure with dividers, the maximum distance across the cross-section surface of the *Longissimus* dorsi from the end next to the spinal process outward along the rib.

1. Length of eye muscle.
2. Depth of eye muscle, i.e. this distance is measured at right angles on the same surface.
3. Thickness of the backfat-over the deepest part of the eye muscle.
4. Thickness of fat over the spinus process.
5. Fat over the rib.
6. Thickness of the muscle over the lower half of the rib and subcutaneous fat at that point.

4. Carcass cuts

Body parts of meat importance are shown in Figs 14.1–14.4.

Leg: Called leg of mutton and includes all parts posterior to symphysis pelvis, i.e. thigh, rear leg, dock, twist, pastern and lower areas (dew claw, foot, etc.).

Loin: From last rib including symphysis pelvis but excluding flanks.

Chop: Is the region from first thoracic to last thoracic. The cut passes through last rib and first lumbar vertebra.

Chuck: Is the region from first cervical to last cervical. It includes neck.

Brisket: Includes fore leg, part of scapula and sternum up to 4th rib.

Flank: Portion behind last rib, below loin and in front of pelvis. It consists of muscles only.

DISSECTION AND JOINTING

The carcass may be dissected on the table in its natural position, i.e. without any stretch on the joints. The following description holds good.

Shoulders: Are detached by severing the muscles attached to the sternum applying slight traction on the arm to remove the shoulder from the thorax, sever *Latissimus* dorsi muscle reaching the midline of the thoracic vertebrae. It is necessary to knife round the scapula to the base of neck cutting through the *Trapezius* to *Brachiocephalic* muscles.

Neck: Sever at the junction of the last cervical and the 1st thoracic vertebra.

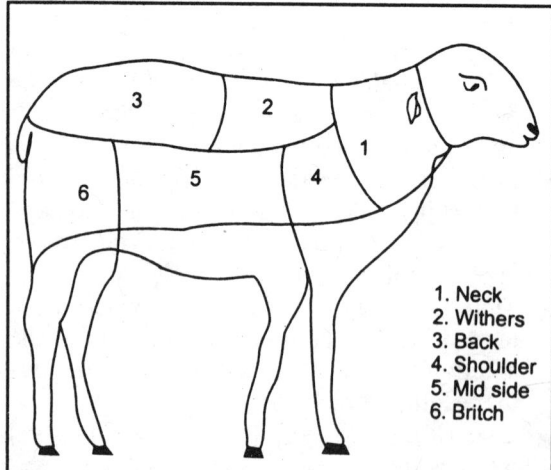

1. Neck
2. Withers
3. Back
4. Shoulder
5. Mid side
6. Britch

Fig. 14.1. External delineation of sheep parts/cuts

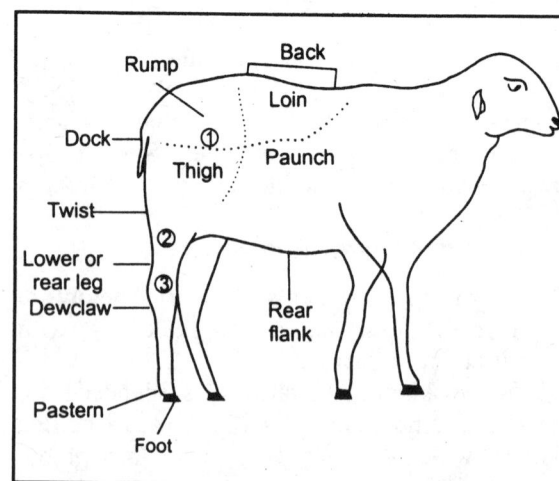

Fig. 14.2. Parts of leg of mutton (1, 2, 3)

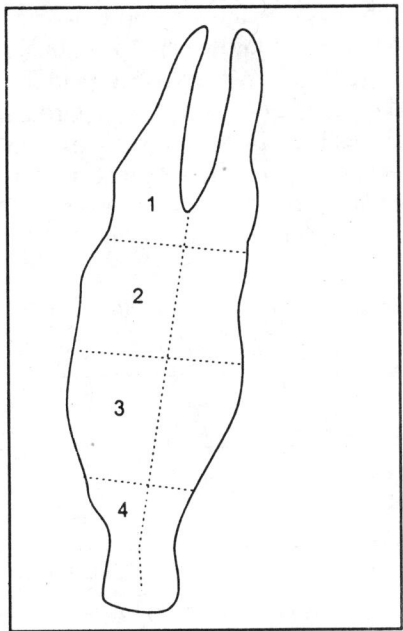

Fig. 14.3. Cuts of a sheep carcass (back view).

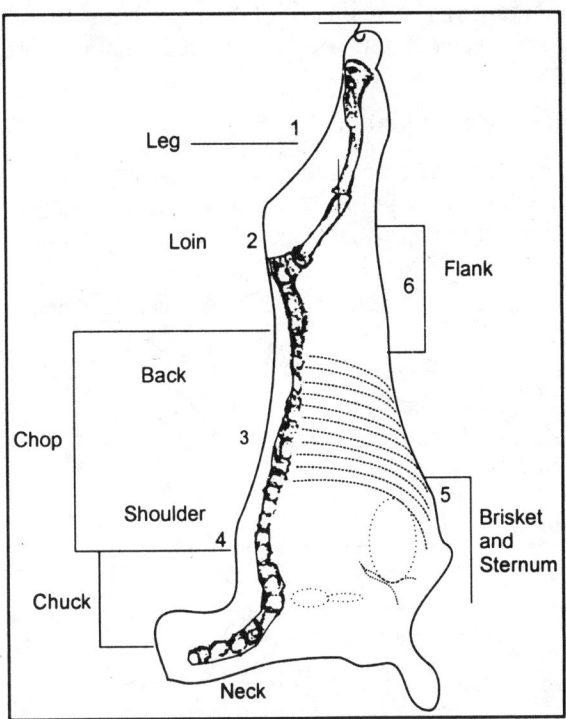

Fig. 14.4. Showing six primary cuts of different joints in a stretched carcass.

Thorax: The last thoracic vertebra which is articulated with the loin is severed by a transverse cut behind the last rib and the first lumbar vertebra. The thorax is then divided into ribs and breast. The rib joint is separated from the breast joint by cutting through the ribs and the sternbrae (sternum).

Loins: The part is separated from the gigots by transverse cut from both sides and at the level of the anterior side of the iliac wing (hip bones). An oblique cut at the iliac wing is then necessary to include the sixth lumbar vertebra in this joint.

Legs: After a transverse cut directly through the muscles, i.e. through the *Rectis abdominis* on each side at the level of anterior edge of symphysis pubis. The two legs are separated by a cut along the posterior medium line on the symphysis ischium. It is necessary to lay bare the surface of the *Gracillus* muscle on each side. The femur acetabulum joint is to be then severed *sagittaly*, working from the symphysis ischium. The Gracillus and *Adductor* muscle attachments are to be separated from the ventral surface of the ischium. The ischial arch and the posterior lateral angle are then followed up to the acetabular branch of the ischium, working as close to the bone as possible and the *Biceps femoris* and semitendinous muscles are severed at their attachments. A circular cut has then to be made from the acetabular femur through the muscles of the thigh to meet the cut previously made at the level of symphysis pubis.

Pelvis: The remaining cut constitutes the pelvis (the tail will have to be separated in the case of long tailed sheep.

Dissection of Joints for meat to bone ratio

Each of the joint is to be weighed separately for recording the weight of:

- Bone alongwith the tendons.
- Edible portion, i.e. muscles together with intramuscular and subcutaneous fat. To study

marbling, the layers of fat will have to be scrapped and its weight recorded separately.

Carcass evaluation

Work on carcass characteristics of Mandya sheep has been reported from various quarters. Scanty literature exists about other breeds. The results, whatever available have by no means any comparison to world's known mutton or dual purpose sheep. No doubt the Mandya sheep and cross breds do hold prospects of a sound breakthrough in this field (Tables 14.4, 14.5). Encouraging results have been achieved in growth rate, dressing percentage and feed utilization after crossbreeding the native sheep with exotic mutton sheep.

Table 14.4: Carcass evaluation of some arid zone sheep and their crossbreds

	Malpura	Sonadi	Muzaffarnagri
Dressed weight (kg)	9.33	8.36	–
Dressing percent:			
Live wt. basis	52.10	57.03	48.64
Empty wt. basis	60.50	58.94	56.37

	Malpura		Sonadi		Muzaffarnagri	
	Dorsets	Suffolk	Dorsets	Suffolk	Dorsets	Suffolk
Dressed weight (kg)	10.67	10.98	10.39	10.93	–	–
Dressing percent						
Live weight basis	52.49	52.05	52.21	51.47	49.55	48.01
Empty wt. basis	60.82	60.23	60.38	59.17	56.75	56.92

Source: Basuthakur and Acharya (1981).

Table 14.5: Carcass evaluation of Mandya sheep

Age in months	Av. Live wt.		Carcass weight	Dressing %
	24 hrs before slaughter (kg.)	At the time of slaughter (kg.)		
3 months (5)	9.363 ± 0.876	8.967 ± 0.830	3.563 ± 0.546	47.12 ± 3.81
6 months (10)	13.447 ± 0.721	12.907 ± 0.766	5.680 ± 0.363	58.37 ± 1.93
9 months (10)	13.940 ± 0.764	12.923 ± 0.407	5.840 ± 0.439	53.41 ± 1.02
12 months (10)	18.022 ± 1.444	17.104 ± 2.003	6.627 ± 1.374	53.9 ± 1.4
15 months (9)	20.216 ± 1.322	19.085 ± 1.377	8.931 ± 0.757	56.78 ± 2.46
18 months (8)	19.990 ± 2.504	18.863 ± 2.426	8.566 ± 1.449	55.73 ± 2.69

Source: Nagaraj (1964).

The results of extensive carcass studies carried out at Pune Research Station in the second half of last century on the Bannur lambs (Nagaraj, 1964) provide a better insight into carcass evaluation (Tables 14.5 and 14.6).

The dressed weight of the carcass is affected by the proportion of non-edible organs, viz., head, blood, skin, hooves and pluck, etc. To arrive at meat bone ratio, the carcass is cut longitudinally into two halves. From each of the cuts, the meat is separated from the bones and tendons. From these weights, the meat: bone ratio is expressed as meat wt./bone wt (Table 14.7).

The carcass evaluation of Mandya breed lambs of different age groups have an average live weight of 8.967 kg at the age of 3 months. This increased to 19.085 kg at 15 months and the dressing percentage increased from 47.13% to 56.78%. This is considered the optimum age for slaughter of Mandya lambs. Head, pluck and amount of blood become proportionately smaller with advancing age (Table 14.8).

Feed conversion efficiency

Table 14.9 shows feed conversion efficiency and percent dressing of native and crossbred sheep.

Table 14.6: Relative proportion of various cuts in the carcass of slaughtered Bannur lambs (Nagaraj,1964)

Age	% Leg	% Loin	% Chop	% Chuck	% Brisket	% Flank
6 months (13)	34.83 ± 0.76	7.57 ± 0.88	10.81 ± 0.76	23.82 ± 0.88	17.71 ± 0.86	5.22 ± 0.49
9 months (9)	35.16 ± 0.47	6.57 ± 0.49	10.08 ± 0.55	22.09 ± 0.49	20.99 ± 0.51	5.13 ± 0.19
12 months (16)	35.59 ± 0.33	6.66 ± 0.23	9.36 ± 0.45	23.78 ± 0.69	20.23 ± 0.77	4.43 ± 0.22
15 months (8)	33.98 ± 0.64	7.79 ± 0.76	10.91 ± 0.71	19.72 ± 1.05	20.57 ± 1.10	5.03 ± 0.24
18 months (12)	34.24 ± 0.39	6.50 ± 0.42	10.42 ± 0.57	23.52 ± 0.70	20.34 ± 0.54	5.38 ± 0.23

Note: Figures in parenthesis in column 1 indicate number of observations.

Table 14.7: Meat to bone ratio in various cuts of carcass of Mandya sheep (meat/bone)

Age in months	Chuck Neck, shoulder with 1st four ribs	Chop Ribs from 5th to last but one	Brisket Sternum, elbow and lower portion of ribs	Leg Behind last lumbar vertebra including pelvis	Loin All Lumbar vertebrae
6 months (3)	2.5	2.1	2.0	3.1	2.67
9 months (7)	2.7	2.1	2.4	3.4	2.90
12 months (4)	3.3	2.99	3.53	4.50	3.26
15 months (5)	3.9	3.34	3.26	4.51	3.71

Table 14.8: Percentage of blood, head, skin, hooves and pluck (on live weight basis for Mandya lambs)

Age	Percentage					
	Blood	Head	Skin	Hooves	Pluck	Other parts kidney, kidney fat, liver, spleen, diaphragm
6 months (14)	5.54 ± 0.46	11.32 ± 0.50	12.50 ± 0.45	1.74 ± 0.11	2.53 ± 0.19	3.73 ± 0.18
9 months (4)	5.31 ± 0.30	11.39 ± 1.05	10.42 ± 0.12	1.90 ± 0.03	2.25 ± 0.10	3.34 ± 0.10
12 months (11)	5.23 ± 0.39	7.54 ± 1.49	11.25 ± 0.70	1.93 ± 0.30	2.83 ± 0.31	3.23 ± 0.13
18 months (7)	4.92 ± 0.22	8.68 ± 0.17	10.21 ± 0.15	1.65 ± 0.04	2.28 ± 0.11	4.01 ± 0.11

Table 14.9: Feed conversion efficiency and dressing% of native and cross bred sheep

Breed/Genetic Group	Slaughter age	Efficiency of feed conversion%	Dressing % (pre-siaughter weight basis)
Gaddi	9 months	12.4	45.2
Nali	6 to 9 months	12.2	48.5
Nellore	6 to 9 months	15.06	47.0
Mandya	6 months	9.62	49.3
Muzzaffarnagri	6 to 9 months	13.6	45.6
Dorset × Native Rajasthan sheep	—	15.7 to 18.6	—
Suffolk × Native Rajasthan sheep	—	14.3 to 16.1	—
Dorset × Nellore	—	12.74	44.75
Dorset × Mandya	—	12.33	44.09
Suffolk × Nellore	—	12.21	44.41
Suffolk × Mandya	—	11.95	48.41

Better combining ability of certain exotic breeds with indigenous sheep, e.g. Corriedale × Kashmir valley and Suffolk × Sonadi has been found to result in body gains and efficiency of feed conversion. The latter declined as the age advanced. Possibly the feed energy got diverted to meet production requirements or was stored as fat depots. Taneja (1978) reported an average dressing percentage of 57 and 56% for Mandya and Nellore lambs at 6 months. The dressing percentage was observed equally good at 18 months age. The feed lot cross bred lambs were found to attain a weight of 28 to 32 kg in the stationary flocks in J&K. Those run on semi-intensive system ranged between 22 to 25 kg. A level of 17% FCE and around 50% dressing percentage at 6 months age appears a desirable proposition for slaughter lambs.

SHEEP MILK

In most of the countries mutton is being paid more attention than wool. Sheep skins, fur and manure occupy place next to wool. By and large the milk production is limited and too low in sheep, so as to make dairy sheep rearing an economically viable entity. Its contribution to the sheep production ranks after meat, wool, manure, etc. Therefore, sheep milk is relegated a position last of all in the list of the sheep byproducts. Prolific sheep breeds are known to have better milk production. This enables the harvesting of twin benefits of higher lambing and surplus milk in some countries of the world.

Though sheep milk has least significance in trade, yet to the temperate and arid region nomad and poor tribal shepherd it is good means to carry his bread down the gullet (Fig. 44, PLATE 8). The migratory sheep in the northern states, lamb in spring and a decline in their milk production takes place after four to six weeks. But as soon as these ewes move to rich high land pasture in June, there is invariably a milk flush especially in the crossbreds. The lambs are usually weaned by that time at the state farms. Private flock owners continue the lambs with the mother ewes till that time for augmentation of growth. Lambs are separated in the evening. Ewes are milked next morning for personal consumption. At times the surplus milk is converted into ghee and milk cake by the shepherd during June to August or till next mating. The sheep milk particularly of early lactation is considered by the tribals to possess immunogenic properties against infant gastric ailments. Quite often fresh sheep milk or preserved milk as cake, or cheese is used to cure buccal ulcerations of the children. In Italy and Balkan states sheep milk is converted into cheese by adding rennet.

Milch sheep

Dairy sheep contribute to almost one-third of the total milk production in Bulgaria. Texel and West Friesian sheep breeds in Denmark and Holland are reared for milk; Sardinia and Piedmont in Italy; Sicilian, Zeckel and Bulgarian are other milk breeds of sheep. The highly prolific Romanov and Welsh-mountain breeds of Europe are associated with high milch potential. These sheep produce 2 to 3 litres milk per day with out suckling of lambs. Awassi is a dual purpose sheep of Palestine and Israel.

Lohi and Kutchi (Patanwadi) are two known Milch sheep breeds in India. An average ewe produces half to one litre of milk a day. The number of these sheep in the respective home tract is however, quite limited. Average butter fat is 6.8%. They do well when maintained in a small flock of 5 to 10 sheep and are stall fed. Whereas most of the Indian sheep are poor milkers and usually not milked, a couple of breeds like Malpura, Sonadi, Muzzafarnagri, Jalauni, etc. yield 20 to 30 litre milk in a lactation period of 100 days. Like the northern temperate region sheep, the milk potential of some other Western and Peninsular zone sheep is also tapped by the rearing communities for their family consumption.

Patil and Dave (1982) reported average lactation yield in Patanwadi and Merino x Patanwadi half breds in the three months lactation as 460 and 443 g a day respectively.

Sheep milk composition and comparative evaluation

Though the sheep milk is a boon for the lamb and the shepherd, this does not figure prominently as a commercial commodity in India. Not much work on evaluation and analysis is available. The data indicated by Aggarwala (1953) provide the essentially needed information about various constituents and comparative composition of sheep milk (Table 14.10).

Russian workers (1970) have reported that their sheep contain about 5-6 percent of albumin, 4 percent lactose, 6-7 percent fat and roughly 1 percent salt. Residual 81 to 83 percent is water.

While reviewing composition of milk from various species, Banerjee (1992) indicates that sheep milk contains 5.3% fat, 5.5% protein, 4.6% lactose, 0.90% ash and 16.3% total solids. Since diet is the ultimate source of most of the materials used in milk synthesis, any change in the amount and type of food affects both milk yield and composition.

SHEEP EXCRETA

Importance: Since the start of cultivation of land, the man did realise the importance of animal excreta in agriculture. Sheep being easily

Table 14.10: Comparative average composition of sheep milk *vis â vis* human and other animals milk

Part I

Species	Sp. gravity		Water		Total proteins	
	Average	Position compared to human milk	Average (%)	Position compared to human milk	Average %	Position compared to human milk
Women	1,0298	–	87.23	–	2.01	–
Cow	1.0319	2nd	86.23	2nd	4.41	3rd
Buffalo	1.0319	2nd	82.55	4th	4.15	2nd
Goat	1.0305	1st	86.88	1st	3.76	1st
Sheep	1.0355	3rd	83.57	3rd	5.15	4th

Part II

Species	Fat		Sugar		Ash	
	Average %	Position compared to human milk	Average (%)	Position compared to human milk	Average %	Position compared to human milk
Women	3.74	–	6.37	–	0.30	–
Cow	3.34	2nd	4.40	3rd	0.75	1st
Buffalo	7.12	4th	4.99	1st	0.86	3rd
Goat	4.07	1st	4.64	2nd	0.85	2nd
Sheep	6.18	3rd	4.17	4th	0.93	4th

Part III

Species	Total Solids		
	Average %	Position compared to human milk	
Women	12.42	–	In all cases position 1st
Cow	12.48	1st	shows nearness and position
Buffalo	17.45	4th	4th fartherness of the
Goat	13.12	2nd	constituents from
Sheep	16.43	3rd	human milk

Source: Agarwala (1953)

amenable to folding and herding were found to be the best source of enriching the soil with least labour (Fig. 45, PLATE 8). The owner of a flock not only used sheep dung and urine for better produce from his land but allowed other farmers also to avail the benefit at very convenient terms.

In various parts of India the sheep especially of migratory nature are kept in the harvested lands for the night. The excreta dung and urine voided by the sheep saturate the soil. This manuring is considered to be more valuable and with lasting effects than fertilization or even usual manuring. The sheep-goat dung pellets mix up with the soil over a period of time thereby release the nitrogen and other nutrients slowly. The effects of sheep folding in the crops can be felt for two to three years.

Manure yield

An adult sheep produces almost 0.4 to 0.5 metric ton excreta in a year, where as the young sheep voids 0.2 to 0.3 ton only. The daily defecation of a flock finds dispersal at the following locations:

1. The day time excreta is shed in the grazing ground, pastures and fields after crop harvesting.
2. A part of it is dropped on the sheep paths, road sides, watering sites or at day time resting places.
3. The night soil is collected in the sheltering places, sheds or at the folding sites.

The latter amounts for almost half of the total excreta, the rest normally goes waste in the pasture, particularly under unmanaged paddocks and grazing grounds. Onground experience reveals that sheep not only dibbles the shed seeds of grass and other plants in the pastures by its gentle movements, but also provides manuring and moisture for seed germination during grazing through random defecation and urination.

100 sheep shall manure half a kanal of a field per night. Folding of almost 2000 sheep shall suffice for an acre of farm land. Sheep dung accumulated in sheds or night folding is swept next morning and heaped by the shepherds and farmers by the side of a field. There exists a wrong practice to spread the same directly into the field. This lowers the utility and effectiveness. The best way to preserve it is to prepare compost. For this sake a pit of following dimensions is suggested for proper bacterial action:

2 m wide × 1 m deep × length, depending upon the production of manure and strength of flock. The pit once full is covered with earth or mud plaster to avoid entry of rain water in the pit and to allow decomposition.

In the prolonged and severe winter zones like Ladakh, Lahaul Spiti, Kinnaur, interior mountainous areas of UP and Sikkim the sheep are housed for months together. The dung and urine voided by the sheep and goat get deposited on the kacha flooring, usually over a hay or straw bedding. The excreta is neither removed regularly nor drained. Continuous accumulation and trampling by the animals leads to the formation of a thick cake of 10 to 15 cm in a season. This serves as urine absorbent and a source of insulation from cold for the animals. At the end of the winter season the cake is scrapped and used partly for fuel and partly as manure in the fields. In the lower ranges where fuel or firewood is no problem, the practice is to clean the sheep sheds and folding pens after a few days gap and utilise the manure in the fields directly or collected in heaps where from it is removed and spread in the cultivable lands at the onset of cropping season.

Composition of sheep and goat manure

Animal excreta in solid condition has the composition of main plant nutrients as given in Tables 14.11, 14.12 and 14.13.

Table 14.11: Comparative composition of organic excreta of various mammal species

Kind of animal	Quantity voided per day (kg)	Crop nutrients (%)		
		Nitrogen	P_2O_5	K_2O
Human	0.6 to 0.8	0.80	0.10	0.20
Cattle	7 to 9	1 to 1.1	Traces	0.20
Horse	3.3 to 4.0	1.35	Traces	1.50
Pig	1.5 to 2.2	0.60	0.10	0.50
Sheep	0.5 to 0.7	0.7 to 1.7	0.03	0.3 to 1.0

Table 14.12: The composition of air dried material (%)

Sps.	N_2	P_2O_5	K_2O
Human	5.0	3.80	2.0
Cattle	1.2 to 1.5	0.5 to 1.0	0.7 to 1.2
Horse	1.27	1.15	1.14
Pig	1.7 to 2.4	2.0	1.5
Sheep	0.7 to 1.5	0.4 to 1.3	0.5 to 1.0

Table 14.13: Soil nutrients (%) in liquid urine

Sps.	N_2	P_2O_5	K_2O
Cattle	1.05	0.007	0.21
Sheep	0.69 to 1.68	0.03	0.29 to 1.03

The above composition figures make it evidently clear that the sheep excreta, dung and urine are better balanced in soil and crop nutrients and therefore the farmers have a preference for the sheep and goat organic matter from their experience of ages.

The sheep manure fetches a higher price, which ranges from Rs 150 to 200 per metric ton against Rs 100 to 150 for cow dung manure.

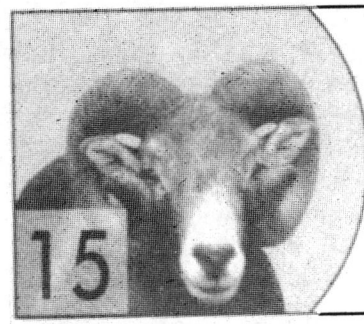

EXAMINATION AND SCORING OF SHEEP

EXAMINATION

Points of sheep

To begin with the physical examination of sheep the learner should be well conversant with the major points of body of the animal. Figure 15.1 provides requisite know-how for practical identification of these points on the body of a standing sheep.

Method

Examination of a ram or an ewe while judging in competition or show rings, and at the time of classing or selection is important. If the examination is thorough and systematic, it matters little which view of the animal is noted first. Normally the examiner or the selecting sheepman should proceed in the following manner.

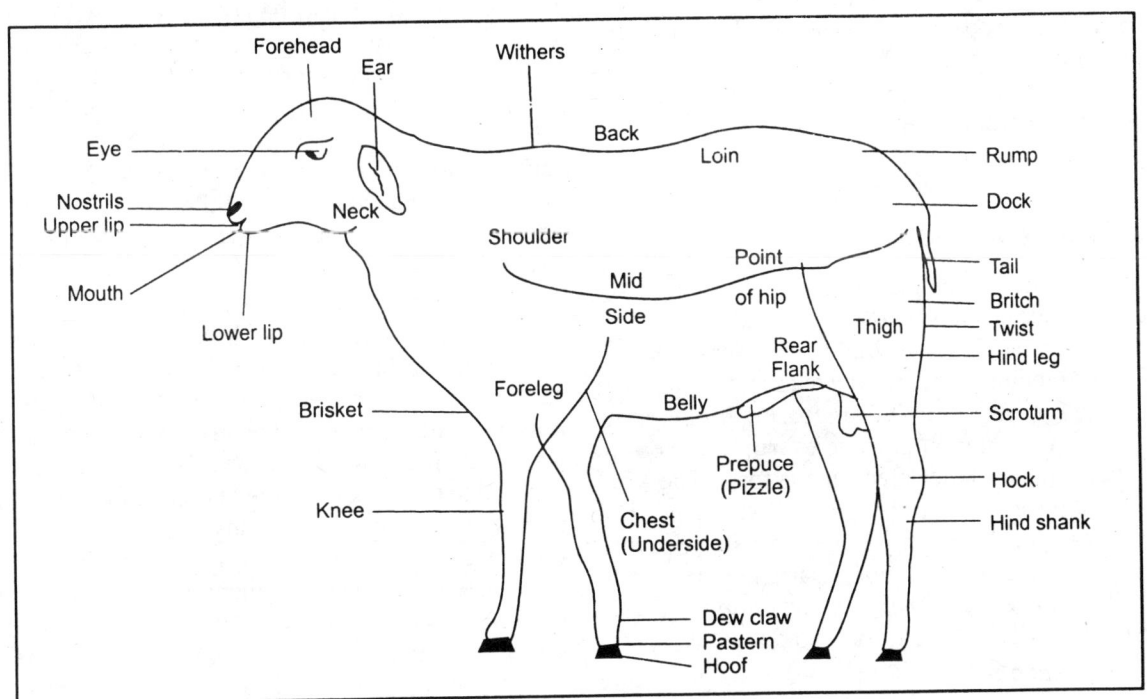

Fig. 15.1. Points of body of sheep (Local breed ram).

Looking over the sheep

Front view: To start with, look the sheep over from a distance. The front view provides fair idea about the form and make up of head, width and depth of brisket and the length, shape and placing of forelimbs. Close attention should be given to the head as its quality is specific for breed specimens and reveals a great deal of what is known as 'breed type'. The development of certain features of the head is indicative of constitution and sturdiness of the animal.

Side: In taking a side view, the size, style and the general setting of the sheep attract attention. A general impression is gained which takes note of length and depth of body, the carriage of head, the length and setting of the neck, the extension of brisket, the evenness and trueness of top and bottom lines, length and shape of legs and lastly the relation of neck, shoulder, middle and rump and to the total length of animal.

Rear: From the rear, the width and evenness in width of body are to be noted. Watch for the development of rump, thighs and twist and placing of hind legs. These aspects are important in mutton sheep and from the point of selecting ewes for breeding.

Physical examination

Visual impressions gained through looking over can further be substantiated by handling. This is necessary because the wool may cover defects in form. Handling is a sure way to assess the amount and quality of flesh. While preparing for the show ring it is a common practice to trim the wool in order to conceal the defects in the form. The wool and skin should be inspected at close range. The manner of handling gives most accurate impression and does not disarrange the wool. Hand should be laid firmly but without undue pressure. Clawing is to be avoided.

1. Rear portion: Proper place and procedure is to begin handling at the rear. A right handed person should stand on the left side of the sheep. The rear includes thighs, twist, dock and rump.

The first thing to feel with the hand is the development of lower thighs. Put the left hand at the back of thigh and right one at the rear of flank. This helps ascertaining flesh on both the outer and inner thighs. The right hand should then press upwards on the twist to estimate the amount and firmness of muscles. To examine the upper thigh, press one hand against the thigh, while resting the other on the top of rump.

2. Middle portion: Includes back, loins and ribs. The loins are examined for width and thickness by placing one hand straight down on either side of it. The covering of loins is judged by placing the fingers flat over the spines and noting whether the bones are prominent or padded with fat and flesh. Width of back is a good point of certain breeds showing the levelness and covering. Ascertain the degree of arch behind the shoulders either by placing the fingers of the hand on one side of spine and the thumb on the other or place one hand on either side of spine. Spring of the last rib should also be noted carefully as the width of a properly shaped barrel increases gradually from shoulder to the last rib along the back. The ribs should be well covered and filled with firm flesh and fat. The *Longissimus dorsii* muscles (the eye muscle) running along the back constitute the main source of fullness. If the spine and ribs are prominent, the covering is poor in both extent and quality.

3. Anterior portion: It includes shoulders, chest, brisket, neck and head. Place one hand on the top of the shoulders. Feel how compactly the shoulder blades are set up against the spine and how well developed is the musculature. Hand should then be moved from sides of shoulder forward to the neck to examine depth of flesh and as how smoothly neck blends with the former. Fullness indicates high condition and well musculated neck. Hand is then placed where the brisket joins the lower parts of shoulders. In the thin animals there is a perceptible depression. The hand should then be run down to the base of brisket and chest to assess the width and fullness, while keeping the other hand on the top of shoulder. The front of brisket is often palpated to have an idea of its extension and contour. Neck in front of shoulders should be grasped with one hand and jugular furrow region with the thumb and fingers of the other hand to know the setting, the size of neck and fullness of sides of neck. Likewise the joining of neck with the head behind the ears is also ascertained. Head may also be handled for examination:

1. In woolly sheep to know the size and width;
2. in polled sheep to see the horn-buttons;
3. to check back or inner side of ears for ticks and tags, etc.;
4. to look at the teeth for age estimation, by parting the lips with the other hand;
5. to examine the eyes and inner canthus.

Examining skin and fleece

Inspection of wool forms an important aspect of judging, classing and assessing wool quality of sheep. The best wool grows on the sides of shoulder and just behind it. The fleece is first opened in that region. This should be done by laying the hands down flat on the surface of fleece and gently forcing it to part so that the density, quality, colour, lustre and condition of wool and colour of skin can be observed. The next site of examination is mid side (last but one rib equi-distance from belly and back) which provides a representative wool producing area, minimum exposed to soiling and weathering.

Thigh wool inspection provides good cues in mutton breeds beside wool examination. The judge may also look for wool quality along the spine, the hip point, dock and belly. For the presence of pigmented fibres, the kemp and dark spots, the fleece should be parted on top of the head, just behind the ears. Similar approach is adopted for examination just above the hocks.

Examination for defects

The judging of ewes essentially involves exami-nation of udder and external genitalia. Instances are on record when hermaphrodite ewes have arrived on importation or some ewes received with cut or permanently impaired teat. Wrinkles under the throat and large lumpy grooves may well go concealed or unnoticed even after trimming unless observed by touch. Beginner judges often fail to notice the over done condition, the presence of soft blubbery fat on the fore limbs and on the rump. To detect it one hand should be placed near the top of the animal and the other lower down and push them towards each other.

EXAMINATION OF BREEDING RAMS

Reproduction capability is the major criterion in which a breeding ram is subjected to examination. This involves the following.

- Manual examination of the reproductive organs of a ram.
- Examination of semen samples.
- A mating trial.

Manual examination

The manual palpation of reproductive organs of ram is an important, practical exercise. It is aimed at knowing abnormalities of genitalia, fertility prospects and soundness as a replacement and for breeding.

While handling rams it is advisable to note whether the scrotum is normally developed. A good breeding ram has usually large springy testicles. They are even in size, shape and resilience. Small, slit or pencil testes is an occasional feature in the Rambouillet and Rambouillet crossbred rams. Such conditions are usually reflected in lack of a masculine head. At times one testicle may be abnormally small, under sized or not descended in the scrotal sac. This testicular retention in abdomen, the monorchid or cryptorchid state is largely discriminated against. No merit or prize should be awarded to such rams.

Handling procedure: The ram should either be handled in standing posture comfortably by an assistant or put in a crate to avoid movements and facilitate palpation, or else may be preferably presented standing in a race, thus obviating extra manpower requirement.

To conduct manual palpation the examiner occupies position behind the ram. Light crutching be accomplished if so needed. Precaution against butting by other rams is also observed.

- Hold the scrotal sac gently but firmly by placing hands on either side of neck, fingers in front and thumb behind scrotum.
- The cords can be now palpated by moving the fingers up and down the lymph glands.
- The head of epididymis be felt then at the upper end of each testicle for any inflammation, abscesses or painful condition.
- The testicles are palpated for size, shape, resilience, fullness, atrophy, cryptorchid conditions and for orchitis, (hot, doughy and painful nature).
- Tail of epididymis should be palpated next, at the centre of the lower end of testicle for evenness and normal size. While maintaining firm grip over neck of scrotum, move fingers of the other hand up and down the central groove and along the inside edge of testicles to detect enlargement, inflammation or abscesses.
- At the end of the manual palpation, examine scrotal skin for mange, ticks, wounds or skin abrasions.

Manual observations should then be corroborated with the laboratory findings of stained semen smears (for Brucella organisms and other bacteria) blood test, complement fixation and sterile semen sample examination.

In short the following conditions need to be taken care of during examination of external genitalia:

1. Varicocele—the varicose veins in the cord.
2. Hernia due to rupture of tissues and a loop of bowel escaping through inguinal canal into scrotum.
3. Enlarged lymph glands.
4. Epididymitis-inflammation or abscesses in the head, body or tail of epididymis.
5. Orchitis-inflammation of the testicles due to Brucella or other infections.
6. Small testicles. In older rams it is a sign of senility or withering after being afflicted due to injury or infection. In young rams lack of

adequate nutrition is attributed for smaller testicles. Various other types of testicular formations, viz. slit, pencil or knob-like conditions are also observed and seem genetic in origin and heritable. Occasionally one testicle may be far less developed than the other.

7. Flabby testicles leading to seminal degeneration and lowered fertility.
8. Cryptorchid, where single testicle is in scrotum and other retained in abdomen. Double rig condition is prevalent in Rambouillet breed associated with polledness as sex linked character. Studies at some of the farms where this breed is maintained reveal that almost 5% of the polled ram lambs have both the testicles absent in the scrotum.
9. Scrotal abrasions or wounds acquired in bushy or spears grass or Nagoora burr infested pastures are common. Small scabs of chorioptic mange, sometimes wide spread, resulting into thickening of scrotal skin is a common feature in private flock rams.
10. Pizzle rot and prepucial adhesions.

Time of examination: The appropriate period for examination of rams through manual palpation is:

1. At about six weeks before mating
2. Just before mating season and
3. After about 2 to 3 months of completion of mating.

Examination of semen samples

Rams retained for breeding must be subjected to examination of their semen before final selection. Semen samples are obtained either by electrical stimulation or by service into an artificial vagina. Broad criteria for semen evaluation are:

- Volume
- Percentage of live sperms
- Motility
- Presence of abnormal cells or infective organisms.

When the rams are suffering from the early stages of seminal degeneration they may be far less fertile than what the semen characteristics indicate. It is advisable to examine two or three semen samples taken several weeks apart.

If both the testicles are flabby, the ram is not fit for mating. Special attention, nutrition and treatment might help restore fertility before mating. Where even one testicle is flabby for no visible reasons, the examination of semen sample for any infection should be considered seriously. The results obtained need to be corroborated further with clinical findings and manual examination of reproductive organs.

If Brucella ovis is the cause for orchitis or soft flabby testicles, the same can be demonstrated by acid fast staining. Prepare a thin semen smear. Dry in air. Stain as follows.

Dilute Carbol fuchsin	10 min
Rinse in water	3 min
Decolourise in 1%	
Acetic acid	4 min
Rinse in water	5 min
Methylene blue	½ to 1 min.

Rinse quickly, drain, and dry and examine under microscope. Brucella organisms are seen as short rods within white blood cells that frequently occur in the semen of infected ram. Agglutination test is another method of diagnosing brucellosis.

Test mating of rams with ewes

The most satisfactory method of proving difference in fertility of rams is to select ewes in heat. The rams to be compared are mated separately with a group of at least 40 ewes of about the same age. Mating be ensured in separate paddocks or through hand service. For appropriate comparison, uniformity is desirable in environment, paddock size, stocking rate, pasture composition, shelter, feed and water availability. Marking fluid or colour block harness is required to be placed on the ram's brisket. Service recording has to be made daily. Ewes, not coming in heat, should be discarded.

After the first oestrus period of 19 to 21 days, the breeding rams be replaced by vasectomised teasers. The heat detected ewes are then hand served by the rams included in the trial.

After conception, normal and identical conditions should prevail during pregnancy in all the sub-flocks. Thorough surveillance till lambing and daily recording of lambing is essential to determine:

1. Ewes conceived as a percent of those joined
2. Ewes lambed as percent of those:
   a. joined (served).
   b. conceived.
3. Lambs surviving up to 3 weeks of neonatal period as percent of those born.
4. Ewes lambing to the recorded service, and
5. Length of the gestation period.

The rams may then be evaluated for comparison of fertility parameters, viz.

- Conception rate
- Successful pregnancy and lambing percentage
- Extent or percentage of surviving lambs in terms of Lbj, Lnj, Lwj and Lwb* components.

When the breeding season is almost terminating, the number of ewes in oestrus or the conception rate decline, a fact that needs consideration.

Replacement

- Ewe-lambs selection for breeding should come from early maturing lambs of approved type
- Ewe-lambs should preferably be from good milking dams.
- Should be of uniform size, appearance, and age and preferably from the first rather than the last lambing.
- While developing a prolific flock it is better to select ewe lambs that were born as twins. This may however, be of not much utility in view of low heritability of twinning.

---

* Lbj - Lambs born per ewe joined. Lnj - Lambs surviving till neonatal age, out of ewes joined. Lwj - Lambs weaned per ewe joined. Lwb - Lambs weaned per lamb born

Proportion of breedable animals retained as replacement depends on a number of factors, like mortality, carrying capacity of the property, culling rates, increasing/decreasing pattern of flock strength, etc.

Sound lambing rate and lamb marking percentage are essential for good replacement levels. When the lambing is around 90 percent which is a usual feature for flock in India, 2 to 4% ram lambs and 25 to 33% ewe lambs are selected as replacement stock. The general assumptions for this are 10 to 12% mortality, 10 to 15% annual culling rates and one ram for every 40 to 50 breedable ewes.

The ewes should be available for at least 4 to 5 pregnancies and successful lambings in life time, and better if ewes are mated more often than once a year. To ensure that sufficient ewe lambs are born to replace the original ewes, the formula given in Chart 15.1 below is used to indicate the mean number of matings necessary for a group of ewes entering the breeding flock.

Tips for the farm-man

- The sheepman should like sheep and understand their habits and peculiarities.
- The farm and pastures should be fit for sheep production providing congenial environment and feed.
- Proper estimation of labour requirements is desirable. These tend to increase at lambing time, shearing, breeding or shifting.
- Determination of flock size shall depend on availability of feed, labour, pasture, shelter and equipment.

- While starting a good flock, the cheapest way is usually to buy good young ewes and good rams as foundation stock.
- Personal likes, market trends, cost of available stock and environmental conditions are important factors in selecting a breed.
- Selection of foundation stock should be based on body conformation, production record and pedigree, Suitable ones are those, that produce a good fleece and carcass.
- Sheep from a flock of high prolificacy, milking ability, growth, fleece and carcass quality are likely to be better than from those flocks where production records have been of least consideration.
- Age, dental condition and udder soundness are important in selecting breeding animals.

SCORING BODY CONDITION

Objectives and gradation pattern

The objective of assessing body condition of sheep is to:

- Understand changes which elude or mask visual appraisals,
- To know the main deterioration or loss in body condition,
- To ascertain body weight trends,
- To assess effect of nutrition and to adopt suitable line of nutrition, and
- To maintain proper condition of sheep.

For accurate body condition scoring, the common yard sticks employed are:

- Feel back bone behind last rib region for sharpness and prominence of spinous pro-

Chart 15.1: Replacement formula

$$\text{Replacement} = n \times \frac{m}{200} \times \frac{(100-d)}{100} = 1$$

where, n — is for mean no. of matings per head

m — mean lamb marking %

d — mean annual death rate between marking and selection, i.e. till ewe lamb stage cesses. Also palpate loins region with extended palm and fingers.

➟ Accomplish feel of lumbar processes ends, sharpness and fullness with finger tips.

➟ Eye muscle appraisal. The thickness and fat coverage of *Longissimus* dorsi muscle be ascertained between back bone and lumbar processes.

➟ Thickness of skin over back also provides fair idea of condition.

Gradation pattern

Scoring body condition as commonly suggested by experts is on following gradation.

0. Extremely debilitated or approaching death.
1. Poor store condition, i.e. weak, prominent back bone, lumbar processes sharp and discernible, eye muscle lean and thin, no fat, skin very thin.
2. Average store condition, i.e. smooth but prominent back bone, ends of lumbar vertebral processes round and less sharp, eye muscle of medium thickness with little fat, skin thin.
3. Forward score condition, i.e. back bone smooth and slightly rounded at top, lumbar processes covered and smooth, can be palpated under firm pressure, eye muscles full with moderate fat; skin medium.
4. Fat condition, back bone can be palpated with pressure, full eye muscles having thick fat cover, lumbar processes difficult to feel, skin thick.
5. Excellent fat condition. The back bone or the ends of lumbar processes can not be felt even under pressure. Fullness is further evident from thick eye muscles, thick fat cover and thick skin.

Scoring of fine wool crossbred sheep

Invariably Merino, Rambouillet or fine wool Russian sheep breeds are being used in India for cross breeding or up grading of indigenous sheep. The fine wool cross bred sheep so produced acquire skin folds or wrinkles to a limited extent at 3/4th fine wool inheritance. On the basis of these folds which normally mark their appearance in young age or by adulthood, the ewes are differentiated into the following three definite types.

A type: Distinct symmetrical skin fold is present under, neck over top of neck, in the flank or thigh region and base of tail. Wrinkles may be more than one. Number of this type of sheep in the fine wool crossbreds is negligible.

B type: Skin fold in one or more parts of body may be present, but not much prominently.

C type: The body of sheep is free from folds, giving the view of a plain bodied animal. At most of the cross breeding projects the proportion of this type of flock is comparatively higher.

Besides above, information about sex, type, date of birth, sire, dam, body weight, general appearance and breeding, style and activeness and even wool coat is needed to score the animal.

Body scoring

A general practice is to fix a perfect conformation score for true to typeness of each point taking into account its importance and weightage in selection. Appropriate value is assigned against each on examination of the respective point. Final actual score card is worked out to decide the placing of a particular sheep under consideration (Table 15.1).

Fleece scoring

In any wool improvement programme, the appraisals of rams and ewes must rest on unshorn fleece condition (Table 15.2).

Scoring (score card) of mutton type sheep/ dual purpose sheep

Table 15.3 describes the scoring pattern of mutton type/dual purpose sheep.

Phenotype appraisal

The general appearance of the sheep is viewed from some distance and observations recorded with respect to:

Table 15.1

Point	Features	Perfect score	Actual score
Body	Stylish and active, free from folds, symmetrical in outlines, Tending towards muttonous conformation (in C-type particularly). Ewes appearing distinctly feminine; rams strongly masculine; Development sound.	10	
Head	Strongly masculine (in rams) medium length, fore head broad, wide between ears, proportionate to body in female as well, which should distinctly appear feminine in character.	2	
Face	Silky hair, free from coarse chalky hair or kemp, broad nose (bereft of Roman nose character) in rams, muzzle well developed, lips thick, pink in colour, free from dark spots; nostrils large, jaws neither under or over short (a disqualification).	4	
Horns	(applicable to horned strains of rams) Well developed with distinct corrugations, wide spread, but not pressing or piercing neck, jaws or orbital bones. In polled strains absence of scurrs, knobs or horn buttons desirable.	2	
Eyes	Large alert, set prominently; eye lashes not obstructing vision, turned-in eye lashes (entropion) defective. Wool blindness undesirable.	3	
Ears	Broad, thick and relatively short, silk like smooth cover.	1	
Neck	Medium length, merging smoothly with head and shoulders; minimum wrinkles desirable.	3	
Chest	Deep and broad.	3	
Withers	Fairly well rounded and covered, not too prominent.	1	
Topline	Straight, with no drop in front or behind withers (Devil's dip), well covered and carried out at rump.	4	
Back	Medium length, fairly broad loins, wide, blending smoothly with hips.	5	
Ribs	Well sprung and well rounded out, ensuring ample capacity for vital organs.	2	
Rump	Long wide and level, carrying width nicely to tail stump (in neatly docked tail cases).	2	
Leg of mutton	Well filled out, twist deep.	2	
Scrotum	(in rams) enveloping two normally developed testicles, nodular or slit testicles undesirable; cryptorchism a disqualification. In ewes udder sound and well developed.	1	
Legs	Medium length, straight, strong, free from off coloured hair sprinkling and physical or bony deformities, pasterns strong, hoof amber colour, free from excessive pigmentation, abrasions, fissures or over growth.	5	
		50	

Table 15.2

General appearance: Attractive and even, carrying dense fleece of good staple (annual growth basis), light to medium face cover, forehead covered but not to the extent of wool blindness, wool covering extending on legs nearly to hooves; free from undesirable fibres and wool faults.	8
Length of staple (12 month basis) Approximately uniform length over body including body covering; Minimum bare area in flanks and chest region; staple length should be over 8 to 10 cm, on annual basis and not less than 4 cm for individual biannual clip.	12
Fineness and quality: Well defined even crimp extending from base to tip, with uniformity in diameter over the length of fibre; soft and pliable to touch, bright attractive colour, sound through out, fleece free from kemp, minimum unevenness of wool.	15
Density or covering Compact, even, clean, free from foreign material. An open fleece is indicated by open ropy locks with dirt, sand and other foreign particles penetrating almost to the skin along the top line and also along bare area in flanks and chest region. Though midside wool is a better representative, the belly wool with medium density and of staple length is a reliable indicator of density and high yielding qualities.	10
Condition: (conditioning as usually termed) yolk moderate, preferably light to creamy in colour and evenly distributed; heavy dark, clotted yolk objectionable, only minimum amount of sand, dirt, vegetable matter and stained locks.	5
	50
G. Total	100

Conformation: Muttonous conformation is one where there is ample width, depth, compactness and low setness. Topline is straight and full. Symmetry and style are desirable features of form for the market. Blocky animals are preferable.

Weight and size: Fast weight gain is economical. Size and weight are specific for age and breed. Rambouillet crossbred lambs of local sheep are heavier and bigger in size than the local breed lambs age for age.

Quality: High quality is indicative of fineness of fleece, bereft of coarseness. Good form relates to fleshing and fineness of bone. A defined clear cut head with wool is expressive of the quality.

Condition: This term applies to both the
(a) Finish or fleshing
(b) Score card condition: cover over the shoulders, back, loins, thickness of dock, brisket, etc. which indicate fatness or condition, carry due weight.

Dressing %: Finished sheep that are trimmed and light in pelt, dress high. At times the lowered dressing percentage because of heavy fleece is not favoured when the fleece sells lower than the carcass.

Head and neck: In breeding sheep, emphasis is given to head and neck, because of their distinctiveness of the former for every breed. Though this is a major component, yet the weightage on the score card is low. Desirable aspects vary from breed to breed. Short head, face and neck trimmed at the throat is peculiar of Mandya sheep. Other local breeds possess, a medium face, wide forehead, open clear eyes, well carried ears and thick neck.

Table 15.3

General appearance	40
Weight: according to age and market requirement.	
Form: wide, deep compact, low-set, straight top line and underline, stylish and symmetrical.	
Quality: free from coarseness, smooth in form and fleshing	
Condition: degree of fatness, indicated by thick firm covering over shoulder, back, loins and ribs. thick dock and plump breast, no soft loose fat.	
Dressing percentage: high condition, and light pelt.	
Head and neck	5
Muzzle: white strong.	
Eyes: large open, quiet.	
Face: sharp, forehead white.	
Ears: fine, well carried.	
Neck: short, thick, clean through out.	
Fore quarters	7
Shoulder: smoothly joining the neck, wide and smooth, top well covered.	
Legs: straight, sharp, strong, wide apart, forearm thick.	
Body	25
Chest: wide, deep and full at back of shoulders.	
Back: wide deep and thickly fleshed.	
Ribs: well sprung, thickly and firmly fleshed.	
Loins: wide, thick, firm, smoothly covered.	
Hind quarter	15
Rump: long, level, wide to the dock, covered with firm thick flesh	
Leg of mutton: deep, wide, plump, heavy.	
Twist: deep, full and firm	
Legs: straight, short and wide apart	
Fleece	8
Quantity: dense, long, body completely covered	
Quality: fibre medium to fine, uniform, free from pigmentation	
Condition: sound bright, clean, soft, lustrous, moderate yolk, evenly distributed.	
	100

Fore quarters: Ideal shoulders: must join smoothly with the neck, well covered with flesh, wide and smooth on top are considered ideal.

Breast: Should be wide and full. Plump breast is an indication of constitution for purpose of carcass as well as of breeding sheep.

Legs: Fore arm must provide a thick well developed mutton conformation. Front legs should be straight and well set from front and side.

Body: A full, wide chest of depth is desirable as it indicates a strong vigorous constitution. Well sprung up ribs, a straight top line, full back and loins are preferred. Ideal mutton sheep possess thick smooth and fleshy backs.

Hind quarters: The desirable market sheep is one, where rump and the leg of mutton is long, wide to the dock and heavily fleshed. Next to the back and loins it is the leg of mutton that is attached a high score card weightage. The *Quadriceps*, the *Femoris*, the *Gracillus* muscles, etc. provide for the desirable plump rump and leg of mutton. The inner thigh, i.e. the twist, should be firm and full.

Well set hind legs and straight and strong hocks are sound traits of a breeding as well as slaughter sheep.

Fleece: This aspect is of secondary importance in a mutton sheep. Its weight on the score card of mutton sheep is just 8 to 10 percent of the total value.

Once the wool occupied prime value position over mutton, though the position has altered a bit. Better the mutton condition, higher are the returns. Sheepman is appreciative that inferior mutton conformation tends to lower the over all dividends. The judges no doubt consider the quantity, quality and the condition of fleece quite often. A long dense fleece cover of uniform fibres in desirable. It should be clean, white and free from black or brown fibres. In carpet wool breeds a sound, bright, soft, lustrous wool is desirable. It should have desirable quantity of uniformly distributed yolk to prevent matting of the fleece and to protect the wool fibre.

WOOLLY SHEEP *vs.* MUTTON TYPE SHEEP

There is much difference between the woolly and mutton type exotic sheep other than the quality and character of the fleece in the two types. The width, depth, compactness, low setness, straightness of top line and characteristic conformation which typify the mutton sheep are usually lacking in the woolly sheep.

Low backs and droopy rumps are also more common in the wool type. More angularity of conformation is likewise typical of wool type. Thick fleshy conformation is usually missing in the fine wool sheep, while flat ribs, light loins and light thighs are quite common. The mutton conformation as seen in the mutton breeds is seldom visible in the wool type breeds. Yet within this type are many which yield very good carcasses.

Fleece of the fine wool sheep is very compact as well as fine. The outer side of the fleece is dark in colour because of accumulation of dirt and dust. A heavy secretion of yolk is typical of the wool sheep as are the folds or wrinkles in the skin of merino· descendants. Thigh wool inspection provides good cues in mutton breeds beside wool examination. The judge may also look for wool quality along the spine, the hip point, dock and belly.

But for a few special breeds there does not exist any distinct division into woolly and mutton types in the indigenous sheep as is seen in Merino types and English origin Down breeds. Nilgiri, Chokla and Karnah breeds are known to produce medium fine wool, but not a compact fleece; while as Mandya as an exception has a typical muttonous conformation. So are some other sister breeds in the Deccan plateau.

The general conformation of other Indian sheep is that of dual nature. Nali, Magra, Deccani, Marwari, Patanwadi, Muzzafarnagri, Gaddie and many other breeds possess a conformation of this type. Open wool coat (bereft of a fleece), bare face, belly and lower legs; and back thigh, etc. not full of muscle are the other characteristic observations.

Crossbreeding with merino strains on one hand and Dorsets, Suffolks and South Downs on the other in certain regions have tended to produce clear woolly and muttonous crossbred forms. Thus, different genotypes of specific utility emerged, but end utility in all cases continues to be of duality under Indian conditions.

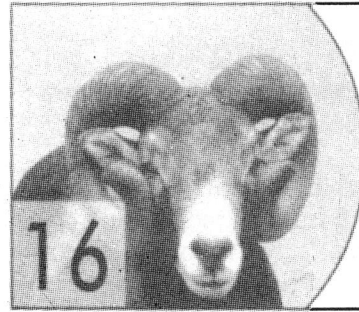

SHEEP CALENDAR AND RECORD KEEPING

PLANNING OF OPERATIONS

To run a sheep flock or a farm successfully it is appropriate to observe the principle of doing the right things at a right time. Unplanned operations lead to inefficient and uneconomic results. Sheep is invariably maintained enflock and thus instead of individual care demand a collective approach in various operations like breeding, feeding and management. While doing so, the favourable climatic conditions, fodder and labour availability have to be kept in view. Breeding is not encouraged in a period, when the resulting lamb crop is endangered by scanty food or adverse weather. Shearing cannot be carried out in a season when exposure or inclement weather conditions prevail. Weather, season and other environmental factors must be considered well before undertaking operations like harvesting, migrations, marketing and disease control measures.

Therefore, it is essential to draw up a programme of the routine operations. Adjustment of these take into account the various phases of sheep husbandry to avoid overlapping.

Mating period: Is the one when the rams are allowed to run with the ewes. Both the rams and ewes should be in a fit condition so that high fertility is possible. Service by rams poses no problems. Flushing of ewes demands some green forage. The appropriate mating period should ensure flushing for achieving fertility. A regular supply of nutritious grass is ensured during advanced pregnancy and lambing time for optimal

growth, and survivability. Vital immunization of the lamb to be born, is conducted by vaccination of mother ewe in late pregnancy.

Lambing phase: Selection of suitable lambing period synchronises with mating phase and must have the ingredients of the following.
- Favourable environment.
- Availability of plenty and rich grazing and sustained milk flow.
- Minimum mortality of lambs.
- Faster growth of lambs.

Whereas lambing time and lactation are the periods of great stress for the ewes these are quite exacting for the tending shepherd too. He should be able to devote sufficient attention to lamb rearing.

The operations of parturition assistance, lamb owning, marking, docking, castration, etc. are smoothly accomplished in dry weather which is bereft of fly strike. The winter months of lambing are therefore preferred over hot summer period to obviate chances of infection.

Lamb weaning: This phase should not coincide with any lean grazing or drought period for the lambs. The gradual decrease of flow of milk is followed by resting or recoupement period for the ewe before next mating. This can be adjusted with a food scarcity period for the ewes.

Classing, culling and selection: Invariably these are yearly but essential operations. The stock is to be classed on the basis of body coat, condition and performance. The records of performance should be available by then about lamb crop. Operation is done at the time of shearing or before it. The low grade animals are culled out on the basis of fleece condition or breeding performance. The culling level depends on replacement levels and carrying capacity of the farm. The disposal of surplus stock is timed with higher trend of the market and should be done before the drought season sets in. This helps in better utilization of feed and pasture resources for other selected and breedable stock.

Feeding and pasture management: While timing various routines the provision of natural feeding, abundance of forage, extra feed and build up of some fodder reserve is necessary. Maintaining a uniform level of physical fitness and growth pattern is of prime importance. Proper harvesting may include maximum collection of fodder as well as generating availability and utilization of dropped crop residues, grains, leaves and the stubbles. Ensilaging or pelleting of surplus fodder helps in easing the problems of scarcity period.

OTHER MANAGEMENT ROUTINES

The operations connected to management may be:
1. Incidental—can be conducted at any time of the year.
2. Fixed—which are time bound and have to be completed at fixed time.

Measurement records

Body weight and body measurement as per stipulated schedule have to be conducted. Birth weight, weekly weight, weaning or subsequent weights have a definite dating, whether under a research programme or otherwise. Being essential, these find priority adjustment in the calender of operations.

Permanent marking and tattooing: This can be carried as a routine task and has not much to do with season, but can not be postponed much longer.

Crutching and shearing: The first operation is adjunct to mating and lambing. The rams and ewes are subjected to crutching while preparing for the mating season. Likewise crutching and udder wool clipping is resorted to in ewes prior to lambing.

Shearing of sheep in India is seasonally irregular operation. It is conducted twice or thrice. The shearing periods vary from zone to zone and also in the migratory, semi-migratory or stationary systems. Best time for shearing is a change in season from winter to spring, prior onset of summers and a change from summer to autumn. At certain flocks, pre-mating shearing is taken up or adjusted as per migration needs. A good grazing and favourable weather is essential to make up for the usual drop of 1–2°C in body heat immediately after shearing. For this important operation the shepherd should be free from other operations. Labour or machinery required if any should also be available. At times the sheepman is forced to make slight alterations in time and duration of shearing operations on reasons of inclement weather, burr catching, etc.

Dehorning, hoof pairing, wigging and other minor operations are routine matters as and when the shepherd or incharge sheepman inspects or observes the flock for any abnormality.

Disease prevention: Hygiene maintenance is getting importance now, especially under housing conditions and is dealt as a routine affair. The cleaning of sheep pens and sheds in the subtropics and even in temperate areas is a routine and essential requirement. To ward off flies and insects the regular and proper disposal of sheep excreta can not be defaulted too.

Dosing, dipping and vaccination operations for the control of internal worms, ectoparasites and diseases due to microorganisms respectively, have to be carried out regularly irrespective of seasonal barrier. These are as such completed as a routine task.

Marketing: Better period for marketing of surplus stock is:
1. When the lambs reach the economic age
2. When the demand for mutton is at its highest.

3. The marketing time should preferably precede the drought period and generally follow a period of abundant forage, prime growth and body weight gains. The migratory tribes in the north temperate region resort to enmasse sales of surplus adult rams and wethers in autumn on their down move from highland pastures. The stock is in excellent condition then. It further limits their number for the scarce feed period of winters.

SEASONALITY OF OPERATIONS

Diverse agro-climatic environment exists in this vast country. The north temperate region has a severe and prolonged winter and less marked summer. This is particularly so in respect of mountainous terrains of Jammu and Kashmir, Himachal Pradesh and Uttaranchal. Sikkim and Arunachal Pradesh are of course no exception. The north western region and northern parts of central India have fairly uniform conditions and contain almost 55 percent sheep population of the country. The peninsular zone, especially Maharashtra, Karnataka, Andhra Pradesh and Tamil Nadu possess sizeable sheep population. Hot and humid climatic conditions prevail for major part of the year. In view of varied seasonality in various parts of the country, the year may be split up roughly into the following seasons.

Spring	March and April
Hot summer	May and June
Hot and humid	July, August and September
Autumn	October and November
Winter	December, January and February

Taking into account the different seasons, peculiar climatic conditions, forage supply and labour availability, the various flock/farm operations are required to be adjusted suitably. For instance the mating of breeding ewes in the temperate region is advantageous from September to November where as February to April is suitable in the northwestern region. This period may be suitable for the fat lamb production provided some supplementary feeds are available to the ewes. As a result the lambs will be ready for market at 9 to 10 month age. The autumn mating in temperate region enables the new born lambs to thrive well in spring when ewes receive ample foliage and grazing flush for an adequate milk flow.

On the other hand autumn mating leading to the spring lambing in the western arid zone faces hot sun and deficient grazing in early season, leading to an adverse effect on the lamb crop. In the autumn months the grasses are still plenty, though dry and less nutritious. The residues and stubbles of kharif crop prove a boon for the lambing, ewe flushing and for conducting shearing operations. The lambs of early spring mating have by late autumn approached weaning, so any drop in the milk shall not affect the lambs at that stage.

Under prevailing marketing practices in India, the economic age for sale of sheep for mature mutton is 14 to 18 months. The lambs born in previous year, age almost 18 months by next autumn in temperate zone and 15 months in the western zone by the onset of winter, when the demand for meat is at peak and the stock is in high condition.

The shepherds have the time tested experience of taking up shearing operations in spring and autumn and additionally* in mid summer in alpines. The rainy season gets avoided. Burry wool problem is minimised. The overlapping of shearing operations with migrations do not occur. For any reduction in number of shearings the adjustment of the calendar of operations should be convincing to the sheepman.

CALENDAR OF OPERATIONS

This is an exercise of identification and laying down of various sheep management routines and

---

* The additional third shearing reduces fibre length, lowers utility and value.

their seasonal adjustment. The practice of framing a calendar facilitates timely implementation of operations and obviates management problems. A sound calendar takes into account the economy in rearing, optimum efficiency in production and behavioural aspects of flock. It varies from institution to institution and area of area. At certain farms a calendar is presented in the form of a diagrammatic model as shown in Fig.16.1.

RECORD KEEPING

Importance

Maintenance of sheep flock record is quite useful and dividend paying at the time of selection, breeding, replacement, marketing and culling. A purposeful system of records for the commercial or nucleus stock animals involves the use of pedigree sheet, extended pedigree, breeding and

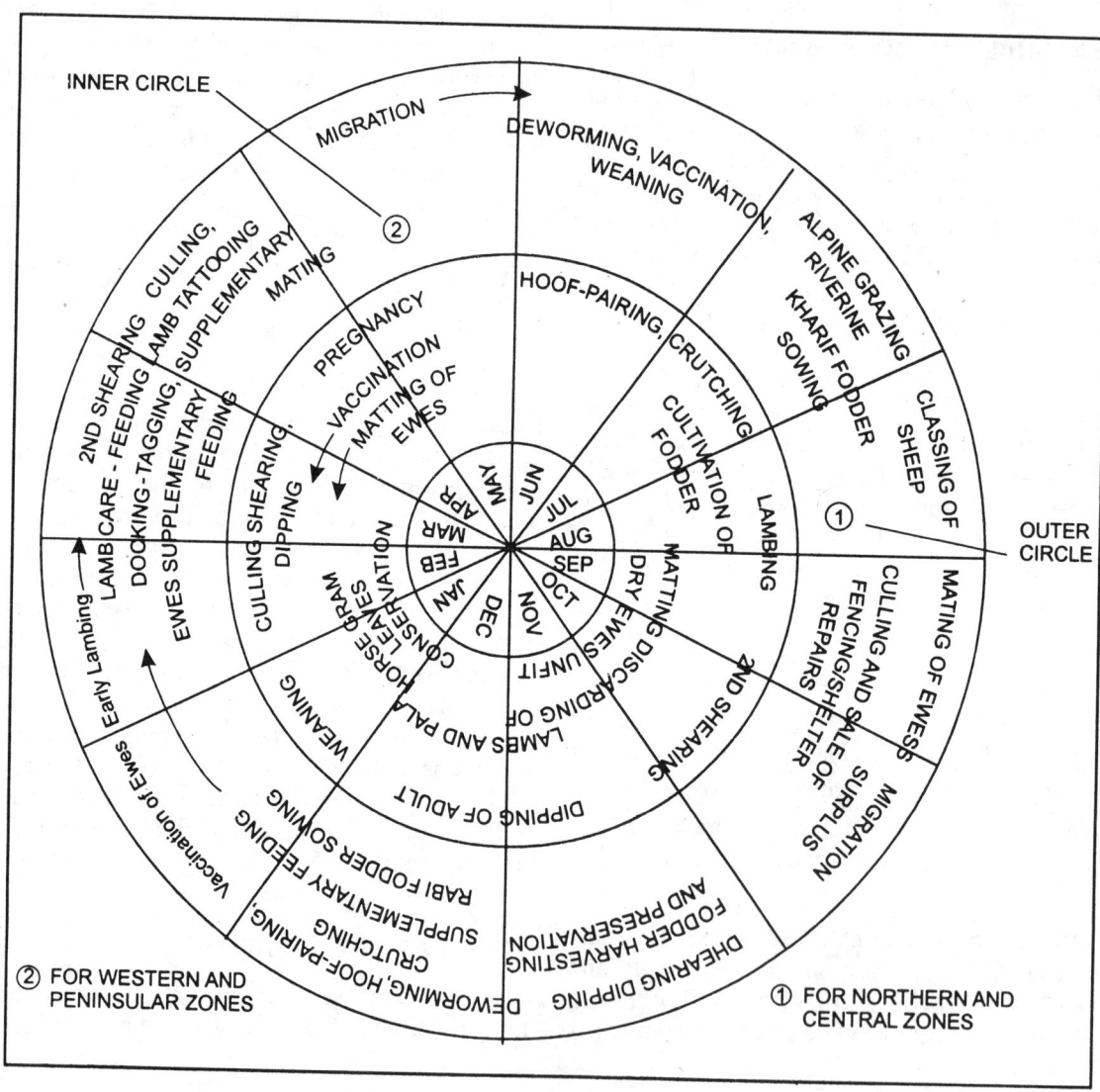

Fig. 16.1. A diagrammatic model of calendar of operations for a sheep farm

production records, etc. Performance of sheep in the farm may be evaluated for a varying period of 1 to 3 years depending on the parameters under consideration. Growth and production records become available at an earlier age than the reproductive performance. These results may then be compared with the standard or usual norms of the breed and with the similar type of animals in other farms or locations. Four types of records are generally constructed.

Growth records comprise of body weight at birth, weekly and then monthly up to weaning, followed by quarterly up to one year. Subsequently 18 and 24 month weight or at shearing and selection time, provide the much needed information. Body measurements particularly length, girth and height at birth, weaning, yearling and maturity stage are relevant. The first record data base starts right at birth.

Production performance: Besides growth data, it is the shearing record and wool analysis results that form the main ingredients of performance as well as pedigree record of woolly sheep. In mutton breeds as in goats, the information about dressing %, meat characteristics finds entry in the record especially in respect of ancestors and collaterals. This lends a fair idea of breed, strain, line or animals within the same pedigree. This data originates automatically from record I when the surviving sheep attain 1 to 1½ year age.

Reproduction performance: Data comprises of age at first mating, age at conception, age at first lambing, lambing interval, abortions, dry periods, repeat breeding, dystocia problems, prolapse or mastitis, etc. in females. Particulars about covering/insemination, parity and lambing are added. The male health may find a mention in data of rams, about libido, ejaculations, semen quality and coverings, etc.

Pedigree sheet: This carries the particulars of animal number, its breed, sire-dam numbers and their breed, date of birth, order of lambing, performance of parents, production and quality (wool) data of the respective animal. Such a record ceases only at death or disposal of the animal.

General: The observations of sheep shows, competitions or prize winning are added to the breeding and pedigree records. Good or bad points/ characteristics of the ancestors are noted. The pedigree may be extended to three generation for the breeding ram or ewe.

Evaluation: The records are subjected to regular updating and periodical analysis and appraisal of performance. This enables evaluation of breeding programme. If required necessary corrective measures can be adopted without further delay for improvement of growth, productive or reproductive performance.

A mention about condition of grazing, type of grazing and hours of grazing needs to be made/ recorded.

Note:

- Besides these records, it is usual to maintain record of daily farm operations, viz. daily diary and weather conditions, lambing register; livestock account of sheep farm/field organisation (weekly/monthly); veterinary aid register, disease prevention (dosing, dipping, vaccination) register, etc. Appropriate formats are devised as per needed information and the requirements of the programme.

- Mating record (iv) and year wise register of service record of rams (viii) combined together serve the purpose of lambing record.

Formats for Maintenance of Records

A. Proforma of pedigree sheet

For Rams
(Card size 30 cm × 20 cm)
(Sheep Breeding Farm)

1. Tattoo/Brand No: of ram Lamb.............

2. Sire.................... Sire.......................

Dam.....................

3. Dam.................... Sire.......................

Dam.....................

4. Breed....................................

5. Date of Birth/Purchase........................

6. Birth wt./wt. at purchase.......................

7. Date of Disposal...................................

Wool Analysis:

Date of shearing	Order of clip	Gr. fl. wt. body skt. total fleece wt.	Remarks

On opposite side of card:

Grade of wool	Date of sampling	Cl. yield%	Fib. diameter (mic)	Fibre/Staple length (mm)
....	....	....	....	....

Density per sq. cm.	Medullated fib. %	% Different fibres			
		hetro	kemp	hair	pure

Crimps per cm.   Remarks

For Ewes
(Card size 28 cm × 20 cm) Information from 1 to 6 as above

Date of service	Ram used	Date of lambing	Sex of lamb born
....	....	....	....

Tag/Tattoo no.	Birth wt.	Weaning wt.	Disposal of lamb
....	....	....	....

Wool analysis	As for ram wool analysis
....	....

On opposite side of card:

Grade of wool	Date of sampling	Clean yield %	Cl. fl. wt. (gm)
....	....	....	....
....	....	....	....

Fib. dia (micron)	Fib. density/Sq. cm.	Medullated fib.%	Staple length cm.
....	....	....	....

Crimps/cm.   *% of different types of fib.*   *Remarks*

hetro   kemp.   hair   pure

B. Sheep biodata and performance records:

(i) *Register for sheep below one year age: (Young stock register)*

S.no.	Tag or tattoo no.	Dam no.	Sire no.	Date of birth
1	2	3	4	5

If purchased

Colour and description	Date of purchase	Approx. age	From whom purchased	Value
6	7	8	9	10

Date of disposal or transfer to adult stock	Mode of disposal	Reason of disposal
11	12	13

If sold

Wt. at sale time	To whom sold	Authority or sanction for sale	Price realised	Remarks
14	15	16	17	18

(ii) *Adult stock register:*

S.no	Tag or Tattoo no.	Dam	Sire	Date of birth	Colour and description (L G Ht)		
1	2	3	4	5	6		

If purchased

From whom purchased	Date of purchase	Approx. age	Value	Date of disposal	Mode of disposal
7	8	9	10	11	12

If sold

Reason of disposal	Wt. at sale	To whom sold	Authority for sale	Price realised	Remarks
13	14	15	16	17	18

(iii) *Weighment register for the young stock:*

Breed.............................. Sex...............................

S. no.	Tag or tattoo no.		Dam	Sire	Date of birth	Birth weight
1	2		3	4	5	6

Weekly wts. up to two months 8 columns	Fortnightly wts. up to weaning 4 col.	Monthly/Quarterly wts. up to 18 months	Remarks
7	8	9	10

Approx. age at weighing be given under each col.

(iv) *Mating register:*

Season of mating: From... to...

Ram no:.. Age:............................... Breed...

S.no.	Tattoo no. of ewe	Breed of ewe	Date of service 1st 2nd	previous service if any	Date of lambing
1	2	3	4	5	6

Nature of lambing single Twin	Abortion	Still birth	Remarks
7.	8.	9.	10.

(v) *Weighment register for adults:*

Ram/ewe...................................

S.no.	Tattoo no.	Monthly weights (kg) (Normally Quarterly or Half Yearly only)						Remarks
		April	May	June	July	August	September	
1	2	3	4	5	6	7	8	9

(vi) *Shearing register:*

Ram/Ewe/Ram lamb/Ewe lamb.....................................

Shearing for.....................Breed...........................

S.no.	Tattoo no.	Date of birth	Date of shearing	Order of clip 1st, 2nd, 3rd	Body wt. at shearing
1	2	3	4	5	6

Greasy fleece wt.					Remarks
Body wool	Britch	Belly	Skirting	Total	
7	8	9	10	11	

Note: In poor yielders col. 8 and 9 may be combined and merged in 10.

(vii) *Sheep mortality register:*

S.no.	Tattoo no. (of deceased) sheep	Breed	Sex	Date of birth	Date of death	Approx. age at death
1	2	3	4	5	6	7

Cause of death	P.M. finding	Book value prior death	P.M. conducted by	Remarks
8	9	10	11	12

(viii) *Year wise register of service record for rams:*

S.no.	Tattoo no of ram	Breed	Age	Dam	Sire	No. of ewes allotted	No. of ewes mated
1	2	3	4	5	6	7	8

No. of ewes repeated	No. of ewes conceived	No. of ewes died before lambing	No. of pregnant ewes sold	No. of ewes aborted
9	10	11	12	13

No. of still birth	No. of ewes lambed normally	No. of twins	No of lambs born
14	15	16	17

Average birth wt. (of lambs) (kg.)		Av. weaning wt. (kg.)		Colour pattern		
18		19		20		
M	F	M	F	White,	Black or black spotted	Brown or brown spotted

No. of lambs died upto weaning (month wise)		Remarks
21		22
M	F	

(ix) *Record of supply of breeding rams from farms/field organisations.*

S.no.	Date of supply	Tattoo no. of ram	Breed	Age	Wt. at the time of supply	Price
1	2	3	4	5	6	7

Person to whom supplied with address	Remarks
8	9

(x) Feed register for the month .... year ....

Type of feed/fodder ....

Date	Quantity in hand (kg)	Quantity received (kg)	Strength of sheep			
			Rams	Wethers	Ewes	Lambs
1	2	3	4	5	6	7

Feeding scale per day per animal (g)				Quantity issued (kg.)				
Ram	Wether	Ewe	Lamb	Rams	Wethers	Ewes	Lambs	Total
8	9	10	11	12	13	14	15	16

Balance (kg)	Remarks
17	18

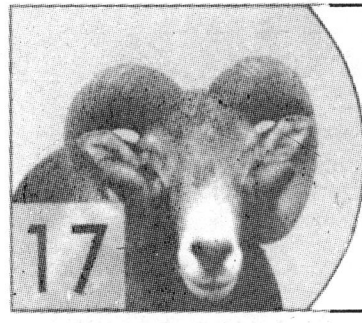

ADDITIONAL INFORMATION

DIFFERENCE BETWEEN SHEEP AND GOAT

Genetic/Anatomical Features	Sheep	Goat
Chromomosomes	2N = 27 (54)	2N = 30 (60)
Vestigial organs	Beard and Tassels are rare. Mostly absent	Tuft of beard hair at the chin region common in males. Tassels (wattles, lorkas) are generally present. It is a vestigial cartilage covered with skin
Presence of glands	Suborbital glands invariably present. The ducts open beneath the inner canthus of the eye. Their secretion is of fatty and sebaceous nature.	Such glands are usually absent in goats
	Inter-digital glands present. The duct opens at the front of foot. Glands are also present in the inguinal region.	Small glands may be present on the fore-foot.
Tail	Short to long one, but always tucked close to the perineum	Short tails, invariably carried high, turned towards back. comparatively tail is thinner.
Horns	Generally angular with transverse wrinkles (corrugations) Grow slightly backwards then foward and spirally outward.	Generally rounded except in Bakerwali where even wrinkles/serrations may be present. Mostly grow slightly back-wards.
Bodycoat	Grows wool, with a breed to breed difference in quality from fine, medium, coarse to hairy nature.	The goat body coat is mostly hairy and bristly, but for some breeds like Mohair (Angora) Pashmina or Chegu goat

(Contd.)

Genetic/Anatomical Features	Sheep	Goat
Conformation	Rounded neck well fleshed withers, Barrel shaped thoracic cavity, udder not well descended. Scrotum is one sac.	Thinner and angular neck. Flattened thoracic region udder more pendulous deviated forward, longer teats. Testicles in bi-fid scrotal sac.
Bones	Radius is just 1.25 times the length of metacarpal bone. Scapula is short and broad. The middle of superior spine is bent back and thickened	Radius is twice the length of metacerpal bone. Scapula has a distinct neck. Superior spine is thick and narrow.
Meat	Called Mutton, Flesh is light to dark in colour. There exist fat deposits in-between various muscles. Sometimes wool fibres sticking.	Called Chevon, has peculiar 'goaty odour'. Meat paler, lesser intermascular fat. Fat is chiefly in the kidney capsule. Sub-cutaneous fat is lean. Practically no fat in between the muscles.Quite often goat hair may be sticking.
Nature	Shy, timid, nervous showing flocking habit, follows a leader. Short on legs	More active, clever, stout, leggy, with leading nature.

SHEEP AND WOOL TERMINOLOGY

Apparel wools	Wool that is used for manufacture of cloth. To the gentry it connotes fine wool for fine cloth or fabric
Bale	A pack of wool in a wool pack in proper order for transportation or shipment The weight of pack varies depending upon the model of baling press used. The one received under UNDP at wool Grading Centres packs 100 kg of wool.
Britch or Breech	Wool from the lower parts of the hind quarters. This is usually coarser than the whole wool fleece.
Branding of sheep	A permanent marking caused by placing/imprinting an identification number on the body of sheep with fast branding fluid or ink. The sites selected for branding are, chest (bare area), inner side of ear, or horn. In the latter case fire branding is the mode. The elaborate system at some farms, is coding for the serial number, year of birth, breed, and farm where produced.
Break-in-wool	A distinct weakness or thinning in a part of wool staple or fibres of a region resulting into break of staple on light stretching or during processing. The cause is a temporary interference in the follicles and growth of wool due to a sudden change of pasture, shortage of food or water, sickness, rise of body temperature, faulty dipping or lambing problems.
Brightness	White colour wool with light reflecting power, usually seen in finer type of wool, viz. Australian merino, Kashmir merino, etc.
Badger lamb	A badger faced lamb is the one having light grey coat with a black belly, black chin, black around eyes, ear tips and tail. Face and limbs may be tan. A reverse badger faced lamb has the light areas below and dark/black above.

(Contd.)

Baldy sheep	A sheep of extensive black wool with patches of white restricted to head, tail and legs.
Boardy fleece	A compact fleece coat not permitting penetration of dust, vegetable matter, etc. as in merino and other dense wool breeds.
Broken mouth	A sheep having some of the incisor teeth fallen/missing or badly worne out as a result of old age or tough nature of grazing. Loose and irregular condition of teeth is also included. Such ewes are generally bred to get one or two more lambings.
Burry wool	Vegetation seeds with spikes, hooks, bristles, etc. particularly that of *Xanthium strumarium* (Nagoora burr), Burr clover and other burr plant species get stuck to the fleece of sheep in the pasture. Such wool containing burry seeds and vegetable matter is called burry wool.
Burr	Hooked, bristly or thorny vegetable matter sticking to fleece. It is a term applied to the by product of wool processing carrying burr material. This waste product is finding some use in the industry and fetches 25 to 30% of the cost of wool, if the burr content is low.
Canary wool	It is yellowing of wool, due to appearance of a stain in the hot, humid region sheep. This is not washable under ordinary scouring processes.
Carbonising	Is the process of removal of burr and other vegetable matter from the burry wool by treating the same with sulphuric acid.
	The chemical chars the vegetable matter which is subsequently removed through mechanical crushing and blowing.
Carding	It is the term applied by industry to wool suitable for the woollen system of yarn production. The carding wool is usually shorter in length than the raw wool used for yarn in worsted system.
	The process of carding is the breaking and opening of lumps/clumps of staples or tangled fibres by teasing with machines, carding brushes or hands to make the wool into an even film, called carded laps (Tumba by weavers). In the woollen factories the wool is passed between rollers covered with close-set fine teeth like spines for teasing and opening of clumps.
Carpet wool	The coarser variety of wool ranging between 28 to 34 micron diameter, which is preferentially and predominantly used for carpet manufacturing and rugs. The wools of Desi sheep of northern temperature and north western arid regions fall in this category. Such wool possessing additional characteristics of desired medullation and lustre are considered ideal carpet wools.
Cast for age (sheep)	Old sheep invariably over 7 to 8 year age that have passed prime lamb production or wool production and are culled on a definite set of reasons. Sheep may be rejected even at a bit earlier age due to defective, worn out or shedding teeth conditions and declared CFA.
Character	The term when applied to sheep implies animals possessing strongly marked distinctive qualities of sheep breed and type. Character with regard to wool means the characteristic trait of good inbred or well bred wool generally showing even, pronounced crimp and staple formation.
Classing	Sheep classing: is an exercise to grade flock into various groups on the basis of definite standards. In other words, it is the process of visual selection and culling applied to the animals of a flock.
	Wool classing: It is the dividing and grouping of fleeces into various lots of a like quality while preparing the wool clip for market.
Clip	Is the wool obtained on shearing by weight or type of wool from a flock of sheep. The term is also applied for total yearly production.

(Contd.)

Clipping	Is the act of shearing of wool from the body of a sheep or rabbit with hand shears or scissors.
Chalky face	The presence of harsh, coarser, white chalky hair cover over the face, also known as Frosty face. Chalky face is characteristic of Polled-Dorset sheep.
Combable or combing wool	Wool suitable for combing process. Standard length for combing is 7.5 cm, but wools with minimum length of 4 cm and above can also be used as combable wool in some of the combing plants. Fibres shorter than this length are not fit for combing and find use in woollen system, hosiery and blending.
Combing	Is the process by which the longer fibres are set parallel through an intermediate process of tops preparation in the manufacture of worsted yarn. The shorter fibres than the stipulated combing length fall through (as noils-I) alongwith tangled naps, larger vegetable matter, etc. The longer ones also get trimmed to required length and short or cut pieces also get retained (as noils II).
Come back	Merino half breds with long wool breeds or derived through further infusion of Merino blood into long wool and tending towards the Merino are known as come-backs. Corriedale, Panama, Columbia, etc.
Come-back wool	Is the wool obtained from such a cross bred sheep. It is usually of 58's quality or above.
Condition	The term condition is frequently applied by:

1. Butcher for carcass-where it implies the degree of fatness and flesh of a sheep.

2. Sheepman for wool. In terms of wool classer, it is qualitative and quantitative expression of extent of wool grease (yolk) and other associated impurities in the fleece coat or raw wool.

3. To the industry or woollman as scoured wool, it is indicative of the moisture present in the wool expressed as yield percent on dry weight basis. Being hygroscopic, the wool may add up as much as 30% of moisture by weight.

Cotted wool	Fleece wool that has partially matted or felted on the back of sheep itself.
Count ('s)	It is the term used to express the fineness or coarseness of wool with reference to spinning quality. For various sheep breeds the count is.

Merino-64's and above.

Rambouillet-60's and above.

Kashmir Merino-60's and above.

Exotic come-backs (C.B.) of Merino 58's and above.

Cross breds of Merino and Rambouillet in India-56's and above.

½ breds-48's and above.

Medium quality wool breeds of North temperate and western arid region-44's.

Deccani-40's, etc.

Higher the count, lower the diameter of wool.

Count is however defined in F.P.S. differently for the worsted and woollen yarn.

Worsted yarn: It is the number of standard hanks of 560 yards each that are spun out of one pound (lb=454g) of wool.

Woollen yarn: The number of standard skeins of 256 yards long each out of a pound (454g) of wool.

(Contd.)

Crimp	It is the natural waviness of the wool fibre. Closer or more are the waves, finer the wool. The number of crimps are expressed per centimeter and measured with the help of a crimpometer.
Crutching	The act of shearing away of wool from hind legs and britch area of sheep.
Culling	Rejecting or discarding of inferior, substandard and lower grade sheep, i.e. culls, from a flock of sheep.
Dead wool	Wool taken out from the pelts of dead sheep after some time.
Devil's dip/grip	A congenital depression appearing just behind withers. It is a serious conformation defect exposing the dip area wool to fleece rot in heavy rainfall zones. Otherwise too the wool produced around the site is of poor quality being short, stained and greasy.
Doggy wool	Wool produced by old sheep is short, lumpy and devoid of usual crimp, lustre and strength.
Elasticity	Power of wool fibres to withstand tension, stretching or compression.
Felting	Interlocking of wool fibres to form an entangled compact mass or mat, under pressure, heat and moisture. In namdah preparation this process finds utility. The knit wool wear felt when beaten or squeezed while washing.
Fell mongering	Is the process of removing wool from the pelts through chemical treatment or bacterial action.
Fleece	The wool coat of the sheep.
Full mouth	The sheep around four to four and a half year age when all the incisor teeth have erupted.
Gummy mouth	An aged sheep that has lost its incisor teeth. Gummer condition due to senile changes starts appearing around 6 to 7 years, but may be delayed in certain sheep to 8 or 9 year age.
Hocky	Sheep with inward inclining hocks which rub each other when the sheep is moving. Cowhocks is another term used to define such hocks.
Hogget	A young male or female sheep from 8 month age onwards to the yearling stage.
Joining	Putting the rams with ewes for mating.
Kemp	In certain breeds of sheep, associated with wool fibres are found coarser, much shorter, brittle, opaque, medullated fibres called kemp. They grow for a limited period and are shed automatically, to be observed lying loose in the fleece in the poll and neck region frequently. Kemp fibres are found in many Indian breeds of sheep. Do not take-up dyes.
Lamb	1. Young one of a sheep from birth to suckling stage of 18 to 20 weeks. 2. In mutton terminology, it is the young sheep of five to six month's age slaughtered for meat. In practice under Indian conditions, lamb covers sheep upto hogget stage.
Lamb marking	Is an act of putting an identification mark (like tagging, ear marking, tattooing, etc. Number of lambs alive at weaning is also expressed as lamb marking (%)
Lanolin	Is the refined yolk derived from wool grease, finds use in various superior cosmetics and is an adjuvant for medicinal preparations.
Leggy sheep	Sheep having comparatively longer legs than the usual standard for the breed. Or a breed of sheep that possess longer legs vis-a-vis the body barrel. It is almost the opposite of a blocky sheep, a term used for mutton sheep which besides a muttonous conformation have normally shorter legs.
Lustre	The glossy shining appearance of a wool peculiar to English long wool breeds, the Lincoln, Romneys, etc. Bikaneri wools also possess lustre, but is lesser in other Indian sheep.

(Contd.)

	Lustre wool is preferred for carpet manufacturing in order to provide better sheen and brilliance.
Maiden ewe	A grown up female hogget or two tooth age ewe lamb that has not been served or that has yet to bear its first lamb. Age of maiden stage varies from breed to breed or even in the animals of the same breed. Quite often desi ewes conceive at 10 months age and drop a lamb before attaining two tooth age. The cross bred ewes have however been found to bear a lamb at two year age or above only.
Medullation	Existance of medulla, a medullary canal or core of air filled sac inside the fibre. Medullated fibres when examined under the microscope or micro projector, ermascope, etc. appear hollow, spongy. These fibres are coarse, hairy and harsh to handle. Such fibres do not take up dyes uniformly.
Mohair	Hair (fibre) growing on the body of the Angora goat.
Naps	Small knots of tangled fibres removed in the combing process.
Noils	Fibres dropped/removed from the wool during combing which may either be shorter than the required length or are cut-pieces from the longer fibres, trimmed for uniformity. It carries vegetable matter to some extent.
Pedigree card	A statement or table depicting ancestral lineage of a living being, animal or man.
Pie wool (slipe wool)	Wool removed from the carcass of dead sheep other than slaughtered as soon as the fibres become loose in the skin. Plucked/pulled wool is better type of dead wool, as it is recovered from pelts of slaughtered sheep.
Prepotency	The genetic power of an individual sire to impress its own traits of likeness upon a larger proportion of its progeny.
Regain	Percentage of moisture in wool or any other such material, expressed in terms of clean dry weight.
Rig	Is a condition in male when one testicle does not descend in the scrotal sac and remains lodged/retained in the abdominal cavity.
	Rig is also termed cryptorchid. Double rig condition is associated with polledness in Rambouillet rams. This defect is also observed in Mandya sheep.
	Such rams are rejected for breeding as there may be defective/impaired spermatogenesis due to higher abdominal temperature and improper growth of testicles.
Scouring or scoured wool	Washing of wool in a series of bowls containing soap alkali and water at certain temperatures is known as scouring. In the process most of the grease is removed. The wool is then oven dried and weighted to get clean (sample) fleece weight. Scouring loss or clean fleece weight is then expressed in percent.
Scur	Rudimentary horn. Also called horn buttons at times.
Sheep cote/ sheep pen	An enclosure for sheep
Sheep fold	A place where sheep are collected, a sheep pen
Sheep run	A tract or area for feeding sheep
Sheep walk	A pasture for sheep
Shoddy wool	The wool recovered from old woollen clothes, garments, woven rags, etc. after tearing and teasing. Shoddy trade has come up in a big way because of re-use of shoddy wool for felting, blanket making, etc.

(Contd.)

	A part of by-products produced in the combing process earlier to noils is also named shoddy wool.
Skirting	The inferior portion of fleece particularly from britch, legs, belly, tail or head region as removed during shearing or separated out at the wool sorting table.
Stag	A male sheep castrated after attaining maturity.
Steely wool	Wool lacking character and possessing a characteristic steely sheen. Pastures deficient in trace elements like Co, Cu give rise to steely wool. An identical type of defective wool is known as mercury wool, giving appearance of glassy beads and curls. The fibre in both cases is weak and poor in quality.
Stocking rate	It is the number of sheep that a hectare of pasture can carry, on rotational basis without detriment to the pasture. Poor pastures accommodate just one or two sheep where as well managed ones may have a carrying capacity of 5 to 6 sheep per hectare or even more.
Strong wool	Wool having greater fibre thickness or diameter than is usual for a particular breed or type of sheep/wool. Kashmir Merino with 20-21 micron fibre diameter is finer where as the one with 23-24 range is a strong wool. Same is true of Rambouillet and Rambouillet cross breds. Even within Chokla breed there exist finer and strong wool sheep.
Suint	It is the water soluble portion of the yolk.
Teaser	It is an approned or a vasectomised ram used for detecting ewes in heat. A teaser can also be prepared by deviation of penis method.
Tippy wool	Where the wool fibres of a staple are not of uniform length. The staple thus appears tapering to a tip. Usually observed in the fleece coat of old sheep. The lamb wool also gives an appearance of tippy wool until shorn.
Tops	A uniform and continuous strand of untwisted fibres made parallel by combing which removes noils, the shorter fibres and even trims the longer ones to the standard length of the combable lot.
Top knot	Tuft of wool on the poll or fore head of the sheep. Top knot is characteristic of merino sheep.
True to type	An animal possessing marked resemblance of all the peculiar characteristic features to that particular type or breed.
Warp	Twisted thread or yarn used along length wise (Taana) on a loom to fabricate cloth.
Waft	Thread/yarn used in passing under the warp (width wise-Buna) when weaving cloth.
Wether	A male sheep castrated in lamb hood.
Withers	The heighest point of back of a sheep, between and above shoulders.
Wool blindness	Excessive wool growth and cover around the eyes of sheep impeding vision of the animal. Fine wool merino and some other breeds are known to develop much wool which interfere with the sight and therefore not preferred much on reasons of grazing and mating problems.
Woollen system	It is the method of yarn production from carded wool fibres but not out of combed ones. The fibres do not lie parallel to each other.
Worsted system	Is the system of yarn production from wool fibres which have been combed to prepare tops in the first instance, thus rendering them parallel in the yarn.
Yolk	Is the combined secretion of the sebaceous and sudoriferous glands of the skin containing lanolin, suint, etc. It is removed from the wool by the process of scouring.

FEEDING STANDARDS RECOMMENDED BY NRC (1985) FOR SHEEP

Table 17.1: Daily nutrient requirements of sheep (NRC 1985)

Body weight	Weight change/ day	Dry matter per animal	Nutrients per animal								
				Energy			Crude protein	Ca	P	Vitamin A activity	Vitamin E activity
			(% body weight)	TDN (kg)	DE (Mcal)	ME (Mcal)					
(kg)	(g)	(kg)					(g)	(g)	(g)	(IU)	(IU)
Ewes Maintenance											
50	10	1.0	2.0	0.55	2.4	2.0	95	2.0	2.8	2,350	15
60	10	1.1	1.8	0.61	2.7	2.2	204	2.3	2.1	2,820	16
70	10	1.2	1.7	0.66	2.9	2.4	113	2.5	2.4	3,290	18
80	10	1.3	1.6	0.72	3.2	2.6	122	2.7	2.8	3,750	20
90	10	1.4	1.5	0.78	3.4	2.8	131	2.9	3.1	4,230	21
Flushing-2 Weeks prebreeding and first 3 weeks of breeding											
50	100	1.6	3.2	0.94	4.1	3.4	150	5.3	2.6	2,350	24
60	100	1.7	2.8	1.00	4.4	3.6	157	5.5	2.9	2,820	26
70	100	1.8	2.6	1.06	4.7	3.8	164	5.7	3.2	3,290	27
80	100	1.9	2.4	1.12	4.9	4.0	171	5.9	3.6	3,760	28
90	100	2.0	2.2	1.18	5.1	4.2	177	6.1	3.9	4,230	30
Non-lactating-First 15 weeks gestation											
50	30	1.2	2.4	0.67	3.0	2.4	112	2.9	2.1	2,350	18
60	30	1.3	2.2	0.72	3.2	2.6	121	3.2	2.5	2,820	20
70	30	1.4	2.0	0.77	3.4	2.8	130	3.5	2.9	3,290	21
80	30	1.5	1.9	0.82	3.6	3.0	139	3.8	3.3	3,760	22
90	30	1.6	1.8	0.87	3.8	3.2	148	4.1	3.6	4,230	24
Last 4 weeks gestation (130-150% lambing rate expected) or last 4-6 weeks lactation suckling singles[d]											
50	180(45)	1.6	3.2	0.94	4.1	3.4	175	5.9	4.8	4,250	24
60	180(45)	1.7	2.8	1.00	4.4	3.6	184	6.0	5.2	5,100	26
70	180(45)	1.8	2.6	1.06	4.7	3.8	193	6.2	5.6	5,950	27
80	180(45)	1.9	2.4	1.12	4.9	4.0	202	6.3	6.1	6,800	28
90	180(45)	2.0	2.2	1.18	5.1	4.2	212	6.4	6.5	7,650	30
First 6-8 weeks lactation suckling singles or last 4-6 weeks lactation suckling twins[d]											
50	25(90)	2.1	4.2	1.36	6.0	4.9	304	8.9	6.1	4,250	32
60	25(90)	2.3	3.8	1.50	6.6	5.4	319	9.1	6.6	5,100	34
70	25(90)	2.5	3.6	1.63	7.2	5.9	334	9.3	7.0	5,950	38
80	25(90)	2.6	3.2	1.69	7.4	6.1	344	9.5	7.4	6,800	39
90	25(90)	2.7	3.0	1.75	7.6	6.3	353	9.6	7.8	7,650	40
First 6-8 weeks lactation suckling twins											
50	60	2.4	4.8	1.56	6.9	5.6	389	10.5	7.3	5,000	36
60	60	2.6	4.3	1.69	7.4	6.1	405	10.7	7.7	6,000	39

(Contd.)

Body weight	Weight change/ day	Dry matter per animal	Nutrients per animal								
				Energy			Crude			Vitamin A	Vitamin E
			(% body	TDN	DE	ME	protein	Ca	P	activity	activity
(kg)	(g)	(kg)	weight)	(kg)	(Mcal)	(Mcal)	(g)	(g)	(g)	(IU)	(IU)
70	60	2.8	4.0	1.82	8.0	6.6	420	11.0	8.1	7,000	42
80	60	3.0	3.8	1.95	8.6	7.0	435	11.2	8.6	8,000	45
90	60	3.2	3.6	2.08	9.2	7.5	450	11.4	9.0	9,000	48

Ewe lambs
Non-lactating-First 1.5 weeks gestation

Body weight	Weight change/ day	Dry matter per animal	(% body weight)	TDN (kg)	DE (Mcal)	ME (Mcal)	Crude protein (g)	Ca (g)	P (g)	Vitamin A activity (IU)	Vitamin E activity (IU)
40	160	1.4	3.5	0.83	3.6	3.0	156	5.5	3.0	1,880	21
50	135	1.5	3.0	0.88	3.9	3.2	159	5.2	3.1	2,350	22
60	135	1.6	2.7	0.94	4.1	3.4	161	5.5	3.4	2,820	24
70	125	1.7	2.4	1.00	4.4	3.6	164	5.5	3.7	3,290	26

Last 4 weeks gestation (100-120% lambing rate expected)

40	180	1.5	3.8	0.94	4.1	3.4	187	6.4	3.1	3,400	22
50	160	1.6	3.2	1.00	4.4	3.6	189	6.3	3.4	4,250	24
60	160	1.7	2.8	1.07	4.7	3.9	192	6.6	3.8	5,100	26
70	150	1.8	2.6	1.14	5.0	4.1	194	6.8	4.2	5,950	27

Last 4 weeks gestation (130-175% lambing rate expected)

40	225	1.5	3.8	0.90	4.4	3.6	202	7.4	3.5	3,400	22
50	225	1.6	3.2	1.00	4.7	3.8	204	7.8	3.9	4,250	24
60	225	1.7	2.8	1.12	4.9	4.0	207	8.1	4.3	5,100	26
70	215	1.8	2.6	1.14	5.0	4.1	210	8.2	4.7	5,950	27

First 6-8 weeks lactation suckling singles (wean by 8 weeks)

40	50	1.7	4.2	1.12	4.9	4.0	257	6.0	4.3	3,400	26
50	50	2.1	4.2	1.39	6.1	5.0	282	6.5	4.7	4,250	32
60	50	2.3	3.8	1.52	6.7	5.5	295	6.8	5.1	5,100	34
70	50	2.5	3.6	1.65	7.3	6.0	301	7.1	5.6	5,450	38

First 6-8 weeks lactation suckling twins (wean by 8 weeks)

40	100	2.1	5.2	1.45	6.4	5.2	306	8.4	5.6	4,000	32
50	100	2.3	4.6	1.59	7.0	5.7	321	8.7	6.0	5,000	34
60	100	2.5	4.2	1.72	7.6	6.2	336	9.0	6.4	6,000	38
70	100	2.7	3.9	1.85	8.1	6.6	351	9.8	6.9	7,000	40

Replacement ewe lambs*

30	227	1.2	4.0	0.78	3.4	2.8	185	6.4	2.6	2,410	18
40	182	1.4	3.5	0.91	4.0	3.3	176	5.9	2.6	1,880	21
50	120	1.5	3.0	0.88	3.9	3.2	136	4.8	2.4	2,350	22
60	100	1.5	2.5	0.88	3.9	3.2	134	4.5	2.5	2,820	22
70	100	1.5	2.1	0.88	3.9	3.2	132	4.6	2.8	3,290	22

(Contd.)

Body weight (kg)	Weight change/day (g)	Dry matter per animal (kg)	(% body weight)	Energy TDN (kg)	DE (Mcal)	ME (Mcal)	Crude protein (g)	Ca (g)	P (g)	Vitamin A activity (IU)	Vitamin E activity (IU)
Replacement ram lambs*											
40	330	1.8	4.5	1.1	5.0	4.1	243	7.8	3.7	1,880	24
60	320	2.4	4.0	1.5	6.7	5.5	263	8.4	4.2	2,820	26
80	290	2.8	3.3	1.8	7.8	6.4	268	8.5	4.6	3,760	28
100	250	3.0	3.0	1.9	8.4	6.9	264	8.2	4.8	4,700	30
Lambs finishing- 4 to 7 months old											
30	295	1.3	4.3	0.94	4.1	3.4	191	6.6	3.2	1,410	20
40	275	1.6	4.0	1.22	5.4	4.4	185	6.6	3.3	1,880	24
50	205	1.6	3.2	1.23	5.4	4.4	160	5.6	3.0	2,350	24
Early weaned lambs-Moderate growth potential'											
10	250	0.5	5.0	0.40	1.8	1.4	127	4.0	1.9	470	10
20	250	1.0	5.1	0.80	3.5	2.9	167	5.4	2.5	940	20
30	300	1.3	4.3	1.00	4.4	3.6	191	6.7	3.2	1,410	20
40	345	1.5	3.8	1.16	5.1	4.2	202	7.7	3.9	1,880	22
50	300	1.5	3.0	1.16	5.1	4.2	181	7.0	3.8	2,350	22
Early weaned lambs-Rapid growth potential'											
10	250	0.6	6.0	0.48	2.1	1.7	157	4.9	2.2	470	12
20	300	1.2	6.0	0.92	4.9	3.3	205	6.5	2.9	940	24
30	325	1.4	4.7	1.10	4.8	4.0	216	7.2	3.4	1,410	21
40	400	1.5	3.8	1.14	5.0	4.1	234	8.6	4.3	1,880	22
50	425	1.7	3.4	1.29	5.7	4.7	240	9.4	4.8	2,350	25
60	350	1.7	2.8	1.29	5.7	4.7	240	8.2	4.5	2,820	25

Indication:

* To convert dry matter to an as-fed basis, divide dry matter values by the percentage of dry matter in the particular feed.

* One kilogram TDN (total digestible nutrients)= 4.4 Mcal DE (digestible energy): ME (metabolizable energy) = 82% of DE.

　Because of rounding errors, values in Table 17.1 may differ.

* Value are applicable for ewes in moderate condition. Fat ewes should be fed according to the next lower weight category and thin ewes at the next higher weight category.

　Once desired or moderate weight condition is attained, use that weight category through all production stages.

d Values in parentheses are for ewes suckling lambs the last 4-6 weeks of lactation.

* Lambs intended for breeding; thus, maximum weight gains and finish are of secondary importance.

f Maximum weight gains expected.

OTHER COMMON FODDER TREES AND THEIR FEED VALUES

Table 17.2: Feed values (composition) of other important fodder trees (Singh, 1985)

Sl. no.	Botanical name	Local name	Cr. protein	Cr. fibre	NFE	Ash	C	P
1.	Acacia nilotica	Kikar, Babul	13.90	9.20	69.90	7.10	1.50	0.19
2.	A. leucophloea	Safed Kikar, Rinj	15.28	18.81	55.80	7.28	1.12	0.21
3.	Ailanthus excelsa	Ardu	19.56	13.52	47.74	15.50	2.42	0.17
4.	Albezia labbek	Sirin, Sirisha	16.81	24.47	35.99	7.11	1.10	0.14
5.	Celtis australis	Khirak	14.47	19.45	42.65	11.66	3.47	0.18
6.	Ficus bengalensis	Barh, Bargad, Alada	11.50	38.60	42.60	11.68	0.25	3.80
7.	F. religiosa	Pipal, Ashvatha	9.02	15.93	39.04	13.96	2.25	0.14
8.	Grevia optiva	Dhaman, Bhimal	16.0	18.88	41.73	9.60	2.70	0.14
	G. elastica	Biul						
	G. oppositifolia	other varieties of Dhaman						
9.	Leucaena leucocephala	Koo-babul	24.20	13.30	46.70	10.80	1.98	0.27
10.	Morunga oleifera	Suhanjana	15.32	17.89	48.71	11.80	3.22	0.27
11.	Prosopis cineraria	Khejri, Jand	13.90	17.52	53.24	3.80	1.90	0.20
12.	Quercus dilatata	Moru, Tilonj	9.56	29.06	51.75	5.11	1.61	0.11
13.	Q. glauca	Fanat, Bani, Banj, Rein	9.62	29.04	49.60	7.60	1.87	0.23
14.	Q. leucotricophora	Banj, Rein, Chhidar	10.20	31.43	46.74	5.13	0.90	0.11
15.	Robinia pseudoacacia	Robinia, Hill Kikar	25.50	17.20	46.50	7.50	1.50	0.32
16.	Tamarindus indica	Imli	13.43	15.93	46.01	7.94	1.65	0.25
17.	Terminalia arjuna	Arjun, Koha	10.10	13.54	56.76	10.97	2.08	0.16

Loppings of following fodder trees are also utilized in various zones either as routine feeding or during scarcity.
1. Butea monosperma (Palas, modunga, flame of forest)
2. Butea utilis (Bhuj patra)
3. Flacourta indica (Kukoa, Klku)
4. Mangifera indica (Aam, mango tree)
5. Melia azedarach (Drank, Bakain)
6. Morus alba (Mulberry-Shahtoot)
7. Putranjiva roxhburgii (Putrangan, Putranjiva, Putajan)
8. Salix acmophylla (Bisu)
9. S. alba (willow, Bisa)
10. S. babylonica
11. S. daphnocides (Veer, Bedi, Shrub type)
12. S. wallichiana (Bhains, Bhainsora)
13. Quercus ilex (Irri, Bre)
14. Q. lanata (Rainj, Reein)
15. Rhododendron arboreum (chiu, fire of the jungle)
16. Ulmus lencifolia (Manuk, Lapi) Found in eastern Himalayas upto 1800 m.
17. U. villosa (Marin, Marn) Northwest Himalayas, upto 2200 m
18. U. wallichiana (Bren, Bran, Punj, Mareen)

A GLOSSARY OF PASTURE VEGETATION AND FORAGE RESOURCES (ACHARYA, 1982)

The Northern Temperate Region

Grasses: Agropyron spp, Agrostis spp., Andropogon spp, Apluda mutica, Aristida spp., Arundinella nepalensis, Arthraxon lancifolius, Bothriochloa pertusa, Calamagrostis emodensis, Chrysopogon spp. Cymbopogon spp., Cyonodon dactylon, Dicanthium spp., Digitaria spp., Eragrostis spp:, Eremopogon foveolatus, Festuca valesiaca, Heteropogon contortus, Ischaemum indicum, Iseilema laxum, Koeleria cristata, Microstegium ciliatum, Oropetium thomaeum, Oryzopsis lateralis, Panicum spp., Paspalum spp., Perotis indica, Phalaris spp., Phleum alpinum, Poa spp., Polypogon fugaz, Saccharum spp., Setaria glauca, Sporobolus spp., Themeda anathera, Tripogan spp., Trisetum spicatum.

Shrubs and trees: Acacia spp. Adhatoda vasica, Adina cordifolia, Albizia spp. Bauhinia spp., Berberis spp., Butea monosperma, Carissa spinarum, Cassia spp., Cotoneaster microphylla, Dodonaea viscosa, Grevia spp., Holoptelea integrifolia, Hypericum mysorensis, Juniperus macropoda, Madhuca indica, Mallotus philippinensis Morus spp., Murraya koenigii, Pinus spp., Pogostemon spp., Prinsepia utilis, Rhododendron spp., Tectona grandis, Terminalia spp., Viburnum foetens, Zizyphus spp.

The Eastern Region

Grasses: Agropyron canaliculatium, Agrostis spp. Andropogon Spp., Apluda mutica, Aristida spp., Arthraxon spp., Srundinella spp., Bothriochloa pertusa, Calamagrostis emodensis, Chrysopogon spp., Cymbopogon spp., Cynodon dactylon, Dactyloctenium aegyptium, Desmostachya bipinnata, Dicanthium spp., Digitaria spp., Dimeria spp., Echinochloa colonum, Eragrostiella spp., Eragrostis spp., Eremopogon faveolatus, Erianthus rufipilus, Festuca spp., Heteropogon contortus, Ischaemum spp., Imperata cylindrica, Iseilema laxum, Koelaria cristata, Leersia

hexandra, Microchloa indica, Microstegium ciliatum, Narenga porphyrocoma, Oropetium thomaeum, Oryza rufipogon, Oryzopsis lateralis, Panicum psilopodium, Paspalum spp. Perotis indica, Phleum alpinum, Poa spp., Polypogon fugaz, Saccharum, spp., Sehima nervosum, Setaria glauca, Themeda anathera, Tripogon filiformis, Trisetum spicatum.

Shurbs and trees: Acacia catechu, Adhatoda vasica, Adina cordifolio, Albizia procera, Anacardium accidentale, Anona squamosa, Bauhinia sp., Berberis sp., Butea monosperma, Calamus spp., Cassia auriculata, Cotoneaster microphylla, Cryptomeria japonica, Dendrocalmus strictus, Dodonaea viscosa, Emblica officinalis, Erythrina variegata, Euopatorium coloratum, Holoptelea integrifolia, Ilex dipyrena, Madhuca indica, Morus alba, Phoenix spp.; Pueraria hirsuta, Pyrus spp., Rhododendron spp., Rosa spp., Salamalia malabarica, Shorea robusta, Tectona grandis, Terminalia tomentosa, Trewia nudiflora, Zizyphus numularia.

The Southern Peninsular Region

Grasses: Andropogon spp., Apluda mutică, Aristida spp., Anthraxon spp., Arundinella spp., Bothriochloa pertusa, Brachiaria ramosa, Cenchrus spp., Chrysopogon aciculatus, C.fulvus, Cymbopogon coloratus, Cynodon dactylon, Dactyloctenium aegyptium, Desmostachya bipinnate, Dicanthium annulatum, Digitaria spp., Dimeria orinithopoda Echinochloa colonum, Eragrostis spp, Eremopogon foveolatus, Heteropogon contortus, Imperata cylindrica, Ischaemom indicum, Iseilema laxum, Microstigium ciliatum, Oropetium thomaeum, Penicum spp.; Pennisetum clandastinum, Perotis indica, Poa annua, Saccharum spp., Sehima nervosum, Steria glauca, Themada spp. Tripogan spp. Urochloa panicoides.

Shrubs and trees: Acacia spp., Adina cordifolia, Albezia amara, Anacardium accidentale, Bauhinia spp., Berberis aristata, Butea monosperma, Capparis decidua, Cassia auriculata, Dichrostachys cinerea, Dodonaea viscosa, Grewia spp., Holoptelia integrifolia, Indigofera gerardiana, Madhuca indica, Mimosa rubicaulis, Phoenix sylvestris, Prosopis cineraria, Prosopis juliflora, Tectona grandis, Terminalia tomentosa, Zizyphus mauritiana.

The Northwestern Arid and Semi-arid Region

Grasses: Andropogon spp., Apluda mutica, Aristida spp., Arthraxon spp.; Arundinella spp.; Bothriochloa pertusa, Brachiara ramosa, Cenchrus spp.; Chloris barbata, Chrysopogon fulvus, Cymbopogon sps.; Cynodon dactylon, Dactyloctenium spp.; Desmastachya bipinata, Dicanthium annulatum, Digitaria spp.; Dimeria spp.; Eleusina spp.; Eragrostiella spp.; Eragrostis spp.; Eremopogon foveolatus; Heteropogon contortus, Imperata cylindrica, Ischaemom indicum, Iseilema laxum, Lasiurus indicus, Microstegium ciliatum, Oropetium thomaeum, Panicum antidotale, Perotis indica, Poa annua, Saccharum spp.; Sehima nervosum, Setaria glauca, Sporobolus marginatus, Themeda spp.; Tragus biflorus, Urochloa panicoides.

Shrubs and trees: Acacia spp.; Adhatoda vasica, Adina cordifolia, Albizia spp.; Bauhinia spp.; Berberis aristata, Butea monosperma, Carissa spinarum, Cassia auriculata, Dichrostachys cinerea, Dodonea viscosa, Gravillea robusta, Grewia asiatica, Holoptelea integrifolia, Madhuca indica, Mimosa rubicaulis, Morus alba, Prosopis cineraria, P.Juliflora, Shorea robusta, Tamarix dioica, Tectona grandis, Terminalia tomentosa, Trewia nudiflora, Zizyphus spp.

Herbs: Aerva tomentosa, Alysicarpus spp., Artemisia spp.; Atylosia spp.; Cassia tora, Crotalaria prosterata, Desmodium spp.; Heylandia latebrosa, Indigofera spp.; Phaseolus spp.; Rhyncosia capitata, Rhyncosia minima, Tribulus terrestris, Trichodesma indica, Vernonia cinerea, Vicoa indica, Zornia diphylla.

The Southern Peninsular Region

Aerva lanata, Alysicarpus spp.; Atylosia Spp.; Cassia tora, Crotolaria prostrata, Dasmodium floribundum, Heylandia latebrosa, Indigofera spp.; Justicia betonica, Phaseolus spp.; Rhynchosia minima, Tribulus terrestris, Trichodesma indica, Vernonia cinerea, Vica indica, Zornia diphylla.

The Eastern Region

Abelia triflora, Ageratum conyzoides, Alpinia spp.; Alysicarpus spp.; Atylosia spp.; Carex condensata, C.foliolosa, Cassia tora, Centella asiatica, Crotolaria prostrata, Cyperus spp.; Desmodium spp.; Eriocaulon spp.; Galium triflorum, Indigofera spp.; Junus sp.; Lespedeza sericera, Mimosa pudica, Moghania stricta, Oldenlandia corymbosa, Phaseolus spp.; Plantago major Polygala mollis, Polygonum spp.; Potentilla mooniaca, Thymus serpyllum, Trichodesma indica, Tridax procumbens, Trifolium spp.; Urasia picta, Zornia diphylla.

The Northern Temperate Region

Abelia triflora, Alysicarpus spp.; Atylosia spp.; Cannabis sativa, Carex spp.; Cassia spp.; Crotolaria spp.; Desmodium spp.; Fregaria spp.; Galium triflorum, Indigfera spp.; Lespedeza zericea, Morina longifolia, Phaseolus spp.; Plantago major, Polygala mollis, Polygonum spp.; Trichodesma indica, Trifolium spp.; Thymus serpyllum, Zornia diphylla.

Some Other Common Low Vegetation of Different Regions

Abelia triflora, Aerva spp.; Alysicarpus spp.; Artemisia spp.; Atylosia spp.; Cassia spp.; Crotalaria spp.; Desmodium spp.; Heylandia latebrosa, Galium triflorum, Indigofera spp.; Phaseolus spp.; Polygonum spp.; Rhyncosia spp.; Tribulus terrestris, Trichodesma indica, Trifolium spp.; Vernonia cineria, Zornia diphylla, etc.

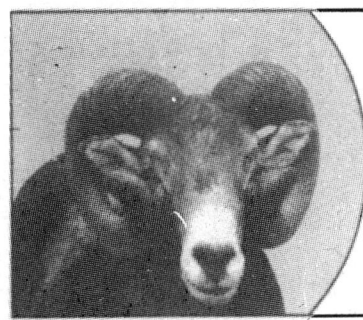

APPENDIX

ABBREVIATIONS AND SYMBOLS USED

ARC	–	Agriculture, Research Council (of UK)
aver	–	average (mean)
B.SE	–	Bovine Spongiform Encephlopathy
B.wt	–	Body weight
CAE	–	Caprine Angio Encephlomyelitis
CAZRI	–	Central Arid Zone Research Institute (Jodhpur)
Cl.fl.wt.	–	Clean fleece (Wool) weight
CGRI	–	Central Goat Research Institute (Makhdoom)
CP	–	Crude Protein
CSWRI	–	Central Sheep and Wool Research Institute Avikanagar
DCP	–	Digestible Crude Protein
DM	–	Dry Matter
DP	–	Digestible Crude Protein
DM	–	Dry Matter
DP	–	Digestible Protein
ECU	–	European Currency Units (Euro)
Est.	–	Estimates
ETT	–	Embryo Transfer Technology
EXIM	–	Export Import
EYC	–	Egg Yolk Citrate
EYG	–	Egg Yolk Glycerol
F	–	FAO estimates
FAO	–	Food and Agricultural Organisation of the United Nations.
GI sheets	–	Galvanised iron sheets
GI tract	–	Gastero-intestinal tract
Gr. fl. wt.	–	Greasy fleece weight
hec	–	hectare
ICAR	–	Imperial Council of Agricultural Research
	–	Indian Council of Agricultural Research
IGFRI	–	Indian Grassland and Fodder Research Institute (Jhansi)

ISSGPU	–	Indian Society for Sheep and Goat Production and Utilization (Jaipur)
IVRI	–	Indian Veterinary Research Institute (Izatnagar)
IU	–	International Units
KG/kg	–	Kilogram
KG/AN	–	Kilomgram per animal
KG/HA	–	Kilomgram per Hectare
Lbj	–	Lambs born per ewe joined
Lnj	–	Lambs surviving till neonatal age out of the ewes joined
Lwj	–	Lambs weaned per ewe joined
Lwb	–	Lambs weaned per lamb born
m	–	million
	–	metre
mcg	–	microgram
mg	–	milligram
mi	–	micron (μ)
MSL	–	Mean sea level
MT	–	Metric ton
mth	–	month
NCA	–	National Commission on Agriculture
NES	–	Not elsewhere specified or included
NPN	–	Non-Protein Nitrogen
NRC	–	National Research Council (of America)
Ramb./R	–	Rambouillet
μ	–	micron
	–	mean
SE	–	Starch Equivalent
TDN	–	Total Digestible Nutrients
ug	–	microgram
wt.	–	weight
*	–	Unofficial figures
*	–	Indication of Reference/Clarification
–	–	Figures/Data not available

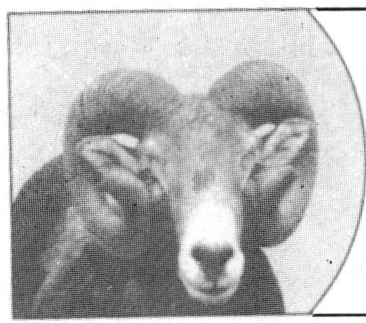

BIBLIOGRAPHY

(Literature Consulted and References Cited)

Acharya, R.M. (1981)   Status of Sheep Production in India. Key Note address, 1st Proceedings of the Society and National Seminar on Sheep and Goat Production and Utilisation (ISSGPU-CSWRI) Jaipur.

Acharya, R.M. (1982)   Sheep and Goat breeds of India. FAO Animal Production and Health paper. Oxford and IBH Pub. Co. Ltd. New Delhi.

Acharya, R.M. Arora, C.L.; Malik RC and Sahni, M.S. (1972)   Genetic Aspects of Performance of Indian breeds of sheep and their crosses with Exotic Wool Breeds. Review of Res. in S and W Prod. CSWRI.

Acharya, R.M. and Saksena S.K. (1972)   Economics of Sheep Rearing in India Review of Research in Sheep and Wool Prod. CSWRI.

Acharya, R.M., Misra R.K; and Patil V.K. (1982)   Breeding strategy for goats in India. ICAR, New Delhi 1-III.

Aggarwala, A.C. (1953)   A Laboratory Manual of Milk Inspection (3rd Ed.) M/s Gulab Chand Kapoor and Sons Jullundur City/G.B. Road Delhi.

Agricultural Research Council ARC (1980)   The Nutrient Requirements of Ruminant Livestock. Commonwealth Agri. Bureaux, Farnham, Royal Slough, U.K.

Agricultural Research Council ARC (1984)   The Nutrient Requirements of Ruminant Livestock. Commonwealth Agri. Bureaux, Farnham Royal Slough, U.K.

Arora, C.L. (1981)   Genetic Basis for improving Sheep fo Mutton Production Ist Proceedings of the Society and National Seminar ISSGPU (CSWRI), Jaipur.

Arora, C.L. and Garg, R.C. (1998)   Sheep Production and Breeding. International Book Distributing Co. Charbagh, Lucknow (India)-226004.

Bandey, G.A. (1975)   Communication to farm managers. Slow growth and delayed mating of sheep. Directorate of Sheep Husbandry (J&K).

Bandey G.A. (1981)   Constraints in Sheep Development in India-and possible solution. 1st Proceeding of National Seminar of ISSGPU (CSWRI) Jaipur, India.

Banerjee, Ajit Kumar (1989)   Shrubs in Tropical Forest Eco-system UNESCO, Publication.

Banerjee, Ajit Kumar (1989)   Shrubs in Tropical Forest Eco-system UNESCO, Publication.

Banerjee, G.C. (1992)   A Textbook of Animal Husbandry (7th Ed.) Oxford and IBH Publishers Co. Pvt. Ltd. New Delhi.

Basuthakur A.K.   Sheep Research, Production and Marketing in India. Inter India Publication, D-17 Raja Garden Extn. New Delhi-110015.

Basuthakur, A.K. and Acharya, R.M. (1981)   Breeding Sheep for Fine Wool Prod. Ist Proceedings of the Society and National Seminar of ISSGPU (CSWRI) Jaipur.

Bell, H.M. (1978)   Rangeland Management for Livestock Production. 2nd Ed. University Oklahowa Press, Norman.

Belschner, H.G. (1965)   Sheep Management and Diseases 8th Ed. Angus and Robertson, Sydney, Australia.

Bernhard Smith, A (1993)   Poisonous Plants (of all countries) Vinod Publishers and Distributors, Pucca Danga, Jammu, J&K (India).

Botkin, M.P.; Ray, A Field and Johson, C. LeRoy (1988)   Sheep and Wool Sci. Production and Management Deptt. of Ani. Sci. University of Wyoming (USA). Prentice-Hall, Englewood Cliffs, New Jersy-07632.

Brijendra Singh (1985)   Application of Genetic Principles in sheep breedings. Proceedings of Workshop-cum-Seminar on Sheep Management (CSBF-Hissar) Directorate of Ext. Min. of Agri. and Rural Dev. G.O.I. New Delhi.

Carles, A.B. (1983)   Sheep Production in the Tropics. Oxford University Press, Walton Street, Oxford.

Chabra, A and Arora, S.P. (1985) — Effect of Zinc deficiency on Serum Vit. A level, tissue enzymes and histological alterations in goats. Livestock Production Sci., 12; 69-77.

Charray, J; Humbert, J.M. and Levif, J. (1992) — Manual of Sheep Production in the Hummid tropics of Africa. Pub. CAB International Wallingford Oxon (UK).

Christopher, K James (1990) — Plant poisoning in animals. Pashudhan (Bangalore) Vol. 5:8 pp.3.

Coop, I.E. (1982) — Sheep and Goat Production, Elsevier Scientific, Amsterdam (Holland).

Choudhary A.L.(1981) — Breeding sheep for Carpet wool Prod. Ist Proceeding of the Society and National Seminar ISSGPU (CSWRI) Jaipur.

Choudhary S.R. (1985) — Economics of Sheep Rearing for Marginal Farmers and Landless labours in India. Proceedings of the workshop-cum-seminar on Sheep Management CSBF (Hissar) Directorate of Extn. Min. of Agri. (GOI).

CSWRI (1987) — Sheep Bulletin, Vol. 1:2.

Chopra, S.C. (1971) — Animal Breeding-Lectures to P.G. Faculty, Ani. Sci. HAU Hissar.

Chopra S.C. (1985) — Import of Sheep in India and their importance on sheep improvement. Proceeding of workshop on Sheep Management CSBF Hissar Directorate of Extn. Min. of Agri. GOI.

Davendra, C. and Faylon, P.S. (1988) — Sheep Production in Asia. Proceedings of Workshop. International Development Research Centre, Philipines.

David, C.Henderson (1990) — The Veterinary Book for Sheep Farmers Publishers-Farming Press Book, 4, Frears Courtyard, 30-32 Princess Street Ipswich, IPI, UK.

David Croston and Geoff Pollott (1994) — Planned Sheep Prod. (2nd Edn), Blackwell Scientific Publications 25, John Street, London WCIN 2BL.

Dhamale S.P. and Mooley R.C. (1963-64) — Sheep and Wool Production and Management-Lectures. P.G. Institute of Sand W Prod. ICAR, Pune.

Duthie, J.F. (1978) — The Fodder grasses of Northern India. Scientific Publishers, Man Bhawan Ratanada Road Jodhpur (India).

Elliott, R.G.H. (1985) — Hides and Skins improvement in developing countries; FAO Agricultural Services Bulletin, 67. United Nations, Rome.

Ely, D.G. (1991) — Livestock Feeds and Feeding (3rd Edi.) Prentice Hall, Englewood Cliffs N.J.

Ercanbrack, S.K. and Knight, A.D. (1996) — Responses to selection for lamb production. J. of Animal Sci. pp. 527.

Falconer, D.S. (1981) — Introduction to Quantitative Genetics (2nd Ed.) English Language Book Society, Longman.

FAO (1985) — Production Year Book Vol. 39. Food and Agricultural Organisation of the United Nations Rome.

FAO (1995) — Production Year Book Vol. 49.

FAO (1997) — Production Year Book Vol. 51.

FAO (1999) — Production Year Book Vol. 53.

FAO (1998) — World Statistical Compendium for Raw Hides and Skins. Commodities and Trade Div. of the United Nations, Rome.

Fayez, M.Marai and Owen, J.B. (1987) — New Techniques in Sheep Production. Butterworths and Co. Publishers Ltd. London.

Fraser, Allan (1965) — Sheep Farming (7th Edi) Crosby, Lockwood London.

Fuller, M.F. (1969) — Climate and Growth. Growth and Nutrition by E.S.E. Hafez and I.A. Dyer Publishers Lea and Febiger. Philadelphia.

Ghalsasi, P.M.; Gray, G.D. and Nimbkar, B.V. (1993) — The Garole microsheep of Bengal. Animal Genetic Resources Information, 12, 73-79.

Ghalsasi, P.M.; Nimbkar B.V. and Gray, G.D. (1994) — The Garole Prolific microsheep of West Bengal (India). Proceedings of 5th World Congress on Genetics Applied to Livestock Production Guelph, Ontario, 20, 456-459.

Godfrey, R.W.; Gray, M.L. and Collins, J.R. (1995) — Estrus Synchronisation of sheep in Tropics. Jr. of Animal Science 73 (Supdp-1) p.232.

Gupta, J.L. (1964) — Growth performance of Deccani sheep and its crossbreds with Merino and Rambouillet P.G. Dissertation submitted to ICAR (Pune).

Gupta, J.L. (1972) — Inheritance of some Economic traits in Gaddi and Poonchi sheep and their crosses with Rambouillet sheep M.Sc. Thesis; HAU-Hissar.

Gupta, J.L. (1977) — Sheep transportation by truck. An observation. Reported to Directorate of Sheep Husbandry J&K.

Gupta, J.L. (1978) — Performance of Mandya sheep and its scope for exploitation in mutton development in Jammu Division Report sent to Govt. of J&K.

Gupta, J.L. (1992) — Sheep Development in J&K State. Proceedings and Souvenir of Golden Jubilee (1942-1992) Conference; Sheep Husbandry Deptt.

Gupta, J.L. (1993) — Sheep and Goat Breeding Strategies in J&K. A review at 2nd Regional workshop of Task Force, Min. of A.H. and Darying G.O.I.

Gupta, J.L (1994) — Sheep Development in Temperate Region (1st Edi.) CBS Publishers and Distributors 485, Bhola Nath Nagar, Shahdara Delhi-110032 (India)

Gupta, J.L. (1996) — Emerging Trends-Production of Prime Quality Wool. Proceedings of Workshop on Sheep Development, S.H. Deptt J&K.

Gupta, J.L. (1999) Development of Small Ruminants. Achievements and Challenges, Proceeding of Technical Workshop on S and G Dev. Directorate of Sheep Husbandry Jammu.

Gupta, J.L. (2001) Management of Small ruminants and pastures in J&K Hills. Proceedings of 5th Agri Sci. Congress on Sustainable Development of Hill Mountain Agriculture, NAAS, AAU Gowahati.

Gupta, J.L. and Chopra S.C. (1974) Comparison of body weights of Gaddi, Poonchi sheep and their crosses with Rambouillet. Indian Jr. Animal Sci. 44(7): 447-51.

Gupta, J.L. and Chopra S.C. (1975) A note on body measurements of Gaddi, Poonchi Sheep and their crosses with Rambouillet Indian J. Animal Sci. 45 (9): 700-703.

Gupta, J.L.; Chopra, S.C. and Dhamale, S.P. (1974) Effect of mating seasons on growth of Deccani Sheep and their crosses with Merino and Rambouillet HAU J. Res. Hissar, Vol. IV: 2 pp:158-161.

Gupta, O.P. (1984) Scientific weed management. Today and Tomorrow Printers and Publishers, 24 B/5 Desh Bandhu Gupta Road New Delhi-110005.

Gupta, R.D. (2003) Managing Grass land ecosystems in Jammu and Kashmir. Daily Excelsior Sept. 22, 2003.

Gupta, R.D. (2003) Managing degraded lands in J&K Daily Excelsior Magazine Nov. 10, 2003.

Gupta, S.C. (1998) Sheep and Goat Development in J&K Seminar Proceedings. Sheep Husbandry Deptt. Jammu.

Hafec Consultants (1978) Perspective Plan 1980-95. Integrated Development, Govt. of J&K, Rajouri Distt. Vol. II, Chap. VIII p-19.

Hafez, E.S.E. (1980) Reproduction in Farm Animals (5th Edi.) K.M. Varghese Co. Post Box 7119, Mumbai-400031

Hart, Edward (1994) SHEEP-A Guide to Management. The Crowood Press Ltd. Ramsbury, Malborough Wiltshire.

Hazel, L.N. and Lush, J.L. (1942) J.Hered, 33: 393-9 Quoted by Turner and Young (1969).

Ian Gordon (1997) Controlled Reproduction in Sheep and Goats Vol. 2. Univ. Press Cambridge.

IDWP (1984) Mineral, trace elements and Vit. allowances for ruminant livestock. Recent Advances in Animal Nutrition. Haresign, W. and Cole. DJA Eds. London.

Indian Agriculture (1999) Indian Economic Data Res. Centre (IEDRC), B-713 Panchvati, Vikaspuri New Delhi.

Jarriage, R. (1989) In Ruminant Nutrition, Recommended Allowances and Feed Tables. Institute National de la Rechercha, Agronomique, Paris, p-365.

Kassem R; Owen J.B. and Fadel 1 (1990) A note on the characteristics of oestrus and ovulation in Awassi ewes. Animal Production, 50, 198-201.

Kaul, D.N. (1943) Sheep and Wool Survey Reports of Jammu and Kashmir State.

Kaul, M.L. (1973) Open penning of imported Russian sheep in snowfall conditions at Daksum farm, J&K. A personal communication.

Kaushish, S.K. (1994) Sheep Production in Tropics and Sub-tropics. Scientific Publishers, Jodhpur.

Kempthorne, O (1957) An Introduction to Genetic Statistics. John Wiley and Sons, New York.

Khajuria, R.R and Singh, K. (1967) Studies on the chemical composition and digestibility of Dhaman (Grewia elastica) tree leaves. Ind. Vet. J. 44: 929-34.

Khan, G.M. (1972) Performance of Kashmir Merino and Stevropol breeds of Sheep. Thesis submitted to Agra Univ. in fulfilment of M.V.Sc. degree requirement.

Khot, S.S. (1962) Bhed aur Oon. Ministry of Food and Agriculture, GOI New Delhi.

Kumar, S. (1992) Economic Survey Reports of Sheep units compiled for the Deptt of A.H. and Dairying GOI.

Lall, H.K. (1956) Breeds of sheep in Indian Union. Misc. Bulletin ICAR. 75(ii).

Lush, J.L. (1940) Quoted by Falconer. (1981).

Lush, J.L. (1945) and Chopra (1971).

Lush, J.L. (1948) Genetics of populations, Dept. of A.H. Iowa State College, Ames. Quoted by Turner and Young (1969) and Chopra (1971).

Lynch, J.J; Hinch, G.N. and Adams, D.B. (1992) The behaviour of Sheep. CSIRO Publications, Victoria, Australia.

Malicot, G. (1948) Quoted by Falconer (1981) and Chopra (1971).

Mali, P.C; Badekar, A.R. and Patnayak, B.C. (1981) Growth and Nutrients utilization in Sheep and Goat Fed Z. nemularia (Pala leaves) Ist Proceedings of the National Seminar of ISSGPU (CSWRI), Jaipur.

Malik, C.L. (1990) Report of Technical Committee of Direction for improvement of A.H. and Dairying Statistics; Deptt of A.H. and Dairying, Min. of Agri. GOI.

Margaret, M and Martin, A (1998) In practice Hand Books. Sheep and Goat. W.B. Saunders Co. Ltd. 24-28, Oval Road, London.

Maxwell, W.M.C. (1984) Reproduction in Sheep. Current Problems and future potential of A.1 programme (pp. 291-97) Cambridge Univ. Press Cambridge.

May, Neil D.S. (1970) Anatomy of Sheep-dissection manual (3rd Edi.) St. Lucia Univ. of Queenslands, Australia.

Min. B.R.; Barry, T.N.; Attwood, G.D. and McNabb, W.C. (2003) The effect of condensed tannins on the Nutrition and Health of ruminants fed fresh temperate forages...a review. Animal Feed Sci. and Tech. 3-19.

Modi, N.J. (1983) Textbook of Medical Jurisprudence and Toxicology. N.M. Tripathi Pvt. Ltd. Booksellers, Publishers, Princess Street Mumbai-2.

Mohammed, F. Fahmy (1996) Prolific Sheep. Research Branch Agri. and Agri. Food Canada Pub. CAB International.

Morrison, F.B. (1956) Feed and Feeding 22nd Edi. The Morrison Publishing Co. Ithaca, N.Y.

Mudliar, ASR (1981) Increasing Prolificacy. Lambing percentage in Sheep. 1st Proc. of National Seminar on S and G. ISSGPK (CSWRI) Jaipur.

Mushtaq, A Memon and Karl, M. (1992) Gene manipulation in Goat through Biotechnology. Pre-conference Proceedings, V-International Conference on Goats, New Delhi.

Nagaraj, M (1964) Effect of Age on quality and quantity of Bannur Meat. P.G. Dissertation, ICAR Sheep and Wool Production and Management Training Centre Pune (Maharashtra).

National Research NRC (1985) Nutrient Requirements of sheep. National Academy of Sciences, Washington.

Nina, Hyde (1988) Wool Fabric of History. National Geographic J. Vol. 173 No: 5,552-591.

Olesan, I. (1993) Effects of Cervical Insemination with frozen semen on fertility and litter size of Norwegian sheep. Livestock Production Sci. 37: 169-184.

Osamu Ishikawa (2003) Report from Nasu Safari Park, Tokyo, Japan. Don't be an ass, I am a Zenkey T.O.I. August. 28, 2003.

Owen John B. (1981) Sheep Production. A Bailliare Tindall Publication, 35, Red Lion Square, London.

Patil, J.M. and Dave, A.D. (1981) Milk Production ability of Pattanwadi × Merino half bred ewes and Pre-weaning Growth response. Ist Proceedings of ISSGPU (CSWRI), Jaipur.

Parotra, K.K. (1993) Wool quality traits of Sheep in Jammu Region and its economic aspects of utilisation. WOOLWAYS. Vol. 3 No: 4.

Patnayak, B.C. (1981) Research in India on Nutrient Requirements for sheep. 1st Proceedings and Seminar ISSGPU CSWRI, Jaipur.

Patnayak, B.C. (1992) Production and Marketing of Raw wool. A report of Sub-Committee Mini. of Agri. GOI.

Patnayak. B.C. (1994) An overview of Animal Fibre Prod. Research in India. WOOLWAYS Vol. 4, 7-12.

Patnayak, B.C. and Manohar Singh (1972) Sheep Nutrition Research in India. Review of Res. in Sheep and Wool Production (CSWRI).

Patnayak, B.C. and Singh N.P (1985) Nutrition problems of sheep in arid and semi-arid regions of India. Proceedings of workshop-cum-seminar on Sheep Management Ministry of Agri. and Rural Dev. GOI (ND).

Paula Simmons (1995) Raising Sheep, the Modern way. A Gardenway Publishing Classic, Storey Communications Inc. POWNAL VT.

Piper, LR. and Bindan, B.M. (1982) Genetic Segregation for fecundity in Booroola Merino Sheep. Proceedings of World Congress on Sheep and Beef Cattle Breeding. Dunmore Press, Palmarstan North (NZ).

Pond, W.G; Church D.C. and Pond, K.R. (1995) Basic Animal Nutrition and Feeding. Johnwiley and Sons, New York.

Prasad, J (1996) Goat, Sheep and Pig production and management Kalyani Pub. Ludhiana.

Prasad, J (2000) Goat, Sheep and Pig Production and Management Kalyani, Ludhiana KVK Bathinda (Punjab). (2nd edn).

Proceedings (1979) Summer Institute on Goat Production (1979) Central Institute for Research on Goats (ICAR) Makhdoom-Mathura (UP).

Proceedings (1981) 1st Proc. of Soc. and National Seminar on Sheep and Goat Production and Utilization CSWRI Jaipur.

Proceedings (1985) Workshop-cum-Seminar on Sheep Management CSBF Hissar, Ministry of Agri. and Rural Dev. GOI (ND).

Proceedings (1992) Golden Jubilee of Sheep Dev, J&K Deptt. of Sheep Husbandry J&K, Jammu.

Raina A.K. and Raina R.K (1997) Lantana Toxicosis in Sheep and Goats. Paper presented in seminar on Sheep and Goat Management S.H. Deptt. Jammu.

Radostits, D.M.; Blood D.C. and Gay, C.C (1994) Veterinary Medicine (8th Edit) ELBS London, UK.

Ranjan, S.K (1989) Nutrition values of common fodder tree leaves.

Ranjan, S.K. (1997) Animal Nutrition in Tropics. (Revised) Vikas Publishing House, Pvt. Ltd., 5 Ansari Road, N.D.-110002.

Ranjan, S.K; Singh C.P; Nadgir, S.R. and Talpatra, S.K. (1959) Studies on some high protein green feeds of Uttar Pradesh (*Carthamus tintorius*) Ind. Vet. J. 36: 267-72.

Rao, K.L; Vishishta M.S; Goswami, S.K. and Bihani D.K. (1985) Meat Inspection in Indian States. L.D. Prakashan, Purani Ginani, Bikaner-334001.

Reports (1965 to 1968) Annual Reports Govt. Sheep Breeding and Research farm Billawar/Sarthal J&K State.

Reports (1974 to 1978) Annual Reports, Govt. Sheep Breeding and Research Farm Reasi/Banihal. J&K State.

Report (1975-76) Land Use Pattern. Ministry of Agri. and Coop. G.O.I.

Report (1987) Task Force, GOI, Ministry of Agriculture Deptt. of Agri. and Coop. New Delhi. To evaluate the impact of sheep and goat rearing in Ecologically, fragile zones.

Research Centre Tech. Report (1992) Texas A and M Agri. Res. and Extn. Centre at San Angelo-Improvement of Sheep through selection-The ROM Index.

Richardson, C (1972) Pregnancy diagnosis in Ewes. A Review. Veterinary Record, 90, 264-275.

Ross, C.V. (1989) Sheep Production and Management PRENTICE HALL, Englewood Cliffs, New Jersey-07632.

Roy, R.S. (1999) A Report on Trade Promotion and Public Relations. Central Wool Dev. Board WOOLWAYS, Vol. 9:1.

Ruth, M.Gatenby (1995) The Tropical Agriculture, SHEEP CTA MACMILLON Publishers, London.

Ruth, M.Gatenby and Humbert, J.M (1991) Sheep CTA MacMillon Publishers London.

Sahni, K.L. and Tiwari, S.B. (1972) Review of Research done in applied Reproduction and A.I of Sheep in India CSWRI Avika Nagar (Rajasthan).

Sahoo, A; Sharma, R.K; Kurade, N.P; Bhat, T.K. and Singh, B (2002) Effects of tanniferous top feed on parasitic load in calves. Proceedings Xth Int. Congress, Asian-Australian Association of Animal Prod. Societies, New Delhi, p 105-106.

Scott, W.N. (1978) The Care and Management of Farm Animals Bailliare Tindall London.

Sharma, J.P. (2003) Biological control of *Parthenium hystrophorus* weed at Panthal Farm (J&K) A personal communication.

Sharma, R.K.; Singh, B and Sahoo, A. (2002) Ruminal availability of nitrogen from some promising tree forages. Proceedings IV Bi-annual conference. Animal Nutr. Assoc. Kolkatta, Nov. 20-22, pp 35-36.

Sharma, R.K. and Samantha, A.K. (2003) Impact of Feed Tannins in Animal Production. A review-SKAUST-J Journal of Research Jammu (J&K).

Sharma, R.K; Singh, B; Soodan, J.S; Kotwal, S.K and Rashid, A (2000) Tannin contents of common tree leaves of Jammu region and their role in Ani. Nutri. Tech. Conference on Sheep and Goat Dev. Jammu March, 2000.

Sheep Breeding in Russia (1970) Russian book translated to English by Indian National Sci. Documentation Centre (INSDAC) New Delhi.

Sheep Council of Australia (1990) Feeding standards for Australian Livestock, Ruminants CSIRO Australia pp. 266.

Sheep Industry Dev. (1992) Handbook, Sheep Industry Development, Denver Co.

Showkat, Parvaiz, Qureshi, M.Q. and Mohd. A, (2000) Studies on wool quality in crossbred Merino Sheep in Kashmir WOOLWAYS. Vol. 10:1.

Singh, B and Tannins revisited. Changing perceptions of their effects on animal systems Animal Nutrition, Feed Tech. 1:3-18.

Singh, R.N. (1998) Sheep Production and Improvement in India-A perspective. WOOLWAYS Vol. VII No: 2 and 3.

Singh, R.V. (1985) Fodder trees of India. Oxford and IBH Publishing Co. New Delhi.

Stan Dorman (1995) Information about evolved Sheep Breeds of Australia, DRT (Dale River Transplants, Animal Breeding specialists and Consultants) Beverly (W.Aust.) Through Australian High Commission, New Delhi.

Statistical Abstract India (1997) Vol. I and II Central Statistical Organisation. Deptt. of Statistics, Ministry of Planning and Programme Implementation G.O.I.

Srivastava, R.K. and Chaturvedi, M.L. (1971) Determination of pasture consumption Ind. Vet. J 48: 958-62.

Taneja, G.C. (1978) Technical Report on Sheep Farming in Russia (Stavropol area) by Jt. Comm. Sheep to G.O.I.

Taneja, G.C. (1978) Sheep Husbandry in India Orient Longman Ltd., 3/5 Asif Ali Road, New Delhi.

Thakur, S.S. and Patnayak, B.C. (1981) Comparative Intake and Digestibility of Nutrients in non-pregnant and pregnant ewes–1st Proceedings of ISSGPU Seminar (CSWRI) Jaipur.

Toshinwal, S.N. (1969) Reproduction and A.I. in Sheep. A compilation of Lectures for P.G. Trainees, Jaipur (Rajasthan).

Turner Helen Newton (1969) Genetic Improvement of Reproductive rate in Sheep A.B.A. Vol. 39, No: 4 pp. 545.

Turner H.N. and Young S.S.Y. (1969) Quantitative Genetics in Sheep Breeding. Macmillan of Australia.

Turner, H.N. (1982) Quoted by Ghalsasi et al (1994).

Turner, H.N. (1993) Quoted by Ghalsasi et al (1994).

Umberger, S.H; Jabbar, Gand Lewis, G.S. (1994) Seasonally an-ovulatory ewes fail to respond to progesterone treatment in absence of gonadotrophin stimulation. Theriogenology 42, 1329-1336.

University of California (1996) Sheep Production and Management in a Mediterranean Climate. A publication of small ruminant collaboration, Res. Support Programme; Davis, USA

Verma, D.N. (1995) A Textbook of Animal Nutrition. Kalyani Publishers, New Delhi.

Vikas Singhal (1999) Indian Agriculture. Indian Economic Data Research Centre, B-713, Panchvati, Vikaspuri, New Delhi.

Vidyarthi, O.P.(1997) Wild and Cultivated plants of Jammu, Kashmir and Ladakh, Directorate of Social Forestry Project (J&K).

Wani, G.M.; Risam, K.S and Nowshahri M.A. (1988) Effect of Synchronisation of Oestrus on lambing in Corriedale ewes. I.J. of Ani. Sci. 58(7), 800-801.

Wani, G.M.; Sinha N.K. and Khan, B.U. (1987) Oestrus synchronisation with Progestagens in Muzzafarnagri ewes. Ind. J. of Ani., Sci. 57(2): 1296-98.

Werner Von Bergen (1965) Wool Handbook. Vol. I (3rd Edi.) J.P. Stevens and Co. Inc. Consultants Inter-science Publishers, New York.

Wright, S. (1921) Genetics 6: 111-161. Quoted by Turner and Young (1969).

Wright, S. (1940) AM. Nat: 74:232-48 Quoted by Turner and Young (1969).

Agarwal, S.K. (1981) Oestrus Synchronisation with "Estrumate" (Synthetic Prostaglandin) Ist. Proc. of ISSGPU's National Seminar on S and G. Prod. and Utilization, CSWRI, Jaipur. pp 400.

Zanwar, S.G and Aggarwal, S.K. (1981) Artificial Insemination with reference to conception rates in Sheep. Ist. Proc. of ISSGPU's National Seminar on Sheep and Goat Production and Utilization, CSWRI, Jaipur.

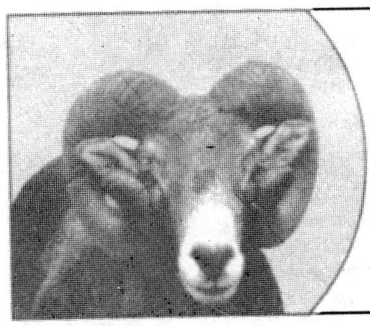

INDEX